CENTRES OF MEDICAL EXCELLENCE?

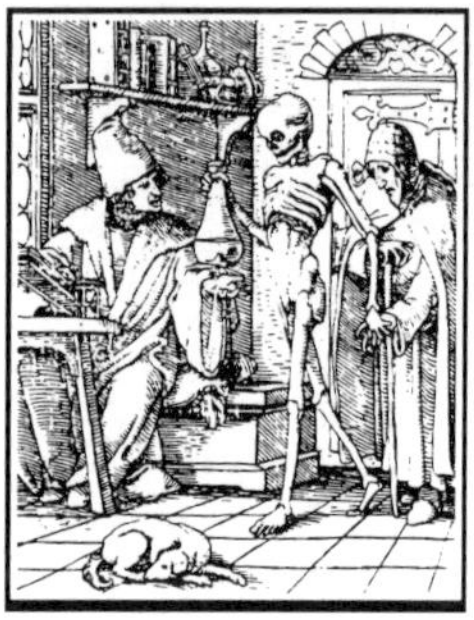

The History of Medicine in Context

Series Editors: Andrew Cunningham and Ole Peter Grell

Department of History and Philosophy of Science
University of Cambridge

Department of History
Open University

Titles in this series include

The Anatomist Anatomis'd
An Experimental Discipline in Enlightenment Europe
Andrew Cunningham

Crafting Immunity
Working Histories of Clinical Immunology
Edited by Kenton Kroker, Jennifer Keelan and Pauline M.H. Mazumdar

Before My Helpless Sight
Suffering, Dying and Military Medicine on the Western Front, 1914-1918
Leo van Bergen

Negotiating the French Pox in Early Modern Germany
Claudia Stein

Ireland and Medicine in the Seventeenth and Eighteenth Centuries
Edited by James Kelly and Fiona Clark

Centres of Medical Excellence?

Medical Travel and Education in Europe, 1500–1789

Edited by

OLE PETER GRELL
The Open University, UK

ANDREW CUNNINGHAM
University of Cambridge, UK

JON ARRIZABALAGA
Institución Milà i Fontanals (IMF), Spain

ASHGATE

Published by

Ashgate Publishing Limited
Wey Court East
Union Road
Farnham
Surrey, GU9 7PT
England

Ashgate Publishing Company
Suite 420
101 Cherry Street
Burlington
VT 05401-4405
USA

www.ashgate.com

British Library Cataloguing in Publication Data

Centres of Medical Excellence?: Medical Travel and Education in Europe, 1500–1789.
– (The History of Medicine in Context)
1. Medical education – Europe – History – 16th century. 2. Medical education – Europe--History--17th century. 3. Medical education – Europe – History – 18th century. I. Series II. Grell, Ole Peter. III. Cunningham, Andrew, Dr. IV. Arrizabalaga, Jon.
610.7'114-dc22

Library of Congress Cataloging-in-Publication Data

Centres of Medical Excellence: Medical Travel and Education in Europe, 1500–1789 / [edited by] Ole Peter Grell, Andrew Cunningham and Jon Arrizabalaga.
p.; cm. – (The History of Medicine in Context)
Includex index.
(hardcover : alk. paper) 1. Medical education – Europe – History. I. Grell, Ole Peter. II. Cunningham, Andrew, Dr.. III. Arrizabalaga, Jon. IV. Series: History of Medicine in Context.
[DNLM: 1. Education, Medical – history – Europe. 2. History, 16th Century – Europe. 3. History, 17th Century – Europe. 4. History, 18th Century – Europe. W 18 C4235 2009]
R771.C46 2009
610.71'14–dc22 2009046530

ISBN 9780754666998 (hbk)

Mixed Sources
Product group from well-managed forests and other controlled sources
www.fsc.org Cert no. SA-COC-1565
© 1996 Forest Stewardship Council
FSC

Printed and bound in Great Britain by
MPG Books Group, UK

Contents

PART III: THE CENTRES OF EXCELLENCE

Acknowledgements

This book is built on the invited papers of an international conference organised by the Renaissance and Early Modern Research Group at the Open University, Milton Keynes, UK and the Department of History of Science at the Consejo Superior de Investigationes Científicas, Institución Milà i Fontanals (CSIC-IMF), Barcelona, Spain, and organised by Jon Arrizabalaga, Andrew Cunningham and Ole Peter Grell. It was held at the CSIC-IMF Barcelona, 6–8 September 2007.

For their generous funding for the original conference we thank the Wellcome Trust, the General Direction of Research of the Spanish Ministry of Science and Innovation (grant HUM2006-27920-E/HIST) and the Spanish National Research Council (CSIC).

We are grateful also to the Direction and administrative staff of the Institución Milà i Fontanals, CSIC, Barcelona for their support in organising the conference, and to the Institut d'Estudis Catalans (IEC), on whose premises the conference was held. Finally, we would like to thank Dr Reis Fontanals, head of the Historical Archives Section at the Biblioteca de Catalunya, for facilitating our visit to the premises of the former Hospital of Santa Creu i Sant Pau, where this library is housed and for the exhibition on archival sources of the hospital that she arranged along with Dr Teresa Huguet-Termes (CSIC-IMF) for the participants of the conference.

We, the organisers and editors, also wish to thank our contributors for their enthusiastic scholarly help in providing the wide and coherent coverage of the topic that we had initially envisaged. The conference originally had the title 'Centres of Excellence', but following extensive and lively discussion at the conference our contributors persuaded us to add a question mark to the title of this resulting book.

Contributors

Jon Arrizabalaga, Consejo Superior de Investigationes Científicas, Barcelona

Laurence Brockliss, University of Oxford

Andrew Cunningham, University of Cambridge

Helen Dingwall, University of Stirling

Mário Sérgio Farelo, University of Lisbon

Toby Gelfand, University of Ottawa

Ole Peter Grell, The Open University

Cynthia Klestinec, Georgia Institute of Technology

Rina Knoeff, University of Leiden

Hilde de Ridder-Symoens, University of Ghent

Catrien Santing, University of Groningen

Hubert Steinke, University of Bern

Elizabeth A. Williams, Oklahoma State University

Illustrations and Legends

PART I
Where to go and How to Get There

Chapter 1

The Bartholins, the Platters and Laurentius Gryllus: the *peregrinatio medica* in the Sixteenth and Seventeenth Centuries

Andrew Cunningham

The peregrinatio medica

Caspar Bartholin the elder (1585–1629) went on a *peregrinatio medica* or foreign medical travel, and gained much medical knowledge, but only 'at great expense, by continual application, and with frequent peril of his life'. That is how he described how he had acquired the knowledge he was presenting in his 1611 book, *Anatomicae Institutiones*, or 'Anatomical basics' as it might be translated.[1] Bartholin came from Copenhagen, and after his *peregrinatio medica*, he went back to Copenhagen, where he was soon made professor of medicine in the university and taught anatomy. When he recalled his *peregrinatio* in this way, he was paying tribute to the anatomy teachers whose personal teaching he had experienced and whose published works he had used in his present little book, especially Felix Platter and Caspar Bauhin of the university of Basle, and Hieronymus Fabricius and Julius Casserius of the university of Padua.

Students notoriously always vote with their feet, seeking out the best, the most innovative (and sometimes also the zaniest) teachers of their subject. The most ambitious students have been travelling long distances for their education since universities were first founded in the late twelfth and thirteenth centuries, making their own educational foreign tour or *peregrinatio*. They hear the news on the grapevine, and then set off. The choices that different generations of students have made have led to some teachers becoming famous and others notorious, and to the flourishing of some universities and even to the decay of others.

With the Renaissance of the sixteenth century, and the new wealth that came with it, more and more students were making their medical journeys, often

[1] I use the 1633 edition published in Oxford. I have not seen the first edition, which was probably published in Wittenberg. '… Atque ita ad operis, quod diuturnis per varias Europaei orbis Academias peregrinationibus, magnis sumptibus, studiis et vigiliis continuis, non raro cum vitae periculo et discrimine edoctus sum, publico bono non invidebo: ne fraudetur juventus; si diutius supprimo, et occulto Euclionis novi instar hanc lare secreto aulam …', C. Bartholin, *Anatomicae institutiones corporis humani*, 1633.

travelling for weeks at a time to sit at the feet of a particular master. In medicine this meant that, over the period c.1500 to 1789, a succession of universities became the medical school of choice for ambitious students: Padua and Bologna in the 1500s, Paris, Leiden and Montpellier in the 1600s and Leiden, Göttingen and Edinburgh in the 1700s.

The arrival of foreign students brought wealth to the university towns, and this significant economic benefit meant that the various governors of these universities tried to ensure the defence of freedom of religion and freedom of speech, thus providing the best conditions for the promotion of new views and innovation in medicine and other subjects. In all the best medical schools – above all in Padua under the guidance of the Venetian Senate, in Leiden under its city council, and in Edinburgh also under its city council – there was the practice (if not the terminology) of something like *Lehrenfreiheit* and *Lehrfreiheit*: freedom of learning and freedom of teaching. For, then as now, it was a definition of the best university that the students were free to take whatever courses they cared to pay for, and also free to complain about them as loudly as they liked. Similarly, the teachers in these universities were allowed – even encouraged – to teach the truth as they saw it, without concern for ancient authority, religious scruples or student preferences.[2]

While we know a fair amount about medical education in the past, historians have mostly dwelt on the *content* of the standard teaching, as with the contributors to *The history of medical education*, edited by O'Malley in 1970, or the more recent volume on medical education in Britain, edited by Nutton and Porter in 1995.[3] The only work I know of that puts the medical student and his choices at the centre of the story in this period is Lisa Rosner's excellent book on Edinburgh in the eighteenth century.[4] Similarly, there has been extensive work on travel for education and on student enrolments at different universities across Europe, but there has been little on travel for education for medicine in particular, except in the case of France.[5]

---

[2] On which see H.S. Commager, 'The university and freedom: *Lehrfreiheit* and *Lehrenfreiheit*', *Journal of higher education*, 1966, 34, 361–70.

[3] C.D. O'Malley (ed.), *The history of medical education*, Los Angeles, 1970; V. Nutton and R. Porter (eds), *The history of medical education in Britain*, Amsterdam, 1995.

[4] L. Rosner, *Medical education in the Age of Improvement: Edinburgh students and apprentices 1760–1826*, Edinburgh, 1991.

[5] The most extensive treatment is in the series under the general editorship of Walter Rüegg, *The history of the university in Europe*, Cambridge, 6 vols, of which vol. 2, *Universities in early modern Europe*, ed. H. de Ridder-Symoens (1996) is the most pertinent, and Professor Ridder-Symoens' own contribution (Chapter 10) 'Mobility' the most valuable for our present concerns. The other important studies both deal with France and French students: D. Julia, 'La pérégrination académique en France'; and D. Julia and J. Revel, 'Les étudiants et leurs etudes dans la France moderne: Les étudiants en médecine',

Yet medicine was the subject where foreign travel was most valuable, especially when one came to set up a practice at home. As Thomas Bartholin (son of Caspar) commented in 1674: 'In our age such great usefulness redounds to the physician from his travels that no one puts much faith in the authority of a physician who has not set foot outside his native land.'[6] Fortunately for us, a number of medical travellers did commit their travelling and learning experiences to writing, and sometimes even had their work published. The present chapter deals with the accounts of their medical foreign travels produced in the sixteenth and seventeenth centuries by three generations of the Bartholin family of Copenhagen, two generations (in effect) of the Platter family of Basle, and Laurentius Gryllus of Ingolstadt. All these travellers came home and became professors in their home universities. I first use the better-known accounts by the Bartholins and Platters to deal with several large topics of the *peregrinatio medica*, especially the 'how' of student life, travel and survival. Then I turn to the account by Gryllus which, though it has been in print since 1566, has not received much notice hitherto from historians. It deserves attention, as it is quite full on the 'where' and the 'who' of an ambitious medical student's travels. I offer a translation-cum-paraphrase of parts of the travel section of Gryllus's *Oration*. Together, these accounts cover the period from about 1548 (Gryllus) to about 1670 (Thomas Bartholin).

Centres and Periphery

The present volume deals with the *peregrinatio medica* primarily from the viewpoint of the travelling students: who went where; what were they expecting; what did they find when they arrived; what did they take back with them from their studies? While there was certainly always much migration of students from one university to another within geographical regions – for instance, within Italy, or Germany, or the Iberian peninsula – the most important effects of the *peregrinatio medica* came about when students from the periphery, that is, generally the north of Europe, came back imbued with enthusiasm for what they had learnt at one or other of the 'central' universities. William Harvey, for instance, came back to London in 1602 from his medical education in Padua. He then continued to engage in the kind of anatomical research he had witnessed there in the teaching of Fabricius. Harvey was probably the only person in England at that time – the first three decades of the seventeenth century – engaging in anatomy at all. By putting into practice precisely the approach to anatomy he had learnt there at the 'centre' – Padua – he was enabled – out there on the periphery, London – to discover the circulation of the blood in animals. Thus, even a single individual could transform

in Julia and Revel (eds), *Histoire sociale des populations étudiantes*, Paris, 1989, 2vols, vol. 2, pp. 66–76 and 243–302.

6 Thomas Bartholin, *On medical travel*, in *On the burning of his library and On medical* travel, tr. C.D. O'Malley, Lawrence, Kansas, 1961, p. 50.

medical studies, research or practice back home on the periphery by trying to reform teaching and practice the way they had seen it at the best universities that they had visited on their own medical pilgrimage.

Travel Logistics

What were the logistics of student travel in this period? One of the fullest and most engaging of the surviving accounts of travel for medical education that have been published is that written up in 1612, some 50 years after the event, by Felix Platter of Basle. It is also the most detailed about the basic mechanics of travel and its hardships, and his quirky observations enable one to see something of student life at the time, such as when his fellow students gave him a farewell dinner where the meat on Felix's plate turned out to be cat. Felix seems to have had an eye to posterity in all this record keeping, for he also encouraged his aged father, who was a teacher, to write his autobiography, and his much, much younger brother Thomas also to produce a travel journal when he, in turn, went on his travels for his medical education in the 1590s. Unfortunately, the younger brother hardly mentioned his medical studies in those parts of his diary that have been published, seemingly being much more interested in travelling around as a tourist.[7] Another printed source I shall be using is from almost a century later and is by the son of Caspar Bartholin: it is Thomas Bartholin's *On medical travel*, published in Copenhagen in 1674 in Latin. This is addressed to his own two sons, Caspar the younger and Christopher, and his nephew, who were about to embark on their own *peregrinatio medica*.

'Today there are many travellers; indeed, it seems as if the whole of Europe is on the move.' So recalled Thomas Bartholin in the 1670s, looking back to his own time travelling for his medical education.[8] There were three basic forms of travel. One could travel on horseback or by horse-drawn vehicle, by boat, or on foot. Where it was possible, travelling by boat was far faster for longer journeys. Thomas Bartholin remarked that 'Today pedestrian journeys are not very common except among soldiers, workmen, and students of intelligence but of very slender fortune. From time to time, however, for lack of horses we are compelled to go on foot, as I well remember happened to me and to my brother Caspar Bartholin ... when we were travelling from Provence through Nice, Monaco, Mentone, Vintimiglia, Finale, Nola to Genoa ...', a distance of over 150 kilometres.

Let us start with Felix Platter (1536–1614). Platter was a Calvinist. He set out from Basel on his *peregrinatio* in October 1552, intending to enrol at Montpellier University, which at that time had a high reputation for medicine. He did not study

---

7 The story of Thomas, Felix and young Thomas Platter has been retold by Le Roy Ladurie in *The beggar and the professor: a sixteenth-century family saga*, tr. A. Goldhammer, Chicago, 1997.

8 Thomas Bartholin, *On medical travel*, p. 47 (note 6 above).

at Basle University, but disregarded his father's advice and went to Montpellier. He was 15 years old. He bought a little horse for the journey. With his companions he took a total of 20 days – virtually three weeks – with 15 days actually spent travelling, during which they passed through Berne, Fribourg, Lausanne and Geneva in Switzerland. Crossing to Lyons, they travelled south, following the course of the Rhone through Vienne, Valence, Montélimar, Orange and Nîmes, to Montpellier. They spent five days on the way relaxing and sightseeing, including dropping in to hear Jean Calvin preach in Geneva and to visit the physician and botanist Guillème Rondelet in Lyons.

When Felix arrived in Montpellier his accommodation was already arranged for him, for he was a sort of 'exchange student'. He stayed with an apothecary and his family, who were Jews whose predecessors had fled Spain in 1498. They were officially Christians, but known as 'Marans', and Felix records that their celebrations of Christian feasts was not always conventional, and that they had other ceremonies unique to themselves, which they carried out discreetly. The apothecary and Felix's father had agreed to, as it were, swap their sons for the duration of their studies. Not only did this save money, for each family provided the visiting student with everything for free, but it also meant there was someone there literally *in loco parentis* to look after the young man and to report back to his parents how he was progressing. Felix made a very good impression on his host family.

Letters to and from Felix and his family and his host were conveyed by travellers or merchants. Merchants were also crucial for the transfer of money. The roads were dangerous, and Felix more than once just escaped being robbed. Lyons had the special royal privilege of holding four fairs a year. Felix's time in Montpellier coincided with the great flourishing (1520–80) of these fairs. Textiles of all kinds were traded, as were spices, metals, books and leather goods.[9] The merchants of Europe who attended these fairs carried out their business using letters of exchange, to avoid having to send money, and students too could have money from home sent this way. 'You will only need to find a merchant in Montpellier to supply your needs', Felix told his younger brother in the 1590s, 'and I will repay him here [in Basel] on your note.' 'And this is what I did throughout the whole of my stay in Languedoc', the younger brother wrote, 'I had not taken any [money], either when I left Basel or at Geneva, because of the insecurity of the roads.'[10] The merchants also provided a relatively safe escort for a traveller against the brigands on all the roads.

Foreign students continued to be attracted to Montpellier right to the end of the sixteenth century and beyond. In fact, it has been calculated that up to around a

[9] R. Gascon, *Grand commerce et vie urbane au XVI siècle: Lyon et ses marchands (environs 1520–environs 1580)*, Paris, 2 vols, 1971, passim.

[10] Thomas Platter, *Journal of a younger brother: The life of Thomas Platter as a medical student in Montpellier at the close of the sixteenth century*, tr. S. Jennet, London, 1963, pp. 27–8.

third of the medical students at Montpellier were foreigners.[11] In the period 1615–17 the English student James Primrose recalled that among his fellow students at Montpellier were Spaniards, Germans, Poles, Danes, Swedes, Swiss and Scots.[12] Thomas Platter recorded: 'In ordinary times there are more than a hundred foreign students here [in the faculty of medicine], attracted by the opportunities offered by the faculty. One of the most prized is that students may accompany professors and doctors on their rounds in the town, visiting the sick. In this way one may study diagnosis, prescription, and the effect of the medicine. It is a great honour for a doctor to be followed in the street by a crowd of students.'[13] So the travelling students were not isolated, but members of cohorts who (then as now) would tend to fraternise with other foreigners who spoke the same vernacular language – all teaching and official matters at the universities being conducted, of course, in Latin. At the universities most popular with foreign students they were often organised into semi-self-governing 'nations', as at Montpellier and Padua.

Religion and Medical Degrees

From the beginning of the Reformation in 1517 there were riots and wars over religion. When Felix Platter was in Montpellier in the 1550s he witnessed many hangings and burnings of heretics – on this occasion Protestants. When his younger brother Thomas was there in the 1590s the town was as Protestant as it was Catholic, and it was hard to tell who was the heretic, though the burnings continued. Yet the travelling students were protected from these local religious battles of life and death as long as they did not try to participate, proselytise or make a show of their own religious observance. Thus Felix recalled how he and his fellow German-speaking Protestant students learnt to cook eggs secretly in paper held over the fire, since the Catholics of Montpellier would not allow any pots or pans to be used during Lent. Discretion is the better part of valour: Protestant customs are continued by the foreign students even though in an atmosphere of Catholicism, but continued discreetly.

In some of the universities attempts were also made to make it possible for foreign students of a different religious persuasion to be able to study and take degrees, in opposition to the local religious authorities. As Hilde de Ridder-Symoens says, 'These were the Universities of Padua, Siena, Leiden, Franeker, Utrecht, Montpellier, and even Basle, to quote only those giving courses in medicine.'[14] The Venetian Senate used a series of sleights of hand to enable

---

11 Julia, 'La pérégrination académique en France', p. 30 (note 5 above).

12 James Primrose, *Academia Monspeliensis ... descripta*, Oxford, 1631, p. A4r. This work also contains all the examination questions Primrose was posed, together with his answers, for all the stages of his degree.

13 Thomas Platter, *Journal of a younger brother*, p. 36 (note 10 above).

14 H. de Ridder-Symoens, 'Mobility', p. 430 (note 5 above).

Protestants to graduate in medicine at Padua, including empowering the Venetian Collegio dei Medici to grant degrees after strict examination, thus evading the veto on Protestants which would have been exercised by the Catholic Church through the local bishop.[15] Sometimes Protestant students would study medicine in a Catholic university, but actually take their degree in a Protestant one which had next to no requirements needing to be fulfilled, except the payment of fees. The university of Angers, for instance, provided many Protestant English medical men with their degrees, but no one would even think of going there to learn medicine![16] However, the increasing confessionalisation of the mid-sixteenth century onwards progressively closed some universities to anyone not of the local faith.[17]

But where you actually took your medical degree had other significances. Felix Platter's father wrote to him: 'Beloved son Felix ... It would be the greatest honour [if you] took the doctorate itself in Basel.' And Felix reasoned to himself: 'If I did take my degree in France, there would always be someone to insinuate that I did not dare to face the superior school in Basle. Everyone knew the saying about the French universities: "Accipimus pecuniam et mittimus stultos in Germaniam", that is to say, "We take their money and send them back to Germany as ignorant as before".'[18]

Other Sites of Learning

The universities were not the only place for the travelling student to learn about medicine. When lecturing on abscesses of the liver in London in 1616, William Harvey recalled: 'These things I have examined both in the Hospital [of Saint Bartholomew in London] and in the Italian hospitals with much nausea and loathing and stench and I remember them, but many I have forgotten.'[19] Thomas Bartholin tried to encourage his sons and nephew, as they set out in the 1670s, that 'There is vast delight and pleasure in gazing upon foreign lands and fields ... observing the different conditions of the sick in homes and in hospitals with their great number of beds ... examining the methods for treating the patients, enjoying the conversation of learned men and calling forth their experiences, and visiting the laboratories, the furnaces of the chemists, the pharmacies and unguent shops ... Furthermore, in the more celebrated cities the hospitals will provide him with

---

15 H. de Ridder-Symoens, 'Mobility', p. 426, 'Tolerant universities' (note 5 above).

16 On these 'venal' universities in France, especially Orange, see Julia, 'La pérégrination académique en France', pp. 38–40; and on Reims as 'venal' university for Scottish and Irish students in the eighteenth century, see pp. 46–8 (note 5 above).

17 Julia and Revel, *Les étudiants et leurs etudes*, pp. 57–61 (note 5 above).

18 Felix Platter, *Beloved son Felix. The journal of Felix Platter a medical student in Montpellier in the sixteenth century*, tr. S. Jennet, London, 1961, p. 120.

19 Cited from Harvey's *Praelectiones* by G. Keynes, *The life of William Harvey*, Oxford, 166, pp. 31–2.

much practical anatomy, offering through the use of diseased cadavers an easy introduction to knowledge of the affected regions [of the body] and the causes of diseases.'[20] Thomas Bartholin had seized such opportunities himself, especially in the ten years he had spent in the south of Italy, in Naples, Salerno, and Messina and Catania in Sicily, meeting all the famous medical men he could and learning their special techniques and recipes.

Outcomes

One of the outcomes of Felix Platter's *peregrinatio medica* – apart from his professorship – was his book *Praxeos medicae* ('The practice of medicine'), first published in 1602. Platter occasionally says 'as I have seen' of some event or fact, such as when he writes about a girl suffering from St Vitus Dance mania in Basel, but (unfortunately) he does not give a systematic account of what he had learnt from his teachers and travels. However, the title of a 1662 English translation of this work puts it right into the context of the value of experience gained in years of travel – boasting of no less than 31 years of travel! This was *A golden practice of physick. In five books and three tomes. After a new, easie, and plain method; of knowing, foretelling, preventing, and curing, all diseases incident to the body of man. Full of proper observations and remedies: both of ancient and modern physitians. Being the fruits of one and thirty years travel: and fifty years practice of physick. By Felix Platter, Cheif [sic] physitian and Professor in Ordinary at Basil. And R.W. [and] Abdiah Cole, Doctor of Physick, and the Liberal Arts [and] Nich. Culpeper, Gent. Student in Physick, and Astrology.* As Platter died in 1614, in fact most of the travel experience seems to be that of the translator, Abdiah Cole (or perhaps of Culpeper); for instance, where he writes (p. 150, col. 2) 'I saw in 1644 in a woman that I opened of a dropsie …', or 'I observed a grievous and wonderful palpitation of the heart in the year 1627, in a noble Virgin of Narbo [sic = Narbonne] in France'.

The Medical Foreign Travel of Laurentius Gryllus, c.1548–56

The first account of a *peregrinatio medica* which appeared in print was the Oration given by Laurentius Gryllus, in Latin, in Ingolstadt University in 1556. Gryllus came from Landshut in Bavaria and had matriculated at Vienna University in 1540 as 'Laurentius Grill', which is what I shall call him. The first part of this Oration will illustrate many of the points made above about the *peregrinatio medica* of the time, especially since Grill spent so much time and money seeking out the best teachers that the whole of Europe had to offer. This *Oration about foreign travel undertaken for medicinal study, and about the greatest value of that part*

[20] Thomas Bartholin, *On medical travel*, pp. 50–52 (note 6 above).

of medicine which expounds the properties of simple medicines, was published in Prague by a colleague in 1566.[21]

This first published account of a *peregrinatio medica* reveals that it was deliberately planned to improve medical teaching in the north, the periphery – Ingolstadt – by sending students to seek out the best and most up-to-date medical knowledge from elsewhere in Europe, especially the centre, which at that time was of course Italy and France. Grill was to spend 'seven years' travelling in Italy, France and Germany. Seven years is of course the classical term for the period spent learning a special craft or skill or becoming an adept in some field, and does not necessarily refer to a precise period of time. But in fact, if you count up the periods that Grill mentions that he spent in various towns, they come to close to seven years. Grill's travels were paid for generously by Johannes Jacobus Fugger, a member of the banking family who had made a great fortune by cornering the market in guaiacum wood as a remedy for the pox. After his return to Ingolstadt, Grill was made professor, thus enabling him to share with his northern students all that he had learnt about medicine in the south.

Unfortunately for Grill, but fortunately for us, he had broken his leg a few days before he was due to deliver his inaugural oration, and this meant he had to change his plans. He excused himself from presenting a splendid and elaborate Oration, since, the mind and the body being so closely linked, he could not think straight from the effects of the accident. 'I will speak therefore about private matters and those pertinent to the present purpose, and especially about the reasoning behind my plans, efforts, foreign travels and studies, which I have followed up to now in learning Medicine.' Then he would then go on to talk about materia medica and simples (that is, the simple ingredients, usually plants, of compound medicines), since that was his assigned field as a new professor at Ingolstadt. Together with his own predilection and personal enthusiasms for plants and medicines, this professional role accounts for Grill's concentration, in his account, on the learning of plants and the materia medica.

Grill's account starts with his boyhood years:

> Since, after the years of my childhood, I had made some progress in Greek and Latin studies in the school at Vienna and in this one at Ingolstadt, and afterwards throughout my youth I had tasted something of the liberal disciplines, finally I turned to the more serious studies of Philosophy, having as teacher the famous Philosopher Jacobus Scheckius (Scheck) in Tübingen University. At that time there was careful discussion about deciding on my future way of life, both by me and my parents and friends. And because of my fragility of body and frequent poor health and other reasons, it seemed sensible to everyone that I should select the profession of medicine for the rest of my life, a little time after which, to the study of wisdom [viz. philosophy] I began to join medicine.

---

21 Published at the end of Gryllus' *De sapore dulci et amaro libri duo* [*Two books on the sweet and bitter flavours*], Prague, 1566.

> I laid the first fundamentals of this art under Leonhard Fuchs [at Tübingen], a man most diligent in training up beginners, and famous everywhere for his various publications. I was with this teacher for two years, and under his tutelage I became familiar with several parts of medicine, and I was especially helped by him in the study of plants. Afterwards I returned to Ingoldstadt, and over two years I heard with no little profit the outstanding physicians of this University, that is Johannus Veltmüller, the most worthy Dean of our College, highly skilled in the art, doctrine and use of medical matters; then also the most learned Johannes Ammonius Agricola, who by his spirit and industry and by his researches, has both improved and enhanced our art and gained for himself immortal fame among the learned.
>
> In the meantime Johannes Jacobus Fugger, a man indeed fortunate by the affluence of his resources, but much more fortunate in his virtue, spirit and prudence, and never truly adequately praised, began in his most prudent deliberations to think of training up one or two medical students in Italy and elsewhere, so that whatever appeared to be lacking in Germany for learning medicine completely, should be brought back for other students, and especially the knowledge and personal experience [*autopsia*] of medicines of foreigners and of the plants which do not grow under our skies. Then they could also hear the judgements, thoughts and the sharp and ingenious thinking of other important physicians in places and disputations outside Germany about the difficulties and problems of this science. Finally, they might prepare for themselves the use and experience of things, which they call *praxis*, and what in Germany is denied by their own Teachers to various patients they may (as it were) be led by the hand – and not just from books, but from inspection and with the thing present – learn, and observe by continued use, what things pertain to curing the sick …

At Fugger's expense, Grill was sent on his seven-year trip to medical teachers and institutions through the whole of Italy, 'the parent of the wise and of all good arts', all of France and everywhere in Germany and the Low Countries. As he crossed the Alps he took careful note of all the special plants; at Venice he studied all the foreign medicines brought from the East, frequently visiting the busy market. He met the best physicians of that town and discussed and disputed with them about tricky points of the medical art. Leaving Venice, he went to Padua, where he spent 22 months to the great improvement of his knowledge. The medical teachers there included Johannes Baptista Montanus of Verona, who Grill thought was far better than Montanus's own teachers Manardus and Leoniceno, and could even be compared to some of the Ancient physicians. Not only did Grill hear Montanus's lectures for two years, but he also consulted him privately and was Montanus's companion in visiting the sick of the town, and he learnt much about both the theory and practice of medicine from him. He also heard the great Basianus Landus, who succeeded Montanus. He followed Aloysius Bellacatus for several months in his town practice, and witnessed innumerable cases in the town's hospital under Antonius Francazanus. He diligently witnessed numerous public and private dissections. Nor did he neglect the study of herbs.

> For the most venerable Senate of the Venetians have constructed inside the walls of Padua a most ample garden and one worthy of the wealth and magnificence of the Venetians, in which are planted foreign herbs, fruits and trees of every kind, unknown to the vulgar, which have been acquired from all parts of the globe by the voyages and wealth of the Venetians. I used to visit this garden with no less joy than profit, and I committed to memory the kinds, forms, images and variety of the plants, and I collected examples of them gathered live.

Then it was on to Ferrara, where for several days he heard Antonius Brasavolus lecture, and to Bologna, where he met Benedictus Faventinus, who had been practising medicine for 60 years, and he spoke there also with Helidaeus Medicus. Moving on to Florence, he spent several days visiting the hospital and meeting with the doctors and pharmacists. In Siena he spent five months, spending much time with Bartholomeus Boninsignius and Julius Verius, two most skilled physicians, the first of whom took him round the town to visit his patients, and the other trained him in the hospital, even letting him have five to seven patients as his own. By October Grill was in Rome, making friends with the most important physicians, such as Gysbertus Belga, whose services the pope himself employed. Again, he attended the hospital and the shops of the pharmacists, studying the compositions and prescriptions of the physicians. Rome of course is the city in which Galen had practised, so Grill paid attention to why Galen had said the city was in such an insalubrious site, and on his way to Naples Grill also looked out the Italian medicinal plants that Galen had used. He found the pharmacists of Naples very skilful and knowledgeable. Galen had particularly recommended the wines of the Naples region, and Grill dutifully looked them out and tasted them, so that he would be able later to recognise ones with similar qualities for medicinal use. Turning back north, Grill went to Pisa, where he spent nine months under excellent teachers, such as Johannes Argenterius and Vidus Vidius, onetime royal professor in Paris and the restorer of Hippocratic surgery. There he also met Simon Portius, the Neapolitan philosopher, Gabriel Fallopius, the highly skilled anatomist, and finally, Luca Ghini, 'who in the knowledge of herbs and the whole materia of simple remedies is second to no one in Italy'.

Now, as he says, having got what he came for in Italy, he turned to France, so that he might listen to the learned men of that region and add to his knowledge.

> For when I was in Italy and with Italian patients I was used to a certain Italian rationale of cure, and if I had gone back directly to Germany, using those things on German bodies would have got me into trouble, so everyone thought it would be a good idea if I visited the physicians of France and observed their rationale of cure in French bodies. For in their customs, education, state of the air and way

> of living, the French are similar to the Germans, whereby very similar diseases arise and the rationale of cure is the same.

He took a boat from Genoa and arrived at Marseilles, where he found the Mediterranean flora very striking. Stopping at Arles, Grill made the acquaintance of Franciscus Valleriola, whose medical publications Grill had found valuable. Then he was off to Lyons, where he spent two months with great benefit, before going to Montpellier, where 'for nearly six months, nothing that I needed for helping and adorning my medical studies was wanting. For that school is dedicated to the study and practice of medicine alone.' The main teachers were Squironius, Saporta, Honoratus and Guilliemus Rondelet, in whose house Grill lived as lodger, friend and disciple. Rondelet was busy finishing his book on fishes.

> In this School there are the best exercises of our art. Frequent disputations about controversial points, the best facilities for herbalising; frequent anatomical dissections. Opportunities for learning about fish and marine animals. Frequent practice, both of surgery and of the rest of medicine. Pharmacy is established in such a way that neither Masters nor servants are admitted who cannot give an account of their art in Latin.

Then Grill set off on a tour of the regions of France, ending up in Paris, where he stayed for 15 months.

Even after all the splendid facilities and outstanding medical men Grill had encountered thus far, Paris was special:

> I stayed there for 15 months in a row, to my great benefit. I heard Jacobus Sylvius, the Physician, most outstanding in years, authority, doctrine and experience. As a kind friend I also had Johannes Fernel, soundly learned in Medicine and Philosophy, as his most careful writings witness. I was friendly also with Jacobus Gupylus, who gave much work and labour to restoring and establishing the writings of the ancients which were partly damaged and partly full of defects. Also Jacobus Hollerius, a physician of great reputation, and other Greek-speaking physicians were known to me. With them I always had what I wanted. In such a multitude of persons there occurred both varied and unknown examples of diseases and varied cures. I also saw rare and notable Surgical cases, and of the French disease, which in that town occupies the whole place like some tyrant, I saw various cures, some of the Empirics, some of the Physicians, and some of the literate Surgeons, amongst whom my very good friend Nicolaus Lambertus excelled the rest. And indeed that town is never immune from pestilential fevers; recommendations and effective remedies were communicated to me against the severity of many of them. We also dissected the bodies of many of those who had died of uncertain diseases, so that we might detect the hidden cause of the disease and inspect it with our eyes.

Grill was constantly busy in practising the art in Paris, meeting as many French and German physicians as possible, learning all he could about medicines, and even how to prepare medicines by chemical distillations.

Next, Grill moved to Belgium, visiting Bruges and Ghent on his way to Amsterdam, 'which is the principal of all the markets of Europe'. He stayed here two months, familiarising himself with all the medicines and plants brought in from the East in their pure state, so that he could later recognise whether such exotic drugs had been adulterated – knowledge not obtainable at home in Germany. Grill over-wintered in Louvain and Brussels, where he spent two months meeting all the practitioners, especially Cornelius and Andreas Vesalius. Then he was off to Germany and the Netherlands again. Later he went to Magdeburg and Wittenburg, 'so that I might learn the new method of teaching which has emerged there'. Then 'I came at last to the most learned and outstanding Georgius Agricola at Chemnitz', who gave Grill seven days of his undivided attention, showing him all the minerals he had collected over many years. Next Grill went to Zwickau, where he met Janus Cornarius, the translator of the works of the Greek physicians. On his way home Grill spent 15 months in Salzburg at one of the Fugger pox-hospitals, the 'Fuggerei', established by the Fugger family to treat the poor who had the pox (or the French disease) with guaiacum wood. These are the same Fugger family who had been supporting Grill throughout his seven-year travels for his medical education, and he celebrates their generosity.

Grill's account of his *peregrinatio medica* is very impressive. He certainly seized all his opportunities of meeting the most famous teachers and practitioners in Italy and elsewhere, including even Andreas Vesalius. I can think of hardly any celebrated teacher of the period that Grill did not meet and seek friendship with on his journey. Their courtesy to him, and their generosity in introducing this ambitious young German student to their facilities, also speaks well of them. In introducing his Oration, Grill had said that how much progress he had made in medicine through his medical travel was for others to judge. Unfortunately, they did not have long to do so. For these years of expensive education did not, in the event, have much of an outcome, as Grill died only a few years later, in 1561, still working on a commentary on the ancient guide to medicinal plants written by Dioscorides.

When discussing different kinds of knowledge, and their relative desirability and trustworthiness, philosophers and theologians often compared *speculative* knowledge with *experiential* or *experimental* knowledge. While all agreed that speculative knowledge is ultimately firmer and more trustworthy and teaches true *scientia*, yet some thought that experiential knowledge is actually preferable and ought to be sought first. As one English theologian wrote in 1606, such knowledge 'is like the knowledge of a traveller which can speak of experience, and feeling, and hath been there and seen and known the particulars'.[22] And as Grill himself wrote, the main point of all this medical travelling for himself was just that: gaining that *personal experience,* that seeing-for-oneself (*autopsia*), and the familiarity with *the things themselves* in medicine that is called *praxis*. It was a different kind of knowledge – a complementary kind of knowledge, perhaps even a superior kind of knowledge – to that which could be acquired from books and the study of the ancient authorities. Medical travel literally broadened the mind, and made one a better doctor.

[22] A. Dent, *A pastime for parents ... containing the principall grounds of Christian religion*, London, 1606. I owe this reference and this point to a seminar paper by Professor Peter Harrison of Oxford.

Chapter 2
Medical Education and Centres of Excellence in Eighteenth-century Europe: Towards an Identification

Laurence Brockliss

Educational Provision

In the course of the period 1400 to 1700 medicine in most parts of western and central Europe became a corporate profession. Theoretically, practitioners were divided into three groups: physicians, surgeons and apothecaries. The first were learned doctors with degrees, trained in the medical faculties of Europe, who had a monopoly of diagnosis and prescription; the second and third were their subordinates, master artisans who carried out their orders, treating lesions and preparing and administering drugs, and were trained on the job. In reality, medical practice was always much more of a free for all. Learned physicians seldom went into the countryside where most of the population lived, so that surgeons and apothecaries frequently doubled up as general practitioners, while all three branches of the medical community suffered perpetual and sometimes intense competition from untrained part-time healers, quacks and charlatans. Nonetheless, by the end of the seventeenth century the distinction between legal and illegal medical practice was clear cut. In virtually every major city of continental Europe there was a corporation of physicians with the power in law to supervise and control medical services in the immediate vicinity, while even the smallest towns had guilds of surgeons and apothecaries who closely guarded their field of practice against interlopers (trained or untrained). Only in the British Isles, where this corporative structure had failed to take root, was the distinction between legitimate and illegitimate medical practice largely theoretical. Even in Britain and Ireland, though, there were medical corporations in the three capital cities and Glasgow, even if to all intents and purposes they lost their monopoly rights from 1704, when the House of Lords ruled that the Royal College of Physicians in London could not stop members of the city's Society of Apothecaries from practising physic.[1]

[1] The literature on the structure of the medical community in different European countries pre-1700 is now quite extensive: see, *inter alia*, H.J. Cook, *The Decline of the Old Medical Regime in Stuart London* (Ithaca, NY, 1986); Andrew Wear, *Knowledge and Practice in English Medicine, 1550–1680* (Cambridge, 2000); David Gentilcore, *Healers*

In the eighteenth century medicine continued to be a corporative profession and individual corporations and guilds continued to bring interlopers before the courts. The localist corporative structure, however, was increasingly moulded into a state-wide system of medical practice as governments began to legislate for the whole of their territories. The intervention of the French king was limited to insisting, from 1707, that every physician in his kingdom must hold a degree from a French medical faculty, and from 1730 that every surgeon, wherever he practised, must be certified by a surgeons' guild. After laying down the minimum requirement expected of a trained physician or surgeon (rules that in the latter case were significantly revised in 1772 and 1784), the monarch left it to the faculties and the guilds to test candidates' knowledge and skills. In Spain, on the other hand, the faculties might still offer degrees and the guilds certify masters, but the right to practise was only conferred after an examination in front of a central government body or its provincial sub-committees, headed by the king's chief physician, the *protomedicato*. The state, too, began to worry for the first time about the paucity of medical provision in the countryside. In German-speaking territories, even in the smallest towns, physicians were appointed to the stipended posts of *Land-* or *Stadtartz* with the primary responsibility of bringing rapid relief to areas struck down by epidemics or epizootics.[2] Again, only the British Isles held out against this trend. It would not be until 1815 that an attempt was made in law to define the medical community more carefully by forbidding practitioners in England who had not been licensed by the London Society of Apothecaries from dispensing medicines. The British state's only concession before this to the new enthusiasm for government-organised certification was to insist that the unqualified had to take a special army or navy diploma before entering the medical corps of the armed services.[3]

---

and Healing in Early Modern Italy (Manchester, 1988); L.W.B. Brockliss and Colin Jones, *The Medical World of Early Modern France* (Oxford, 1997), pt. 1. For an overview, see Mary Lindemann, *Medicine and Society in Early Modern Europe* (Cambridge, 1999), ch. 7. For the 1704 case, see Peter Elmer and Ole Grell (eds), *Health, Disease and Society in Europe, 1500–1800. A Source Book* (Manchester, 2004), pp. 346–8.

2 Brockliss and Jones, *Medical World*, pp. 486–90; M.C. Burke, *The Royal College of San Carlos. Surgery and Spanish Medical Reform in the late Eighteenth Century* (Durham, NC, 1977), pp. 28–9, 41; Mary Lindemann, *Health and Healing in Eighteenth-Century Germany* (Baltimore, 1996), *passim*.

3 Irvine Loudun, *Medical Care and the General Practitioner 1750–1850* (Oxford, 1986), ch. 7; Laurence Brockliss, M. John Cardwell and Michael Moss, *Nelson's Surgeon* (Oxford, 2005), pp. 13–15; Marcu Ackroyd, Laurence Brockliss, Michael Moss, Kate Retford and John Stevenson, *Advancing with the army. Medicine, the Professions and Social Mobility in the British Isles 1790–1850* (Oxford, 2006), pp. 23, 152–3. The Apothecaries Act of 1815 effectively meant that general practitioners had henceforth to be licensed. Those holding a medical degree, a licence from one of the surgical colleges or an army and navy diploma were exempt. The army and navy diplomas were awarded by the colleges of

The traditional structure of medical practice was muddied further in the eighteenth century by the growing belief that surgeons and, to some extent, apothecaries, should also receive formal training in order to be better understand their craft. This was not an entirely new belief, for several faculties of medicine in the seventeenth century had put on courses for the physicians' subordinates, notably the Paris faculty, where the practice had been established before 1550.[4] But it was only in the eighteenth century, when there were clear signs of progress in a number of surgical interventions such as lithotomy and couching for cataract, that it gained broad consent and began to be championed by the state. As a result, besides the novel courses sponsored by some existing surgical corporations, stand-alone schools or colleges of surgery were established with government money all over the Continent. These provided tuition in the different parts of the art and sometimes offered facilities where students could gain hands-on experience in dissection and surgical operations. In France alone there were 17 on the eve of the Revolution, the first and most famous being the Paris *Ecole de Chirurgie*, founded in 1724.[5] At the same time, it became a commonplace that graduate physicians should not just be knowledgeable in the theory of physic but also be properly informed about the arts of their subordinates (in part, the better to control them). Once more, some faculties had been expecting their students to attend lectures on anatomy and surgery, and botany and pharmacy/chemistry from a much earlier date. But it was generally only in the course of the eighteenth century that these subjects became a compulsory part of the curriculum and were sometimes examined as part of the degree. From 1724 Paris graduands had to sustain a surgical thesis, and from 1735 a two-week practical examination in anatomy and surgical operations.[6] Physicians were even expected to take an interest in midwifery. Not only did some faculties begin to provide classes for midwives from the conviction that they too needed limited formal training, but they also encouraged their students to attend.[7]

---

surgeons. The East India Company also demanded that its surgeons were examined before joining the service.

4 L.W.B. Brockliss, *French Higher Education in the Seventeenth and Eighteenth Centuries: A Cultural History* (Oxford, 1987), pp. 393–4. These courses were distinguished from the proper faculty curriculum by being delivered in the vernacular.

5 Brockliss and Jones, *Medical World*, p. 506 (map); Toby Gelfand, *Professionalising Modern Medicine: Paris Surgeons and Medical Science and Institutions in the Eighteenth Century* (London, 1980), ch. 5; Burke, *San Carlos*, p. viii (only three surgical colleges were founded in Spain.). From 1784 French surgeons had to have undergone two years' academic training.

6 Brockliss, *Higher Education*, pp. 74–5. From 1734 Montpellier graduates had to perform three dissections to gain a degree. There had been a specific chair in Latin surgery at Paris from 1635: ibid., p. 394.

7 There were courses in the vernacular on midwifery in four French faculties by the 1780s. The first was established at Strasbourg and was held by J.J. Fried (1689–1769): ibid., p. 394. Obstetrics was also taught in the surgical colleges. Most midwives, if they received formal instruction at all, were trained by itinerant lecturers, such as the Paris

Just as the range of faculty teaching was extended in the course of the eighteenth century, so too was it availability. There were some 150 universities in Europe in the mid-seventeenth century, but many of them did not have a functioning medical faculty. Far fewer people wanted to be physicians than lawyers. The situation changed considerably in the following decades, in an era when the affluent seem to have been much more willing to invest heavily in their health, so that on the eve of the French Revolution some sort of medical education could be obtained in virtually every university town.[8] The creation of the surgical colleges, however, did not so much extend provision even further as create an alternative network, all the more so in that they were generally founded in faculty towns. On the Continent, the age-old distinction between physicians and surgeons continued to have meaning, even if it was breaking down to some degree.[9] It is unlikely, then, that many medical students attended the surgical colleges or vice versa. Britain once more was a special case. It is clear that at the new medical faculty at Edinburgh, established in 1726, future physicians, surgeons and general practitioners rubbed shoulders together on the faculty benches. But in Britain there was no social stigma attached to such fraternisation, while the Edinburgh College of Surgeons did not support independent courses of lectures before the turn of the nineteenth century.[10]

The one location where physicians and surgeons did congregate together in the course of their training was in the hospital. Europe in the eighteenth century was peppered with charitable foundations for the poor sick, frequently dating from the late Middle Ages – France alone had 2,000; and many more were founded in the course of the century, especially in the British Isles, where a swathe of new

accoucheuse Angélique-Marguérite Le Boursier du Coudray: see J. Gélis, *La Sage-Femme ou le médecin? Une nouvelle conception de la vie* (Paris, 1988), pt. iii.

8 By then there were 184 universities: see Willem Frijhoff, 'Patterns', in H. de Ridder-Symoens, *A History of the University in Europe*, vol. II, *Universities in Early Modern Europe (1500–1800)* (Cambridge, 1996), pp. 78, 90–4 (list).

9 On the Continent, ambitious surgeons frequently claimed the right to practise physic on the grounds that their formal training had given them a good knowledge of medical theory, but they usually regularised their position by taking a medical degree in middle age. Typical was the physiocrat and Paris surgeon Francois Quesnay. On a number of occasions he published pamphlets presenting the case for surgeons being learned, and in 1748 claimed that they should have the right to practise physic. But he himself took a doctorate at the Lorraine faculty of Pont-à-Mousson in 1744: Brockliss and Jones, *Medical World*, pp. 594–8, 601, 607.

10 Lisa Rosner, *Medical Education in the Age of Improvement. Edinburgh Students and Apprentices 1760–1826* (Edinburgh, 1991), ch. 5. The Edinburgh College of Surgeons established an independent chair in surgery in 1804. Two years later the University emphasised its role as a training ground for all medical practitioners by gaining the country's first chair in military surgery: see Matthew H. Kaufmann, *The Regius Chair in Military Surgery in the University of Edinburgh, 1806–1855* (Amsterdam, 2003), esp. pp. 65–8.

voluntary hospitals were established to replace endowed institutions secularised during the Reformation.[11]

Traditionally, the hospital had had no role in training medical practitioners, but in the eighteenth century it became an important and novel site of practical learning. For both tyro physicians and surgeons, it was a place where they gained a deeper knowledge of anatomy and surgical operations by becoming the private pupils of the hospital surgeons. For tyro physicians, the hospital provided unprecedented opportunities for practical experience in patient care. Hitherto, the physician had learnt the art of medical practice after graduation, usually by acting as a locum to an established doctor. By the middle of the century this was no longer considered acceptable. It was felt to be reprehensible, in an age alarmed by the high rate of mortality, that physicians should learn at the expense of their patients, and a new emphasis was placed on learning the ropes in the course of study or immediately afterwards. As it was also believed that this was best done by seeing as many patients and diseases as possible in a short time, the obvious place to gain practical knowledge was an infirmary, which sheltered the sick poor, often promiscuously piled together regardless of their disease. Some faculties followed Leiden's, then Edinburgh's example in establishing a specific ward in the local hospital where students could receive clinical training. In most cases, students were left to attach themselves to a hospital physician for a fee and follow him on his rounds.[12]

The ubiquity of the hospital meant there was no necessity for medical students to seek practical experience in a faculty town. Indeed, since many faculties were located in small towns with perhaps a single infirmary, it made sense to travel to the state capital, where the opportunities for studying patients were likely to

---

[11] London had seven general hospitals (four of them voluntary) and a number of specialist infirmaries by the mid-eighteenth century. Throughout England there were 33 voluntary hospitals in 1800 where there had been only one a century before. In Ireland 37 hospitals were founded in the course of the century, a dozen in Dublin: Susan Lawrence, *Charitable Knowledge. Hospital Pupils and Practitioners in Eighteenth-Century London* (Cambridge, 1996), ch. 2; J. Woodward, *To Do the Sick No Harm. A Study of the British Voluntary Hospital System to 1875* (London, 1974), pp. 147–8; James Kelly, 'The Emergence of Scientific and Institutional Medical Practice in Ireland, 1650–1800', in Greta Jones and Elizabeth Malcolm (eds), *Medicine, Disease and the State in Ireland, 1650–1940* (Cork, 1999), pp. 27–32, 35. For a general overview: Lindemann, *Medicine and Society*, ch. 5.

[12] G.A. Lindeboom, *Herman Boerhaave. The Man and His Work* (London, 1968), pp. 282–305, 363–72; Gunther Risse, *Hospital Life in Enlightenment Scotland: Care and Teaching at the Royal Infirmary of Edinburgh* (Cambridge, 1986); Erna Lesky, 'The Development of Bedside Teaching at the Vienna Medical School from Scholastic Times to Special Clinics', in Charles O'Malley (ed.), *The History of Medical Education* (Berkeley, CA, 1970), pp. 217–34; Brockliss and Jones, *Medical World*, pp. 499–502, 511–14. Many faculties did provide instruction in the practice of medicine, but it is unclear whether students were introduced to real patients during the course. Another important site of clinical instruction were the army and naval hospitals that were established across the Continent in the period: Brockliss and Jones, *Medical World,* pp. 689–700, *passim.*

be much greater. It was for this reason that by the end of the eighteenth century a number of cities that had never had a medical faculty had become important centres of medical education. The best-documented example is London, the largest city in Europe, which had no university before the 1820s but a number of thriving medical schools attached to the leading hospitals. Other examples were Madrid and Berlin, where again there would be no university before the nineteenth century.[13] In the second half of the eighteenth century, moreover, these capital cities, with or without a faculty, usually offered a plethora of private courses in a variety of medical subjects outside the hospitals. Enterprising physicians, surgeons and apothecaries used their own homes or built their own auditorium, as the London surgeon, William Hunter, did in Windmill Street.[14] The thirst for practical, often hands-on, medical instruction seems to have been insatiable.

What then differentiates the eighteenth-century from an earlier age is the profusion of educational provision. The future medical practitioner was confronted with a wealth of choice. In many cases, however, his choices would have been quite heavily constrained. In the first place, many practitioners would have been forced by limited means to train locally in whatever branch of the profession they wanted to enter. Second, even assuming relative affluence, freedom of manoeuvre would have been restricted by the conditions that had to be met to join a favoured corporation or guild. Many physicians' guilds would only incorporate applicants with a degree from certain universities – in the case of the London College, only Oxford and Cambridge. Third, for the really affluent, study abroad could be discouraged by national legislation. Many states followed France in insisting that their nationals had to be certificated at home, but the Spanish king was even wary of letting his subjects leave the country to improve their knowledge.[15] Where to study abroad, too, could be affected by religious affiliation: Europe was still divided confessionally, and Protestants and Catholics preferred to live among their own, even if there was no outright ban on their attending a foreign university. On the assumption, then, that among these many and growing centres of medical

---

13 Lawrence, *Charitable Knowledge*, pt. i; Burke, *San Carlos*, chs. 4–7, *passim*. I know of no detailed study of Berlin in the eighteenth century: its leading teaching institutions were the *theatrum anatomicum* (1717), run by the Prussian Academy of Science and the Charité hospital (1725): see Johanna Geyer-Kordesch, 'German Medical Education in the Eighteenth Century: The Prussian Context and its Influence', in W.F. Bynum and Roy Porter (eds), *William Hunter and the Eighteenth-Century Medical World* (Cambridge, 1985), pp. 180, 196–205.

14 Roy Porter, 'William Hunter: A Surgeon and a Gentleman', and C. Helen Brock, 'The Happiness of Riches', in Bynum and Porter, *William Hunter*, chs. 1 and 2.

15 In 1559 Spaniards had been forbidden to study abroad except at Rome, Naples and Bologna. The possibilities of attending other centres of learning were few before the enlightened reign of Charles III: David Goodman, 'The Scientific Revolution in Spain and Portugal', in Roy Porter (ed.), *Scientific Revolution in National Context* (Cambridge, 1992), p. 172; Antonio Dominguez Ortis, *Sociedad y Estato en el siglo XVIII espanol* (Barcelona, 1990), ch. 25.

education there were particular centres of excellence, it must be realised that most medical practitioners in eighteenth-century Europe would never have had the chance to enjoy their benefits.

Centres of Excellence

It must be said at once that any attempt to isolate the centres of medical education in the eighteenth century that stood out from the rest is fraught with difficulty. Today, we primarily associate excellence in the academic world with innovative and internationally recognised research. This, though, is hardly a criterion that can be used to judge excellence in the eighteenth century. It is easy enough to prepare a list of the most original medical investigators of the period and associate their names with particular cities and institutions – Giovanni Battista Morgagni (1682–1771) at Padua, Albrecht von Haller (1708–77) at Göttingen, Maximilian Stoll (1742–88) at Vienna, and so on. But it must be stressed that research was never part of the remit of any eighteenth-century higher-educational establishment. The role of the professor and the teacher was to transmit the current orthodoxy (or, where there was more than one, what they or their institution judged to be the better informed). They might give that orthodoxy a personal tweak and their adjustments might be the result of their own experimental research, but they were under no obligation to be research active in any modern sense. In the eighteenth century the institutional locus of scientific research, to the extent that there was one, was the learned academy, of which a handful of the hundred or so in existence by 1800 were specifically devoted to medicine.[16] It was usually the case that these academies were established in cities that were also centres of medical education, such as the Paris Academy of Surgery (1731), the Göttingen Royal Society of Sciences (1751) and the Vienna Imperial Academy of Medicine and Surgery (1784). And it was normal for their members to hold chairs in the local faculty or surgical college. But many medical professors and teachers had no connection with learned academies and undertook no research. In fact, the first medical schools to expect their professors to contribute to the development of medical science were the three *Ecoles de santé* set up by the French Revolutionaries in 1794 at Paris, Montpellier and Strasbourg.[17]

---

[16] James E. McClellan III, *Science Reorganised: Scientific Societies in the Eighteenth Century* (New York, 1985); idem, 'Scientific Institutions and the Organisation of Science', in Roy Porter (ed.), *The Cambridge History of Science*, vol. 4, *Eighteenth-Century Science* (Cambridge, 2003), ch.4; and *Encyclopedia of the Enlightenment*, ed. Alan J. Cors (4 vols; Oxford, 2003), iv, 3–19.

[17] [A.F. de Fourcroy], *Rapport et décret de la convention nationale sur les Ecoles de Santé de Paris, Montpellier et Strasbourg*, 14 Frimaire, Year III (Paris, 1794), pp. 17–18. The Paris faculty, along with all the other French universities, had been closed by the Revolutionaries in 1793.

A less anachronistic approach would be to isolate the centres with the widest range of medical courses, be they provided by one or a mix of institutions, be they public or private. As was explained in the previous section, to pass muster in the second half of the eighteenth century, the tyro graduate physician had to have been trained in the theory and practice of medicine, have studied the ancillary medical sciences, and have gained experience in patient care. Arguably, the centres of excellence in the period were the cities that offered the most complete medical *cursus*. This is certainly a sensible way of proceeding in the first half of the century, when many faculty towns provided little or no tuition in the ancillary sciences, few surgical colleges had been created and gaining access to the local hospital could be difficult (in Catholic states in particular, where the regular orders that ran them did not welcome students walking the wards). However, by the last quarter of the century, thanks frequently to state initiative, surgical colleges were springing up all over the Continent and most medical faculties, even in relatively small towns, were given the means to teach a much more extensive curriculum.[18]

The faculties of Spain are a case in point. There appears to have been little or no formal instruction in anatomy or surgery in the Spanish faculties before the 1760s, even if some institutions had for a long time had designated chairs in the two subjects. Spain was definitely one part of Europe where formal medical instruction was still solidly theoretical. But reforms in the reign of Charles III (1759–88) brought the curriculum much more up to date, and on the eve of the French Revolution three faculties, Valencia, Granada and Seville, had a chair in chemistry and two, Valencia and Granada, even provided courses in clinical medicine, just like Edinburgh. There were also attempts to rationalise the provision so as to avoid duplication. Towards the end of Charles's reign, in 1787, most of the faculty chairs of surgery were abolished and physicians were expected to study the subject in a local hospital or surgical college.[19] Clearly, then, simply establishing a hierarchy of

---

[18] The extent of the provision across Europe by the end of the century can be gleaned from contemporary guidebooks. They are not always complete and their authors have an understandable tendency to puff their own institutions, but they are still a useful point of entry: e.g. M.-A. Barras, 'L'Etat actuel des établissements destinés en Europe à l'instruction publique et au progrès des connaissances humaines', in idem, *De l'éducation publique dans la France libre* (2 vols; Toulouse, 1793), p. ii; Friedrich Colland, *Kurz Inbegriff von der Ursprunge der Wissenschaften, Schulen, Akademien und Universitaten in ganz Europa, besonders aber der Akademien und hohen Schule zu Wien* (Vienna, 1796). For a list of such guides in the period, see Willem Frijhoff, 'Les guides universitaires (XVIe–XVIIIe siècle)', in Gilles Chabaud, Evelyne Cohen, Natacha Coquery and Jérome Penez (eds), *Les Guides imprimées du XVIe au XXe siècle* (Paris, 2000), pp. 23–36.

[19] Burke, *San Carlos*, ch.3; G.M. Addy, *The Enlightenment in the University of Salamanca* (Durham, NC, 1966), pp. 43–4, 103–7, 123, 172–7; Salvador Albinana, *Universidad e Illustración. Valencia en la época de Carlos III* (Valencia, 1988), pp. 63–6, 193–7, 232, 241. From 1795, in the reign of Charles IV, all Castilian physicians had to do a two-year course in clinical medicine at the newly founded Royal School of Practical Medicine in Madrid, which was located in the General Hospital; this was united with the

medical provision is insufficient to isolate the real centres of medical excellence. The problem with this approach is that it is not discriminatory enough.

There are potentially two ways in which the approach could be refined. The first is to look more closely at the quality of teaching. The fact that a city provides a complete course in medicine says nothing about the quality of the product. Professors of the different branches of medicine were not full-time teachers. Their lectures and demonstrations punctuated a busy day built around their private practice. Chairs, too, were frequently awarded as patronage plums, while stipends were often derisory; in faculties and colleges where professors were impermanent and chosen by lot from the large pool of local physicians and surgeons, professors taught out of duty rather than choice. Many professors therefore must have been humdrum, inarticulate, inaudible or even absent. Even courses given by private teachers could have been of indifferent quality, if they were simply put on to supplement an inadequate salary. Presumably, the centres of excellence were most likely to be those where the public professors were well paid and chosen by *concours*, and the private professors were teaching out of love of the subject and not just love of lucre. Admittedly, such professors were unlikely to be stimulating in the modern sense of the term. The most common form of teaching was to dictate from a prepared text, which the students took down, then give an impromptu elaboration of what had been first said. The alternative method was to read first from a prescribed textbook.[20] Doubtless, though, good teachers had ways of making the format less dry than it appears, and it must have taken a special skill and a rare empathy to lecture in this way while a dissector or demonstrator performed the operation or experiment that was being discussed. The format was unlikely to be mastered by the uncommitted.

Presumably, too, the centres of excellence were likely to be cities with the best facilities. Professors of theoretical medicine needed no more than a lecture hall and a lectern or pulpit, but professors of anatomy, surgery, botany etc. were unlikely to be very effective communicators unless their lectures were supported by practical demonstrations. They needed purpose-built amphitheatres, laboratories, botanical gardens and spacious hospital wards where their auditors could learn

---

Madrid surgical college in 1799: Burke, *San Carlos*, pp. 143–7. The situation was analogous in Portugal before the 1772 reform of the University of Coimbra.

[20] A move to textbook teaching occurred in many parts of Europe in the second half of the eighteenth century. Sometimes the approved text was the work of a local professor, but there were some, such as Boerhaave's works and the anatomy of Lorenz Heister (1683–1758), which were used across the continent. Both were introduced at Salamanca, for instance, in 1771, despite the fact that their authors were Protestants: Addy, *The University of Salamanca*, pp. 103–6. Even the impromptu exposé cannot have been delivered at speed. The Leiden-trained Gerard Van Swieten (1700–70), chief physician at the Austrian court, who published a six-volume commentary on Boerhaave's *Aphorisms* (1742–76), as a student supposedly took down every word that the great professor uttered: F.T. Brechka, *Gerard van Swieten* (1970), p. 75.

through seeing as well as hearing. Indeed, in an age that emphasised the benefits of learning by doing, the optimum situation was where the medical student could digest what he had heard and seen by repeating the demonstrations himself. It was not sufficient, either, that the necessary 'plant' was in place; it also had to be properly maintained. Botanical gardens could very quickly degenerate unless they were properly cared for and continually restocked. It was easy, then, for medical centres to promise more than they offered.

Take the example of Leuven in the Austrian Netherlands. The town was well placed as a cultural centre, for it boasted the only university in the territory, founded in the early fifteenth century, and a long-established faculty of medicine, where Van Helmont had trained. However, in 1788 the Emperor Joseph II of Austria (1780–90) ordered the faculty of medicine at Leuven to be moved to Brussels. Leuven was certainly not backward in the range of medical instruction it provided. Anatomy had been taught publicly for several centuries in the faculty, chemistry from 1685, while the professors also gave private lectures on anatomy, midwifery and women's diseases. Moreover, 13 years earlier, on the suggestion of one of the professors, Van Rossum, the government had set up a chair in clinical medicine, based at a local hospital. From 1755, furthermore, the four professors had been elected by *concours*. But in a report of 1785 Leuven had been deemed inadequate as a medical centre. It offered no lectures in surgery and midwifery in the vernacular for surgeons, the faculty's anatomical theatre was falling down, its chemistry laboratory and botanical garden were too small, dissectors had difficulty finding bodies, and the clinical course was not a success. Transferring the faculty to a large city, it was believed, would remedy the problem. There would be more corpses and better hospital facilities.[21]

Leuven, though, is a particularly well-documented case. At present we know very little about the quality of the medical provision in the vast majority of medical centres in the eighteenth century. Much more detailed research is required before it will be possible to speak authoritatively about the appointments structure, level of stipend and state of facilities for teaching practical medicine and the ancillary medical sciences Europe-wide. It may be the case, too, that the documentation upon which such a study could be based no longer exists and, even if it did, it would still be difficult to rank medical centres authoritatively. There is, however, another way forward. For the eighteenth century, if not for earlier centuries, the matriculation registers of many if not all of Europe's medical faculties exist. It is a relatively simple process, therefore, to discover which were the most popular faculties in a

[21] C. Brunel, 'Au coeur des reformes: la faculté de médecine de Louvain dans le dernier quart du XVIIIe siècle', in C. Brunel and P. Servais (eds), *La Fondation du médecin: Des lumières au laboratoire* (Louvain-la-neuve, 1989), ch. 2. The transfer did not take place because the Austrian Netherlands rebelled against Joseph II. In 1794 Leuven University was closed by the French when they occupied the territory and annexed it to France. Leuven in the eighteenth century had no corporation of surgeons, and there seems to have been no attempt to establish independent colleges of surgery in the region.

particular state by identifying the number of students starting each year. Given the sheer number of medical centres in Europe and the financial attractions of training close to home, it seems reasonable to assume that faculties in large states that had many more students than their sisters and whose recruitment was nationwide were perceived by contemporaries to be the centres of excellence. Fathers would not have sent their sons far from home at great expense if they had not believed that there was a great difference in the quality of tuition to be found there, all the more so in that most expected their offspring to set up their plate in their local area.

It must be stressed, though, that the study must be based on matriculations, not graduations. As will become apparent, there is good reason for believing that the level of graduations is not a reliable indicator of relative institutional health. In fact, Leuven's own buoyant graduation figures suggest that this must be so. In the final quarter of the century, the faculty licensed 30 physicians per annum, a larger number than its Dutch rival, Leiden. The latter, of course, would normally be on any historian's instinctive list of the centres of medical excellence in the eighteenth century. In the first decades of the century, medical students from all over Europe, especially from the British Isles, flocked to the town to hear the great Herman Boerhaave (1668–1738), the outstanding expounder of iatromechanism of the age.[22] Even if the faculty lost some of its élan thereafter, there can be no doubt that it was always the most important medical faculty in the United Provinces. But the paradox is immediately solved once it is realised that no physician could practise in the Austrian Netherlands without a Leuven degree, while Leiden had no such monopoly in the United Provinces.[23]

The information to be potentially gained from a study of faculty matriculations is evident in the case of France. The kingdom was the biggest state in Europe, with a population of 20 million at the beginning of the century and 30 million at the close. Although it is impossible to know exactly how many graduate physicians there were, it can be estimated that there were about 1,300 in the 1690s and 3,100 in the 1780s.[24] Where had they trained? There were 23 universities in France in 1789 (or 24 if the faculty of Catholic theology at Strasbourg is counted as a separate institution). All but four had the right to offer instruction in medicine, but probably only 17 of the 24 actually did so, and only 15 in the second half of the eighteenth century. Between them on the eve of the French Revolution, they contained about

---

[22] In the years 1701–38, while Boerhaave was in post, 746 English-speaking students matriculated in medicine at Leiden : see E.A. Underwood, *Boerhaave's Men, at Leiden and After* (Edinburgh, 1977), p. 20 (table 1). It is now clear that Boerhaave's attraction lay in his teaching (he taught botany, chemistry and theoretical medicine), not his pioneering development of clinical medicine: see the chapter by Knoeff in this volume.

[23] Brunel, 'Au coeur des reformes', pp. 22–4. Only the licence was required to practise in the Austrian Netherlands, so very few physicians had the higher degree of doctor. Boerhaave himself had a doctorate from the tiny university of Harderwijk.

[24] Brockliss and Jones, *Medical World*, p. 520.

500 medical students.[25] The 15 divide into three groups. The largest – seven in number – had hardly any registered students and seldom recruited more than half a dozen new students per year. Avignon, for instance, never attracted more than 15 new students in any one year, and in the period 1711 to 1789 only recruited more than 10 new students per annum on 10 occasions.[26] A second group of four universities – Besançon, Caen, Nancy and Toulouse – seem to have usually attracted from 10 to 30 new students each year, but only the last consistently welcomed more than 20. Finally, an elite of three – Montpellier, Paris and Strasbourg – attracted a solid clientele. Paris in the third quarter of the eighteenth century matriculated between 45 and 55 new students each year, while Strasbourg in the same period welcomed on average 48, though the number dropped thereafter. Montpellier was apparently even more popular: it was recruiting 65 new students per year in the 1750s and 1760s, and 74 in the last two decades of the *ancien régime*.[27]

The pecking order among French faculties of medicine can be refined further by looking at the geographical origins of their students. Faculties that had few students recruited locally. Hardly anyone at Avignon, for instance, came from more than 40 kilometres away, and the few who did usually had singular histories.[28] Ignace-Vincent Voullone, who began to study medicine at Avignon in 1764, was born in Spain, at Alicante. He was a former Lyons Jesuit, who had just been evicted from his convent with the Order's closure in France and was looking to begin a new career.[29] Even the more dynamic second-tier faculties recruited close to home. Toulouse drew its students from a wider area than Avignon, but it was still a regional faculty whose clients came from the south-west of France and scarcely ever from other parts of the country. If it did educate a handful of Irish students in the last decades of the *ancien regime*, this simply reflected the fact that there was a flourishing college for training Irish Catholic priests in the city. It was commonplace for a number to gain a modicum of medical knowledge before they were sent on the Irish mission.[30] Indeed, even Strasbourg did not have a national

---

25 Brockliss (1987), *Higher Education*, p. 479 (map); R. Chartier, M.M. Compère and D. Julia, *L'Education en France du XVIe au XVIIIe siècle* (Paris, 1976), p. 274.

26 Dominique Julia and Jacques Revel, 'Les etudiants et leurs études dans la France moderne', in eidem (eds), *Les Universités européennes du XVIe au XVIIIe siècle. Histoire sociale des populations étudiantes*, vol. 2 (Paris, 1989), pp. 459–85 (tables). Matriculation registers exist for only 12 faculties and a number are very incomplete. There is some information of total numbers for two other faculties.

27 Information about Paris only exists for 1753 to 1774: see Bibliothèque de la Faculté de Médecine, Paris, MS 2005, register of inscriptions.

28 Archives départementales de Vaucluse, D 64: register of inscriptions. See also the analysis of Angers' medical students in Chartier, Compère and Julia, *Education*, p. 281.

29 Archives départementales de Vaucluse, D. 64, f. 206v.

30 Patrick Ferté, 'L'Université de Toulouse au XVIIe et XVIIIe siècles. Etude quantitative de la population étudiante des ses trois facultés supérieures de 1679 à la Révolution', thèse de troisième cycle, Université de Toulouse-Le Mirail (2 vols, 1978), i.

clientele. As a Lutheran faculty in a Lutheran city, it exerted no influence on Catholics and largely drew its students from the German side of the Rhine.[31]

Only Montpellier and Paris were truly national faculties of medicine in eighteenth-century France. Montpellier was still largely a regional faculty in that 80 per cent of its new students in 1780–84 came from the Midi. But it was in no way dependent on its immediate locality for its students, since only 10 per cent came from Montpellier itself and the surrounding dioceses. Moreover, 14 per cent came from northern France and 6 per cent from abroad. This was a much smaller proportion than in earlier centuries – 35 per cent of its students had been foreigners in 1503–12 – but it was still a significant number: there would always have been four or five foreign nationals beginning their studies at Montpellier each year.[32] Paris, conversely, had a northern bias. In autumn 1773, 63 per cent of its matriculands came from north of the Loire. Again, though, it did not recruit overwhelmingly from its hinterland. Despite the size of the capital (500,000–600,000 inhabitants), less than 10 per cent of its students at this date came from the diocese of Paris. More than 30 per cent, on the other hand, came from south of the Loire and 5 per cent from abroad.[33]

It is not difficult to see why Montpellier and Paris were the dominant French faculties, even if little is known about most of the 15 faculties, even Strasbourg.[34] It had little to do with the excellence of their theoretical teaching. Most of the 15, however lowly, could offer students a series of lectures on medical theory, provided they could afford to hire a professor and the professor was conscientious. The Avignon theory chair, for instance, was filled for 20 years, in the third quarter of the century (1756–74), by the local physician Esprit Calvet (1728–1810), whose lecture course survives. Although it was scarcely up to date – students who

171–3; ii. 420–3; L.W.B. Brockliss and P. Ferté, 'Irish Clerics in France in the Seventeenth and Eighteenth Centuries: A Statistical Study', *Proceedings of the Royal Irish Academy*, Section C, 87: 9 (1987), esp. pp. 564–5.

31 See G. Knod, *Die alten Matrikeln der Universität Strassburg (1621–1793)*, in *Die Matrikeln der medicinischen und juristischen Facultät* (Strasbourg, 1987).

32 Julia and Revel, 'Les étudiants', p. 328.

33 L.W.B. Brockliss, 'Patterns of Attendance at the University of Paris, 1400–1800', *Historical Journal*, 21: 3 (1978), 528: figs recalculated to exclude matriculands whose place of origin was not recorded.

34 In the 30 years since 1980, virtually nothing of significance has been published on individual French faculties of medicine in the eighteenth century, except L. Dulieu, *La Médecine à Montpellier*, iii. *L'Epoque classique* (2 pts. in 2 vols; Avignon, 1983–86). Strasbourg has been the subject of a master's thesis: R. Steegman, 'Le Milieu médical à Strasbourg au XVIIIe siècle', Mémoire de maîtrise, Univ. Strasbourg-II, 1977. But Paris has been completely neglected. The secondary literature of an earlier age is recorded in Simonne Guenée, *Bibliographie de l'histoire des universités françaises des origines à la Révolution* (2 vols; Paris, 1978–81). The most informative old history of a minor faculty is Jean Barbot, *Les Chronique des la faculté de médecine de Toulouse du XIIIe au XXe siècle* (2 vols; Toulouse, 1905).

listened to Calvet would have learnt nothing about vitalism – students would have received a clear exposition of Boerhaavian iatromechanism, even enlivened by a few personal twists.[35] Nor can it have had much to do with the fact that both the Paris and Montpellier faculties could teach the complete medical curriculum much more easily than their sisters, in that both had a professoriate of eight rather than the usual three to five. Neither faculty can have provided first-class *ex cathedra* teaching. Montpellier in the 1770s was staffed with a clutch of fertile and original minds who were at the forefront of the new vitalist medicine, but none taught to their strengths because the chairs were ranked according to the date of their foundation and allocated according to seniority. In consequence, as Napoleon's Minister of the Interior, Chaptal, recalled in his memoirs, 'nobody occupied the right place'. The chemist Gabriel-François Venel (1723–75) taught hygiene, the vitalist Paul-Joseph Barthez (1734–1806) lectured on anatomy (a science that vitalists thought to be next to useless), while the botanist Antoine Gouan (1733–1801), (less preposterously) was responsible for *matière médicale*.[36] The academic stars, moreover, were frequently absent. Barthez disappeared from Montpellier in the last 10 years of the *ancien régime* to serve at court and his lectures were given by a substitute. At Paris there was even less chance of hearing anyone of substance lecturing on their specialism, for the chairs were unendowed and there was no permanent professoriate. The faculty comprised some 150 doctors who were also the city's medical corporation. The members took turns in giving lectures. There was a tendency for the task to be allotted to youngsters, so there was little likelihood of a student being addressed by a medical grandee, such as the anatomist Félix Vicq d'Azyr (1748–94) or the clinician Jean-Nicolas Corvisart des Marets (1755–1821).[37]

What gave Montpellier and Paris the edge was that the two cities offered medical students far better facilities for practical instruction. Only five of the minor faculties possessed their own botanical garden on the eve of the Revolution, and even some of the better-attended had limited provision for anatomy teaching. Thus, Toulouse had no anatomical theatre before 1770, when it received a benefaction from the municipality. Prior to this, anatomies had taken place in the residential Collège de Périgord.[38] Nor was the local medical community of physicians, surgeons and

---

35 L.W.B. Brockliss, *Calvet's Web. Enlightenment and the Republic of Letters in Eighteenth-Century France* (Oxford, 2002), p. 28, and ch. 3, *passim*.

36 Jean-Antoine-Claude Chaptal, *Mes souvenirs*, ed. A. Chaptal (Paris, 1893), pp. 15–16.

37 Professors were appointed for two years. In the last years of the *ancien régime*, no medic of note held a Paris chair, though the faculty boasted a number of prominent medical investigators: see *Commentaires de la faculté de médecine de Paris (1777 à 1786)*, ed. G. Steinheil (2 vols; Paris, 1903), faculty minute book, records of professorial elections, *passim*. Vicq d'Azyr was the head of the Paris Société Royale de Médecine; Corvisart became one of Europe's leading pathological anatomists at the turn of the nineteenth century.

38 Barbot, *Chroniques*, i. 208, 275–82.

apothecaries normally large or enterprising enough to offer private courses of instruction, although it was usually possible to walk the wards with one of the local hospital staff.[39] Even when the minor faculties attempted to provide practical facilities, the results left much to be desired. Caen acquired a botanical garden in 1737, the Callard de la Ducquérie, which had originally been a private initiative owned by a medical family in the town. But the faculty lacked the funds to stock it, and until 1765 at least it was maintained largely at the professor of botany's own expense, as the then professor, Charles-Nicolas Desmoueux (1728–1801), complained. In 1764 the same faculty established a chair in chemistry, but for 10 years the first incumbent, Robert-Toussaint Deschamps (1750–1815), was never paid.[40]

The two leading faculties, on the other hand, were much better placed to fill the new market needs either directly or indirectly. Montpellier was no bigger than Caen or many other French cities with a faculty of medicine, but it had been an important centre of medical teaching for many centuries and had good-quality facilities even by the end of the sixteenth century.[41] Moreover, if the professors did not always teach their specialities or were indifferent lecturers, it was always possible to go to others for private instruction. Pierre-Joseph Amoreux (1741–1824) trained at Montpellier from 1759 to 1762. He had little admiration for the official courses he took, but he remembered with affection the extracurricular tuition. Initially, he attended the private anatomy lessons of two surgeons, Joseph Sarrau (1727–83) and Jean-Baptiste Laborie (1730–96); he then moved on to try his hand at dissecting with a Montpellier physician called Avézard. During his second year, he gained practical experience in patient care by walking the wards with the two physicians attached to the Hôtel-Dieu Saint-Eloi. He also became an enthusiastic Linnean botanist, thanks to the tuition he received from the Montpellier physician, Pierre Cusson (1722–83), with whom he lodged, and the young Antoine Gouan, not yet a professor. Finally, he took a private chemistry course given by Venel in the ampitheatre of the pharmacist Jacques Montet (1722–82).[42]

---

39 E.g. in 1778 Calvet of Avignon was asked to take a Montpellier graduate as a paying pupil at the local hospital of Sainte-Marthe, where he was one of the physicians: Bibliothèque Municipale Avignon, MS 1050, f. 714: letter, 22 Jan. 1778.

40 Brockliss and Jones, *Medical World*, pp. 503–4.

41 Louis Dulieu, *La Médecine à Montpellier*, i. *Le Moyen Age* (Avignon, 1975); idem, *La Médecine à Montpellier*, ii. *La Renaissance (Avignon, 1979)*; idem, *Epoque classique*, pt. 1. The faculty had an anatomy theatre of some kind from 1556 and a botanical garden, France's first, from 1593. In that year the faculty also established a separate chair in anatomy and botany. A chair in chemistry was founded in 1676, and from 1732 a degree could be taken in surgical medicine; there were ten graduates per annum in the subject from 1760–90.

42 Bibliothèque Municipale Avignon MS 1269, P.-J. Amoreux, 'Mes souvenirs ou détails historiques', pp. 26–33.

The Paris faculty, admittedly, had little in the way of 'plant'. Until 1749, when a stone edifice was opened, it only had a wooden amphitheatre, and it never possessed a botanical garden. Nonetheless, students throughout the century were able to attend first-rate practical lectures in botany, anatomy, surgery and pharmacy, given by the elite of the faculty and some outsiders at the Collège Royal and Jardin du Roi. The first was an independent higher-educational institute with four stipended chairs in medicine, three in the practical sciences; the second was a well-endowed royal foundation established in 1635, which boasted the best-equipped amphitheatre in France and offered courses in anatomy, botany and chemistry given by the country's premier men of science.[43] If the Paris medical students, too, were willing to swallow their prejudices and rub shoulders with tyro surgeons, they could also attend lectures in the practical medical sciences at the Paris surgeon's independent Ecole de Chirurgie, which eventually had nine chairs, including specialist demonstrators in obstetrics and opthalmology (established in 1747 and 1765) and a state-of-the art amphitheatre (opened in 1775).[44] Moreover, in the second-largest city in Europe, the official medical community numbered in total some 500 practitioners, and plenty of physicians, surgeons and apothecaries were happy to augment their income by putting on private courses or taking in pupils.[45] The city, too, possessed many hospitals, so there were many opportunities for medical students to accompany physicians on their rounds.[46] By the end of the period, furthermore, they could attend a structured clinical course. The faculty never had a chair in clinical medicine itself, though one was mooted in 1774. But from 1785 a private course was instituted at the Charité hospital by two faculty doctors, Louis Desbois de Rochefort (1750–86) and Corvisart, while another was conducted by the physician Nicolas Chambon de Montaux (1748–1828) at the Salpetrière, a woman's hospital.[47]

---

[43] Brockliss, *Higher Education* (1987), 398–9. The Collège royal was set up by Francis I in the 1530s. The best introduction to the riches of the *Jardin du roi* is Y. Laissus, 'Le Jardin du roi', in R. Taton (ed.), *L'Enseignement et diffusion des sciences au dix-huitième siècle* (Paris, 1963), pp. 287–341.

[44] Gelfand (above, n. 5). See also, C.C. Gillispie, *Science and Polity in France at the end of the Old Regime* (Princeton, NJ, 1980), pp. 130–84, *passim*.

[45] No study has ever been made of the number of private courses on offer, but their profusion is clear from the evidence in the published and unpublished diaries, autobiographies and correspondence of medical visitors to the city.

[46] There were 28 hospitals or hospices in Paris on the eve of the Revolution, see D.B. Weiner, *The Citizen-Patient in Revolutionary and Imperial Paris* (Baltimore, 1993), frontispiece.

[47] Brockliss and Jones *Medical World*, pp. 501, 512–13. At the end of the *ancien régime*, trainee physicians in Paris could also have attended the private courses in clinical surgery, such as the one given at the Hôtel-Dieu by Pierre-Joseph Desault (1744–95). The development of Paris clinical surgery is discussed in depth in Gelfand, *Professionalising Medicine*, pp. 303–56. In France only the Strasbourg faculty ever provided a public course in clinical medicine in the eighteenth century: see E. Wickersheimer, 'La Clinique de l'hôpital

It was the sheer range of extra-faculty tuition available in Paris which made the city a magnet for medical students. Those who chose to study theoretical medicine in the faculty could attend extra-curricular practical courses even while they sat on its benches. One such was the Breton Guillaume-François Laënnec, uncle of the great Laënnec, who arrived in Paris in 1769. Even in his first term Laënnec senior was attending the Ecole de Chirurgie twice a week (though understandably for a physician not an official course) and taking a private lessons in botany. In his second term he opted for the private anatomy course given by Antoine Petit (1718–94), one of the faculty doctors, then in the third he followed another given by Raphael-Bienvenu Sabatier (1732–1811), chief surgeon in survivance at the Invalides, while walking the wards at the Charité with Pierre-Louis-Marie Maloët (1730–180) and François Thierry de Bussy (b. 1719). In subsequent terms, he took a course in surgical operations with Sabatier, further courses with Petit on anatomy, surgery, obstetrics, children's ailments and general maladies, and studied chemistry and pharmacy with the faculty doctor, Bucquet, and the apothecary, Mitouart, one part of medicine which he thought was particularly well-taught at Paris. He also regularly attended courses at the Jardin du Roi, although he thought the botany teachers there went too fast for a novice.[48]

Yet if Montpellier and Paris were the evident twin centres of medical excellence in eighteenth-century France, this would not have been revealed by using graduation records as a point of departure. True, Montpellier's hegemonic position is only confirmed. From the 1730s, if not before, the Faculty bestowed the lion's share of doctorates – more than 60 per annum in the 1770s and 1780s, about 50 per cent of the total. The attraction of Paris, however, could never be guessed from its feeble number of graduates, seldom more than five a year – 10 per cent of the intake in the 1750s, probably even less thereafter. Just as surprising, Reims, a faculty that had hardly any students – six in 1789 – was the second to only Montpellier in the number of doctorates it bestowed. Indeed, before the 1740s it held premier place, graduating 35 per annum in the 1730s.[49]

The explanation for this anomaly lies in the sheer expense in time, energy and money in gaining a Paris degree. A Paris doctorate brought with it the right to practise physic in the capital. As this was a valuable corporative privilege, it was not obtained easily. To qualify as a bachelor in medicine, the would-be doctor had to hold an MA from the University of Paris and to have studied for four years in the faculty's schools, rather than the one laid down in the 1707 crown edict governing medical graduation in France. To become a doctor, he then had to spend a further two years gaining his degree. During that time, he was required to demonstrate

de Strasbourg au XVIIIe siècle', *Archives internationales de l'histoire des sciences*, 16 (1963), 253–76.

[48] Alfred Rouxeau, *Un étudiant en médecine quimpérois (Guillaume-François Laënnec) aux derniers jours de l'ancien régime* (Nantes, 1926), chs. 2–6.

[49] Brockliss and Jones, *Medical World*, p. 517 (table). The exact number of students entering the Paris faculty is not known after 1774: see above, n. 27.

his knowledge and skill in a number of theoretical and practical examinations and contribute some 5–7,000 *livres* (nearly £300) to the faculty's coffers.[50] This was a large outlay – a year's *pension* in the smartest Paris arts college was only 600 *livres* – so most medical students were unwilling or unable to make the investment. Instead, they went off to Reims, which offered three different doctorates – one that required effort for someone who wanted to practise in the city, another for those who did not and that could be obtained in a couple of days, and a third, a 'quicky', for non-natives who merely wanted a piece of paper to impress their clients when they returned home.[51] There they would encounter medical students from all over Europe – many from Leiden – all in search of a cheap and undemanding degree. Students from the British Isles were particularly notorious supplicants, especially in the 1730s, when nearly 20 a year were taking a degree there.[52] But native Frenchmen did not blush to follow in their footsteps – 64 per cent were *régnicoles* in the 1780s. Probably the most famous Frenchman to become a Reims graduate in the eighteenth century was the atheistical *philosophe* La Mettrie, who took his degree there in the early 1730s after five years of study at Paris. La Mettrie wanted to set up his plate in his native Saint-Malo: he had initially no intention of settling in the capital, so had no reason to take a Paris degree.[53]

Paris degrees were also much more demanding than ones from Montpellier, so a number of Paris students, those presumably with more intellectual scruples than La Mettrie, took the long road south. Guilluame-Francois Laënnec studied assiduously in the Paris faculty for three years. At the beginning of his third year he began to think about where he should graduate. Knowing he needed an MA to qualify for the baccalaureate in medicine, wherever he graduated, he got his brother to impersonate him and purchase one from the University of Nantes, where there was no examination – at a cost 14 *livres* 10 *sous*. In December 1771 he told his father he would prefer to graduate at Montpellier rather than Reims, chiefly because he had the good sense to see that a Montpellier degree carried more clout. He duly arrived in the Midi in October 1772. Before that, though, he seems to have made a detour to Freiburg im Breisgau (in the Holy Roman Empire), where he gained a doctorate for an English friend who was too ill to travel. At first he was overwhelmed by the number of *actes* that he had to pass to become a doctor – a Montpellier degree, too, was not given away – but he was consoled by the fact that

[50] Brockliss, 'Patterns of Attendance' p. 530. The 1707 crown regulations required that a graduand had studied medicine for three years, one in the faculty where he was taking his degree.

[51] Julia and Revel, 'Etudiants', pp. 281–5; 333. Frenchmen looking for the second type of degree had to make two visits – once for the baccalaureate and again for the licence.

[52] Brockliss and Jones, *Medical World*, p. 518 (table). A detailed analysis of the cohort from the British Isles is given in Laurence Brockliss, 'Etudiants de médecine des Iles britanniques inscrits en France sous l'ancien régime' (forthcoming).

[53] Kathleen Wellman, *La Mettrie. Medicine, Philosophy, and Enlightenment* (Durham, NC, 1992), pp. 6, 34.

it would only cost 580 *livres*. He knuckled down, therefore, and in March 1773 was duly given the doctoral robe and bonnet.[54]

Limitations and Problems

Enough, it is hoped, has been said to justify the study of faculty matriculation registers as the best way of uncovering Europe's leading medical centres in the eighteenth century. The method, though, is not without its problems. In the first place, ranking faculties by the annual number of matriculands only works perfectly if a student studied in just one faculty. But this was not necessarily the case. Some faculties (like Paris) would only graduate students who had done all their medical studies in their midst. However, this was uncommon and there was nothing to stop well-heeled medics from moving around in search of the best, and taking courses in different universities. This must have definitely happened in the Holy Roman Empire, where the practice of *peregrinatio* was well established, if less pervasive than in the past. The information is not subject specific, but in the German lands it would appear the 'coefficient of matriculation' ran at about 1.3 universities per student in the eighteenth century, as against 1.9 in the early seventeenth.[55]

A faculty, then, with a large annual matriculation that would place it high in the ranking might actually have far fewer students than one lower down the list. In France there was clearly a difference between Montpellier and Paris in this regard. In the second half of the eighteenth century, the total number of registered students at the University of Paris ranged between an average of 77 in the 1750s to one of 102 in the 1780s. In other words, most Paris medical students spent under two years in its schools and might be considered birds of passage. Montpellier students, on the other hand, stayed longer, for in 1790 the faculty had 219 on its books.[56] By this token, therefore, Montpellier was far and away the premier faculty in pre-Revolutionary France. The actual size of a faculty was also affected by the number of years it took to gain a medical degree, and this varied from country to country. In France it was three (unless otherwise specified by the individual faculty), but in Spain and Portugal it was five (or six in Portugal if a doctorate rather than a licence was sought). As a result, the Portuguese University of Coimbra at the end of the century had almost as many medical students on its books as Montpellier. In 1797–98 only 30 students joined the faculty but there were 181 studying in its schools. It is hard, though, to imagine that Coimbra was really one of Europe's

54 Rouxeau, *Un étudiant en médecine*, chs. 6 and 7.

55 Willem Frijhoff, 'Surplus ou déficit? Hypothèses sur le nombre réel des étudiants en Allemagne à l'époque moderne (1576–1815), *Francia*, 7 (1979), esp. p. 201.

56 Brockliss, 'Patterns of Attendance', p. 515; Chartier, Compère et Julia, *Education*, p. 274.

centres of medical excellence, even after the reforms of 1772 established a much more up-to-date curriculum.[57]

The value of the matriculation evidence also has its limits where centres of extracurricular tuition were not located in faculty towns. The matriculation figures for the kingdom of Castile (the larger part of Spain) suggest that none of the country's five medical faculties in 1790 for which figures exist in print was really dominant. They shared out the 150 or so medical students fairly evenly. The oldest and traditionally leading university, Salamanca, had only 19 registered students; the largest, Seville-Cadiz, had 67.[58] But this may reflect the fact that no university town in Castile was an important centre of extracurricular study. In the eighteenth century this role was held by the capital, Madrid, which, we saw, had no university, but by the end of the era boasted a wide range of institutions offering tuition in medicine. These included the General Hospital (founded early in the period, which taught anatomy), the Academy of Medicine (created in 1732), the corporation of surgeons (given the right to teach in 1748), the San Carlos school of surgery (established in 1787) and the Royal School of Practical Medicine (founded in 1795). The capital was also close to the court at El Escorial and was the home of the *protomedicato*. Inevitably, it became the place to pursue medical study *after* graduation. In 1806, after San Carlos and the School of Practical Medicine had been merged, there were apparently 200 crowding into the new college.[59]

There was nothing, of course, peculiar about this. Further study after graduation was commonplace in Europe. If a medical student studied in and graduated from a local lowly faculty, then, if he had the means and did not need to set up in practice immediately, he frequently moved on to a more prestigious institution. A typical French instance would be Esprit Calvet. Son of an Avignon apothecary, Calvet studied medicine in his home town from 1746 to 1749, then took his doctorate. He then spent a further three years studying before entering into private practice in his native town: one year at Montpellier attending the faculty's schools and

---

57 Dr Taveira da Fonseca to the author, letters 20 Dec. 1988 and 24 Aug. 1989. In the early 1770s Coimbra was graduating 35 physicians a year. Dr Fonseca is the leading expert on Portuguese higher education in the eighteenth century.

58 Richard Kagan, *Students and Society in Early Modern Spain* (Baltimore, MD, 1974), pp. 249–54. There were 19 universities in Castile; three definitely did not have medical faculties.

59 Burke, *San Carlos*, pp. 39–39, ch. 5, *passim*, esp. p. 91, and pp. 143–7. San Carlos and the Royal School were merged in 1799; San Carlos had established a clinic in physical medicine in 1795. Barcelona may have performed a similar function in the kingdom of Aragon, though in 1786 there were two very populous medical faculties among the five universities: Valencia (209 students) and Zaragossa (230). At this date there were apparently 704 medical students in the whole of Spain, so presumably Castilians were crossing the border. See M. and J.L. Peset, *La Universidad espanola (siglos XVIII y XIX). Despotismo ilustrado y revolución liberal* (Madrid, 1974), pp. 107–14.Valencia was clearly a well-endowed faculty by this date, but it has been impossible to establish the attraction of Zaragossa.

two at Paris.[60] Even medical doctors who had trained in one of Europe's leading faculties would often decide to taste the delights of another. Thus, La Mettrie, after graduating at Reims in the early 1730s, moved on to Leiden before finally going back to Saint-Malo. This, though, introduces a third limitation to constructing a map of excellence from the matriculation registers. The prestigious faculties' post-doctoral visitors can never be studied quantitatively, for their names never appear. Their presence is known only anecdotally.

This is doubly unfortunate. Not only is it evident that there were large numbers of post-doctoral medical students floating around the leading faculties in the eighteenth century, thus swelling their overall numbers considerably, but it seems likely that post-docs were much more in evidence in one of the leading faculties than in the others. Paris might have had fewer medical undergraduates than Montpellier, but it was the French and, arguably, European post-graduate medical school *par excellence*. *Pace* Laënnec the elder, few Parisian-trained students only ever went off to Montpellier after they had graduated. Montpellier students, on the other hand, frequently took the road to the capital, even those who were intending to set up their plate in the southern city. Pierre-Joseph Amoreux was just one who did so. Having graduated in 1762, he spent a further two years walking the wards in Montpellier's hospitals, then left for Paris, where he stayed for 18 months, continually bumping into his Montpellier classmates.[61] Paris, too, welcomed a continual stream of post-graduate medics from outside the country – Britons, Germans, Italians, Swiss, even Spaniards. Albrecht von Haller was just one of many. Having begun his medical studies at Tübingen in 1723, he had moved to Leiden in 1725, where he took his degree two years later. He then spent 1727–28 in the French capital with a number of compatriots, notably Johannes Gessner (1709–90) of Zurich.[62] Yet, if the anecdotal evidence suggests that in the eighteenth century all medical roads led to pre-Revolutionary Paris, this is not a conclusion that can ever be firmly substantiated.

Post-graduates who came to Paris usually ignored the faculty altogether and concentrated solely on the extracurricular provision. Calvet in 1752–53 attended the lectures of the 80-year-old Jean Astruc (1684–1766) at the Collège Royal, who was an expert on VD and children's diseases. He also followed the private courses

---

[60] Brockliss, *Calvet's Web*, pp. 25–7, 142, 160. At Montpellier, he attended the lectures of two professors who have left little mark on the history of medicine – Antoine Fizes (1690–1768) and Jacques Lazerme. What he wanted to learn more about was the current medical orthodoxy – iatromechanism – and to benefit from Fizes's insights into medical practice. He does not appear to have listened to the lectures of the faculty's young Turk, François Boissier de Sauvages (1706–67), who was the founder of Montpellier's vitalist tradition. He got to know Sauvages but what engaged his interest were the Montpellier professor's experiments in electrotherapy.

[61] Bibliothèque Municipale, Avignon, MS 1269, pp. 36–40.

[62] *Johannes Gessners Pariser Tagebuch 1727*, ed. Urs Boschung (Bern, 1985), pp. 162–5; Gesner himself would later graduate at Basel, ibid., p. 61.

given by a young Antoine Petit.[63] Amoreux 10 years later did much the same. He followed Petit's private courses on anatomy, midwifery and female diseases, and improved his knowledge of botany through the good office of Bernard de Jussieu (1699–1777), who showed him round the Jardin du Roi and took him on walks in the countryside.[64] Much earlier in the century von Haller and Gessner had come to learn more about anatomy and surgery from the leading Paris surgeons, as did many other foreign medical students through the century. In particular, they became the private pupils of Henri Le Dran (1685–1770), first surgeon at the Charité. They also busied themselves in forming their own collections of anatomical samples by snatching bodies and boiling the victims' flesh from the bones in their rooms. The French capital was particularly valued for the availability of its corpses.[65]

Of all the leading centres of medical education, Paris was the most likely to draw an international clientele, especially medics from northern Europe. It was the custom for medical courses (public and private) outside the faculties to be given in the vernacular rather than Latin, an indication of the fact that not only physicians but surgeons, apothecaries and interested laymen could be found in the audience. This inevitably gave Paris the edge, for French was the lingua franca of eighteenth-century Europe. Hardly anybody knew German or Dutch, while there were strong confessional and financial reasons why northern Protestants would think twice before exploring the medical delights of Spain and distant Italy.[66] However, practical instruction in a language that could be understood was not all that a medical student sought in the French capital. It must be remembered that physicians (and a few surgeons and apothecaries) played an important part in the European Republic of Letters in the eighteenth century.[67] The practice of medicine provided their daily bread but their leisure hours were passed in other cultural pursuits: they were agriculturalists, botanists, naturalists, antiquarians, even poets (like Haller), and frequently avid book collectors. What lured so many medical students to Paris besides the medical facilities was its rich cultural life, the possibility of pursuing non-professional interests and making contacts. Paris was

---

63 Brockliss, *Calvet's Web*, p. 142.

64 Everyone seems to have studied under Petit, though he provided no opportunity for hands-on dissection: see Rouxeau, *Un étudiant en médecine*, p. 38. He must have been a particularly inspiring teacher.

65 *Johannes Gessners Pariser Tagebuch*, pp. 89–157 (commentary). Gessner's diary (text pp. 273–372) is the fullest extant description of extracurricular study at Paris.

66 Italy appears to have been the exclusive haunt of gentlemen (and ladies) on the Grand Tour, not seekers after medical enlightenment, a reflection of the low esteem (however unfairly) in which its contemporary science was held: see Françoise Wacquet, *Le Modèle français et l'Italie savante (1660–1750)* (Rome, 1989), *passim*.

67 It has been estimated that 40 per cent of the 2,500 members of France's 30-plus provincial academies in 1789 were medics: see Daniel Roche, *Le Siècle des lumières: Académies et académiciens provinciaux, 1680–1789*, 2 vols (Paris, 1978), i. 243–5.

the cultural capital of Europe, and men and women of many *different* classes and ages flocked there from all corners of the Continent.[68]

Esprit Calvet is remembered today as an antiquarian, naturalist and bibliophile whose fine collections were left to the city of Avignon to create the museum, which bears his name. In Paris in the early 1750s he immersed himself in the city's vibrant culture of collecting. He scoured the bookshops, attended sales and struck up friendships with the antiquarian abbé Jean-Jacques Barthélemy (1716–95), later keeper of the king's coin cabinet, and the ageing naturalist René-Antoine Ferchault de Réaumur (1682–1757). He also brushed up on his Greek by studying privately with the great Greek scholar Jean Capperonnier (1716–75) and attending his lectures at the Collège Royal.[69] Amoreux would become a well thought-of botanist, horticulturalist and agricultural reformer who would enter countless prize-essay competitions in the final decades of the *ancien régime*. When he went up to the French capital 10 years later, he was already constructing a herbarium. The correspondence that he conducted during his visit with another young Montpellier botanist, Antoine Gouan, later professor, suggests that he spent much of his time negotiating with the Jussieu family and the physician Etienne-Louis Geoffroy (1725–1810) for plant and insects specimens at the Jardin du Roi and hunting down books for his friends. Amoreux's correspondence with a young medical student from Châteaurenard near Avignon, Isidore-Dominique Vicary, who was still in the capital after the Montpellier doctor had returned home, would also suggest that he and his friends liked the opera and the theatre, though not uncritically. Michel Sedaine's *Le Philosophe sans le sçavoir* (first staged in early 1766) does not seem to have been a hit with Vicary, even if it is judged today to be a classic of the theatre of bourgeois intimacy.[70]

---

[68] In 1788 a minimum of 676 tourists from the British Isles checked into Paris hotels – they were the largest foreign contingent: see Daniel Roche, 'The English in Paris', in Christophe Charle, Julien Vincent and Jay Winter (eds), *Anglo-French Attitudes. Comparisons and Transfers between English and French Intellectuals since the Eighteenth-Century* (Manchester, 2007), pp. 82–3. For an introduction to a cross-section of Britons in the French capital in 1786, see Michael Allen (ed.), *An English Lady in Paris. The Diary of Frances Anne Crewe 1786* (St Leonards, 2006). Many medical visitors were no different from ordinary tourists: they came for a few weeks to see the sites and merely 'tasted' the medical possibilities. The surgeon Thomas Baker spent less than three weeks in Paris in 1732: see Wellcome Library MS 5780, 'A tour in France made by my grandfather Thomas Baker in the year 1732 (old style)'. The American physician Benjamin Rush was there for only five weeks in Feb.–Mar. 1769: see Pierpont Morgan Library, New York, MS MA 14, 'Account of a journey to Paris 1769'.

[69] Brockliss, *Calvet's Web*, pp. 26–7.

[70] Bibliothèque Nationale, Manuscrits français, nouvelles acquisitions 6571, ff. 253–4: Vicary in Paris to Amoreux (by then back in Montpellier), 1 Mar. 1766. For the correspondence with Gouan, ibid., MS 6570, ff. 189–200. E.-L. Geoffroy was the author of a 1762 *Histoire abrégé des insectes*.

Paris, then, was a medical Mecca because it offered so many different things to do. This was equally true of Europe's largest city, London (population some 900,000 by the end of the century). We are now well aware that the British capital became an extremely important centre of medical education in the second half of the eighteenth century. More and more tyro medical practitioners sought practical instruction in its hospitals and private schools. At the turn of the nineteenth century some four hundred medical students were to be found walking the wards in the London hospitals, compared with a hundred 50 years before (though presumably nearly were all Anglophone, since English was as little known to foreigners as German).[71] But London, like Madrid, would never register in a study based on matriculation records, given that it too had no university. Indeed, a fourth and final limitation to this approach would be that it would seem to exclude any discussion of the British Isles. There were eight universities in the kingdoms of Great Britain and Ireland in the eighteenth century, all purporting to provide medical instruction. But none kept a faculty matriculation register of the kind found on the Continent. The nearest equivalent are the Edinburgh class lists that were kept towards the end of the period, which record the number of students listening to a particular professor. Their survival is fortunate in that Edinburgh was unquestionably the only really vibrant medical faculty in the British Isles at this date, offering a full complement of lectures as well as one of the first public courses in Europe in clinical medicine.[72] However, to date, the class lists have not been used to construct an account of the number of new students per year. Indeed, even if they were, the results would not be strictly comparable with those produced by the Continental registers.

To start with, they are likely to be a much more complete list of the numbers attending the faculty. Edinburgh professors were paid fees by the students who attended their courses, so they had an incentive to register everyone; their salaried Continental peers had limited interest in who was sitting in front of them. In addition, the faculty's clients were different from those of their Continental sisters. From the work done on the class lists, it is clear that, however many medical students

71 Lawrence, *Charitable Knowledge*, p. 111. Important medical works by English authors were read in Latin or translated. Few members of the French republic of letters knew English; Calvet, for one, did not: see L.W.B. Brockliss, 'The French Republic of Letters and English Culture, 1750–90', in Charle et al. (eds), *Anglo-French Attitudes*, ch. 6.

72 Rosner, *Medical Education, passim;* Risse, *Hospital Life*, *passim*; R.B. McDowell and D.A. Webb, *Trinity College Dublin 1592–1952* (Cambridge, 1982), *passim*; C. Webster, 'The Medical Faculty and the Physic Garden', in L.S. Sutherland and L.G. Mitchell (eds), *The History of the University of Oxford* (Oxford, 1986), ch. 25; Michael Moss and Derek Dow, 'The Medical Curriculum at Glasgow in the Early Nineteenth Century', *History of Universities*, 7 (1989), 227–58. The seven other faculties except St Andrews provided lectures in theoretical medicine, but their practical facilities were poor or difficult to access. From the first decade of the nineteenth century Edinburgh ceased to reign supreme as both Glasgow and Dublin developed first-rate medical schools.

there were in Edinburgh at the turn of the century, from two-thirds to four-fifths never took a degree in the faculty and that 70 per cent of these attended for only a year. In the 1790s only 30 per annum took a degree, no more than at the apparently underpowered Leuven. This was partly because taking an Edinburgh degree was demanding – graduands had to write and sustain a thesis of some length in Latin – and it was much easier to graduate at St Andrews and Aberdeen, where degrees could be gained *in absentia*. But it also reflected the fact that many of the auditors were not intending to be physicians. As was noted earlier, the Edinburgh benches were full of apothecary-surgeons, prospective general practitioners, gaining a modicum of formal education in a state where there were no surgical colleges, though some of the students may have been artists boning up on anatomy, or even artisans (brewers, dyers and so on) seeking instruction in chemistry. If many of the auditors were tyro surgeons, then Edinburgh was obviously a faculty *sui generis*. *Prima facie*, the class lists would point to the city being one of the most populous medical faculties in Europe at the end of the period, with perhaps 200 to 300 students, but its numbers were clearly peculiarly inflated.[73]

The Edinburgh anomaly, however, does indicate yet a further limitation in the use of faculty matriculation registers to identify centres of excellence. On the continent of Europe, these tell us nothing about the educational preferences of the large majority of licensed medical practitioners who were not graduate physicians. It is impossible to know how many surgeons and apothecaries there were in any state during the eighteenth century, but they probably outnumbered physicians by a factor of six to one, given that they dominated practice in the countryside.[74] Yet, as we saw in the first section, surgeons in particular were not just encouraged to seek formal education for the first time but often required to do so. Where did they train? Did they choose the nearest surgical college or hospital course, regardless of its quality, and simply go through the motions in order to fulfil state regulations? Or, despite the extra expense, did they embrace the *Zeitgeist* and flock to the one or two cities in states of any size which were already attracting young physicians in considerable numbers because of the quality of their facilities?

This is not a question that can be easily answered with the information to hand. Just like the private courses, there is very little statistical data about attendance at the surgical colleges. If the French evidence is typical, though, the centres of medical excellence were not the sole property of the physicians. Paris had the same allure for surgeons as for physicians. Not only was the Paris college of surgery the best endowed and equipped in the state but it was also by far the most popular. In the third quarter of the eighteenth century, the Paris school had 600 to

---

[73] Rosner, *Medical Education*, ch. 6; Christopher Lawrence, 'The Edinburgh Medical School and the End of the "Old Thing"', *History of Universities*, 7 (1988), 259 and 263. By the 1820s the Edinburgh faculty had grown rapidly and had more than 700 students; by then it graduated 100 per year. Dublin taught 40 students per year in the early nineteenth century; in 1813 Glasgow had 500 on its books.

[74] See the estimates for France in Brockliss and Jones, *Medical World*, pp. 520–1.

700 students signed up for individual courses, while Toulouse eventually had 150 auditors, Montpellier perhaps 100 and the rest (like Rennes) seldom more than 20. It would seem, then, that the Paris college was attracting tyro surgeons from all over France in large numbers. Even if attendance was swelled by the presence of medical practitioners from abroad and some French physicians, such as Laënnec, pursuing their practical studies in the capital, this can only have accounted for a small proportion of the total. On the other hand, in the 1780s at any rate, only about a third of the matriculands in any year were likely to complete the full three-year course. Some 400 new students came to the college each year, but 40 per cent left after 12 months. As in the case of the physicians, Paris was only one, albeit important, staging post in a surgeon's education.[75]

Of course, the French case may be exceptional, especially if Paris really was unique in its international appeal. Ultimately, the question can only be settled by detailed prosopographical study of the educational *cursus* of a selected cohort of medical practitioners. Admittedly, this is virtually impossible to do before the modern era, unless for some reason or other practitioners had to give a full account of their education and qualifications and the documentation has survived.[76] Where an ideal source exists, however, the results are extremely illuminating. During the French Revolutionary and Napoleonic wars, the British army recruited nearly 3,000 medical officers. About 12 per cent had a medical degree and a further 40 per cent had been certificated by one of the three surgical colleges before joining up, but the rest had only passed the army entrance examination. After Waterloo, the Director General of the Army Medical Service, Sir James McGrigor (1771–1858), sent out a questionnaire to all serving medical officers asking them to record the details of their background, education and military service. Their response emphasises how far, in the British Isles at least, formal instruction for all medical practitioners had become de rigueur, even though such study was still not required under the recently passed Apothecaries Act. The army, understandably, attracted young medical practitioners from modest backgrounds and with limited

[75] Brockliss and Jones, *Medical World*, p. 507; Willem Frijhoff, 'L'Ecole de chirurgie de Paris et les Pays-Bas: Analyse d'un recrutement, 1752–1791', *Lias*, 17: 2 (1990), 185–239 (broader than the title suggests). The Paris school only kept a matriculation register from 1784, but there are surviving class lists from the 1750s: see Bibliothèque de la Faculté de Médecine de Paris MSS 54–69. These have never been fully analysed to find the pattern of geographical recruitment, but sample years are studied in Toby Gelfand, 'Deux cultures, une profession: les chirurgiens français au XVIIIe siècle', *Revue d'histoire moderne et contemporaine*,' 27 (1980), 468–84. Between 1784 and 1791 foreigners only formed 3.4 per cent of the intake: Frijhoff, 'L'Ecole de chirurgie', p. 195 (table).

[76] The first problem is to construct the cohort, when there are very few complete lists of medical personnel in a town or region that could be used as the basis for such a study. Even the prosopographical study of medical graduates, using university registers as a point of departure, is very difficult. What can be achieved simply using random archival material is best displayed by Willem Frijhoff, *La Société néerlandaise et ses gradués, 1575–1814* (Amsterdam, 1981).

prospects: no one would have opted for military life if a comfortable civilian billet were available. Nonetheless, almost to a man, they had not simply served their time as medical apprentices but were the beneficiaries of one or two years of formal medical training. Out of a sample of 454 doctors, 432 had attended medical lectures (on average, seven courses each) and 425 had walked the wards.[77]

More importantly, in the context of this present study, their experience confirms the role of Edinburgh and London as centres of medical excellence. Some 260 had paid to listen to private medical lectures in London, 70 alone enrolling in the anatomy class of Joshua Brookes (1761–1833) at his Blenheim Street theatre. A further 200 had attended the Edinburgh faculty, notably the chemistry lectures of Thomas Hope (1766–1844), who had taught 168, and the lectures in practical medicine of James Gregory (1753–1821),who had entertained 160. Roughly the same number had also gained hospital experience in the two capital cities. Of the 244 who had walked the wards in London, the largest group had attended St George's (60 plus); of the 188 who graced the far smaller number of Edinburgh hospitals, the most popular, inevitably was the Royal Infirmary (133). The only other medical centre of significance that the army doctors had studied in was Dublin, where 120 had listened to lectures and 111 spent time in a hospital. Of those who had taken a course in the Irish capital, too, the large majority had attended the Royal College of Surgeons. Only 29 had matriculated in the Dublin faculty.[78]

Interestingly, hardly any of the cohort had studied outside the British Isles before entering the army. The most notable was Michael Lambton Este (1779–1863), who spent five years on the Continent from 1792 to 1797. He had begun his studies at Pavia, a faculty with good facilities, thanks to the munificence of its Austrian rulers, and where the Lausanne physician and medical populariser Samuel Tissot had taught clinical medicine in the 1780s. He had then moved on to Vienna, where his teachers included the clinician Johann Peter Frank, and finally to Berlin.[79] But Este was an exceptional recruit to the army service. His father,

[77] Ackroyd et al. (eds), *Advancing with the Army*, pp. 118–45. Basic information about the 454 doctors is given in appendix 2. The study is based on a sample of one-third of the filled-in questionnaires which are held in The National Archives (WO 25/3904–11). The database containing extensive biographical details of the 454 doctors is held on the University of Oxford mainframe.

[78] The importance of Dublin reflects the fact that one-third of the recruits came from Ireland (see Ackroyd et al. (eds), *Advancing with the Army*, p. 62. The figures slightly exaggerate Dublin's importance. They include courses attended and wards walked after joining the army. When medical officers were stationed in Dublin they often took advantage of their sojourn to explore the city's medical facilities.

[79] Database, no. 250, table 'lectures/courses'. On the first part of the trip he was with his father; see Charles Este, *A Journey in the Year 1793 through Flanders, Brabant and Germany to Switzerland* (London, 1795). For Pavia, see S. Emch-Deriaz, *Tissot: Physician of the Enlightenment* (New York, 1992), ch. 8.

a London apothecary-turned-clergyman, was extremely well connected and the young doctor was immediately posted to a guards regiment.[80] Parents might be able to send their sons to London or Edinburgh, but they could evidently not usually scrape together enough to get them across the Channel, even if this was wartime and the most obvious Continental port of call for Britons, Paris, was closed. It is a salutary reminder that centres of medical excellence in the eighteenth century were really national (or perhaps better, dynastic), not international in character. Even the internationalism of pre-Revolutionary Paris should not be exaggerated. The foreigners who came to its school of surgery in the 1780s were nearly all natives of the Low Countries.[81]

At the very least, it must be assumed that a medical centre with an international reputation could quickly lose part of its clientele if a new national focus of attraction once developed. It was not Boerhaave's death that led English and the Scots physicians to desert Leiden, but the rise of Edinburgh. This is underlined by the equally steep decline in the number of Anglo-Scots graduating at Reims after 1740. Only a half of the Anglo-Scots that took a doctorate at Reims in the Boerhaave era had studied at Leiden. The rest had attended other medical institutions. The fact, then, that over the next 40 years little more than a quarter of the previous number passed through the Champagne faculty (less than a fifth in the case of the Scots) suggests that far fewer were seeking medical instruction anywhere on the Continent than hitherto, now that Edinburgh's reputation was rising.[82] Only the Irish continued to take degrees in large numbers at Reims, normally after studying in Paris. And their behaviour was probably determined by confessional loyalty and had nothing to do with medical considerations. Many, possibly most, of the Irish graduates at Reims were Roman Catholics. Although there were no religious tests discouraging their attendance in the Scottish faculty, Presbyterian Edinburgh would have had a limited attraction, especially when they could take advantage of the scholarships attached to the Paris Irish College to support their studies.[83]

---

[80] Database, no. 250, table 'regiments and garrisons'. Este senior was a friend of Nelson.

[81] Frijhoff, 'L'Ecole de chirurgie', pp. 196–7.

[82] Brockliss, 'Etudiants', tables 1, 3 and 4. While Boerhaave was a professor, 655 Anglo-Scots attended Leiden; during the same time 227 took degrees at Reims, of whom 117 had studied in the Dutch faculty.

[83] Ibid., tables 1–4. Between 1740 and 1779, 248 Irishmen graduated at Reims, as compared with 61 Anglo-Scots. Over the same four decades 65 Irish students passed through Leiden. However, only eight graduated at Reims. That the very large majority of Irish students had been in Paris during this time is evident from the information provided by one of the two extant Reims graduation registers. The register that runs from 1749 to 1793 (Bibliothèque Municipale, Reims, MS 2564) gives details of a graduate's previous medical education. The Irish College at Paris existed to shelter clerics preparing to go on the Irish mission, but a number of the scholarships attached to the college were given to medical students: see Liam Chambers, 'Irish *Fondations* and *Boursiers* in Early Modern Paris, 1682–1793' (forthcoming).

The emergence of national or dynastic centres of medical education, usually in capital cities, clearly distinguished the eighteenth century from the sixteenth and seventeenth, where the handful of centres of excellence were characterised by their mix of provincialism and cosmopolitanism.[84] Arguably, what differentiated the eighteenth-century centres of excellence too was their openness to a much broader medical constituency. Much more work needs to be done here, but the example of Paris, London, Edinburgh and, on a much smaller scale, Dublin, leads ineluctably to the conclusion that a parallel educational *cursus* was gradually emerging for both physicians and surgeons. No better illustration could be had of the way in which the traditional distinctions between the two were breaking down than the fact they both sought educational enlightenment in the same urban space. Outside the British Isles, they probably did not enjoy a common education; physicians and surgeons were largely trained in different institutions; they even probably took separate private courses (though this will never be known). But they were studying the same subjects. It was inevitable, then, that in the Age of Reason, it should be suggested that, for economy of effort, the parallel system should be rationalised and a single *cursus* of institutionalised education established.[85] It was inevitable, too, that this would be the most obvious medical product of the French Revolution, which waged war on hierarchy and privilege and swept away all the guilds and corporations, including, in 1793, all the universities.

In 1803, after a decade of medical anarchy, Napoleon set up a new system of medical practice which retained pharmacy as a distinctive *métier* but ended the age-old distinction between physicians and surgeons. Henceforth, French medical practitioners would be divided into two new tiers: graduate *médecins* (who could specialise in either physic or surgery) trained in the three medical schools (from 1808 called faculties), with the right to practise nationwide, and local *officiers de santé* trained as apprentices or in departmental hospitals.[86] In the following decade the system was carried far and wide in the knapsacks of the Grande Armée and puffed as the height of modernity. In many ways, though, the Revolutionaries

---

[84] See the chapter in this book by Hilde de Ridder-Symoens.

[85] On the Continent, calls for physicians and surgeons to be trained together seem to begin about 1780. See the works cited in L.W.B. Brockliss, 'Before the Clinic: French Medical Training in the Eighteenth Century', in Caroline Hannaway and Ann La Berge (eds), *Constructing Paris Medicine* (Amsterdam, 1998), ch.2, nn. 1 and 3. The most famous was F. Vicq d'Azyr, 'Nouveau Plan de constitution pour la médecine en France', in *Histoire et mémoires de la Société royale de médecine, 1787–88*, vol. ix (Paris, 1790), 1–201.

[86] The decree is published in *Recueil des loix et règlements concernant l'instruction publique, depuis l'édit de Henri IV en 1598 jusqu'à ce jour. Publié par ordre de son Excellence le Grand-Maître de France* (8 vols; Paris, 1814–27), ii. 344–53. For a general account of the developments during the Revolutionary period, see Jacques Léonard, *Les Médecins de l'ouest au XIXe siècle* (reproduced doctoral dissertation, 3 vols, Université de Lille, 1979), vol. I, chs 3 and 4; Jean-Charles Sournia, *La Médecine révolutionnaire* (Paris, 1989).

had not put medicine on a new footing. They had merely given legal expression to a development that was already happening and which had already been taken much further in Great Britain, where London physicians and small-town and rural general practitioners trained together.

It is true that there was more to the French medical revolution than structural reorganisation. Arguably, the heart of this new system, the new Paris school of medicine, established in 1794 in the buildings of the old school of surgery, did more than teach physic and surgery as an integrated discipline. Through its novel dedication to research, the fundamental role it gave to anatomy, its emphasis on learning through seeing and its abandonment of Latin as a classroom language, it offered an entirely new concept of a centre of medical excellence. Arguably, too, existing centres of medical excellence immediately lost their sheen as a result, and in the early nineteenth century Paris reigned supreme as the international beacon of light to which all would rush once peace returned to Europe. Certainly this is what its creators and its most famous historians have claimed.[87]

This, though, is another story and the jury is still out.[88] Suffice it to say that the new Paris school was born at the dawn of nationalism. Some foreign medical practitioners certainly did come to the French capital and marvel at what they saw. The Edinburgh physician-surgeon John Thomson, who toured Europe in 1814, for instance, shamelessly promoted Paris at the expense of his own alma mater in order to initiate curricular reform at home.[89] Many Britons, though, including the army medics who were stationed in the French capital from 1815 to 1818, were mindful that the Paris faculty was the child of the national enemy and went to gawk and carp. The new school, they wrote home, had its strengths, but had little to teach them about medical practice.[90]

---

87 A.-F. Fourcroy, *Rapport et projet de décret sur l'établissement d'une Ecole centrale de santé à Paris* (Paris, 1894); idem, 'Exposé des motifs du projet de loi sur l'exercice de la médecine', *Receuil des loix*, ii. 350–1; Michel Foucault, *Naissance de la Clinique* (Paris, 1963); E.H. Ackerknecht, *Medicine at the Paris Hospital, 1794–1848* (Baltimore. MD, 1967).

88 The myth has been scrutinised critically by a number of medical historians in recent years. For an overview, see the essays in Hannaway and La Berge, *Paris Medicine*. The first chapter in the volume, Ann La Berge and Caroline Hannaway, 'Paris Medicine: Perspectives Past and Present', provides a solid account of the cultivation of the myth since the beginning of the nineteenth century.

89 John Thomson, *Additional Hints respecting the Improvement of the System of Medical Instruction followed in the University of Edinburgh* (Edinburgh, 1826). Thomson had been the first incumbent of the Regius Chair in military surgery. By the 1820s the Edinburgh faculty was coming under attack from outside, though it still drew large numbers of students: see Lawrence, 'End of the "Old Thing"', and the essay by Dingwall in this volume.

90 E.g. Tyne and Wear Archives, Acc. No. 1132, letters home by Joseph Brown, 29 Oct. 1815 and 7–8 Mar. 1817. Brown (no. 6 in the database) later settled in Sunderland and became a local worthy.

Chapter 3
The Mobility of Medical Students from the Fifteenth to the Eighteenth Centuries: The Institutional Context

Hilde de Ridder-Symoens

Till the end of the *ancien régime*, the universities north of the Alps comprised four faculties: arts, theology, law and medicine. By contrast, in Northern Italy arts and medicine together made up one 'faculty' called *universitas* (Appendices 1 and 2). The arts faculty was considered a propaedeutic centre, training students to acquire the essential conceptual and factual knowledge that would give them the competence to follow courses in the higher faculties. Arts faculties regularly complained about the fact that students in the higher faculties had not previously passed through the arts faculty. They wanted the responsible authorities to make this compulsory. They were never completely successful, however, in achieving their goal.

In fact, only the medical faculties succeeded by enacting statutes imposing on its students a preliminary training in the arts faculty, e.g. Montpellier, Angers, Reims, Oxford, Ingolstadt, Louvain (Leuven). At Cambridge the requirement of an arts degree was rescinded in the sixteenth century. In some universities medical students got advantages if they already had an arts degree. In Montpellier and Caen, they could save one year of study before passing the bachelor's exams, in Paris half a year.[1] Until the sixteenth century an average course of medical study

[1] M. Fournier (ed.), *Les statuts et privilèges des universités françaises depuis leur fondation jusqu'en 1789*, vol. III (Paris, 1892), 1595c, 1687; *Cartulaire de l'Université de Montpellier*, vol. I (Montpellier, 1890), 5; H. Denifle and E. Chatelain (eds), *Chartularium Universitatis Parisiensis*, vol. I (Paris, 1889), 453; examples: L.W.B. Brockliss, *French higher education in the seventeenth and eighteenth centuries* (Oxford, 1987), 13; C.D. O'Malley (ed.), *The history of medical education*, UCLA Forum in Medical Sciences, 12 (Berkeley, Los Angeles and London, 1970), 236–7; R. Benoit, 'Entre rénovation et archaïsme: les Statuts de la Faculté de médicine de Reims (24 avril 1662)', *Revue historique de droit français et étranger*, 77, 1 (1999), 42–3; K. Von Prantl, *Geschichte der Ludwig-Maximilians-Universität in Ingolstadt, Landshut, München*, 2 vols (Munich, 1872; reprint Aalen, 1968), 389. On the Louvain general statutes of 20 August 1642, see V. Brants, 'Visite de l'Université; Bruxelles, le 18 avril 1617', in V. Brants (ed.), *Recueil des ordonnances des Pays-Bas. Règne d'Albert et Isabelle. 1597-1621*, vol. II (Brussels, 1912), 331, art. 66; N. Siraisi, 'The faculty of medicine', in W. Rüegg (ed.), *A history of the*

lasted five to six years, two to three years for the baccalaureate and three to four years for the licentiate. In the course of the seventeenth century the whole course of study was reduced to three to five years, and in the eighteenth century to three to four years.[2]

An obligatory arts degree was also imposed, in principle, on theologians, but in some universities the students from the regular religious orders were exempted, as in Louvain, Bologna, Salamanca. In the French theological faculties the practice varied. Half of the law students contented themselves with a short stay in the arts faculty, or they skipped it completely if their training in the Latin school or gymnasium was of a sufficiently high quality (Oxford, Orleans, Bologna).[3]

From the sixteenth century onwards the position of the arts faculty as a propaedeutic faculty changed as a consequence of the emancipation of the Latin schools. The arts faculty, whose main task had been to acquaint youngsters with the liberal arts and to prepare them for one of the three higher faculties (theology, law and medicine), evolved into a real philosophical faculty. In the larger universities or in the universities in the bigger cities, the basic liberal arts were left to Latin grammar schools that often were attached to the university, as, for instance in Paris, Louvain or Cologne. This meant that many students received sufficient liberal arts training in secondary schools to be able to could skip the arts faculty entirely or content themselves with a shorter stay, following classes on the *quadrivium*, which was less taught in the Latin schools.[4]

---

university in Europe, vol. I; H. de Ridder-Symoens (ed.), *Universities in the Middle Ages* (Cambridge 1992), 374–5.

[2] Siraisi, 'Faculty of medicine', 360–87 (note 1); L. Brockliss, 'Curricula', in W. Rüegg (ed.), *A history of the University in Europe,* vol. II: H. de Ridder-Symoens (ed.), *Universities in early modern Europe (1500–1800)* (Cambridge, 1996), 609–18; D. Campbell, 'The medical curriculum of the universities of Europe in the sixteenth century, with special reference to the Arabist tradition', *Bulletin of the History of Medicine*, 36 (1962), 358–67; O'Malley, *History of medical education* (note 1); see also the chapters on medical faculties in the monographic histories of universities as, for example, L.H.D. Buxton and S. Gibson, *Oxford University ceremonies* (Oxford, 1935), 4 and Brockliss, *French higher education* (note 1), 13.

[3] M. Asztalos, 'The faculty of theology', in Ridder-Symoens, *Universities in the Middle Ages* (note 1), 417–8; Brants, 'Visite' (note 1), 331, art. 66; W. De Schuymer, 'Les statuts de l'université médiévale dans les pays romans (Bologne, Paris, Salamanque). Etude historique et lexicologique comparée', Ghent, unpublished Master's thesis, 1996, 69, 82; Brockliss, *French higher education* (note 1), 13; H. de Ridder-Symoens, 'Brabanders aan de rechtsuniversiteit van Orléans, 1444–1546. Een socio-professionele studie', *Bijdragen tot de Geschiedenis*, 61 (1978), 209–13.

[4] J. Sarnowsky, 'Die artes im Lehrplan der Universitäten', in U. Schaefer (ed.), *Artes im Mittelalter* (Berlin, 1999), 68–82. See also M.R. Di Simone, 'Admission', in Ridder-Symoens, *Universities in early modern Europe (1500–1800)* (note 2), 285–325 and M.-M. Compère, 'Les collèges de l'Université de Paris au XVIe siècle: structure institutionnelle et fonctions éducatives', in D. Maffei and H. de Ridder-Symoens (eds), *I collegi universitari*

Still, in the sixteenth century only a limited number of universities had a properly functioning medical faculty. Outside northern Italy only Montpellier and Paris had fully fledged medical educational centres. This phenomenon was connected with the low esteem in which the medical profession was held.[5] Until the sixteenth century medical education was purely theoretical and bookish. The manual activities in the medical profession were the responsibility of surgeons and barbers united in guilds, mostly under the patronage of the saints Kosmas and Damien.[6] Medical studies were considered by students mainly as a preparation for a lucrative medical career. Medical science as such was appreciated by only a happy few.

The situation began to improve in the sixteenth century, thanks to a more pronounced interest in the natural sciences resulting in an increase in scientific and medical discoveries. The growing interest in the *materia medica* and the increasing medicalisation of society called for a better medical education, a better-adapted organisation of health services and a strictly regulated health policy. To realise these goals, *collegia medica* were established in many cities, in cisalpine Europe from the late Middle Ages and in transalpine Europe from the early sixteenth century onwards. The overall aims of these colleges were to verify that all medical practitioners were in compliance with all the regulations and to improve the standards of medical practice. Taking into account the poor opportunities for medical practitioners to attain a high standard of practical training during their studies, many colleges offered courses of all kinds.[7] Some confusion is evident in the literature concerning the usage of the term *collegium medicum*. It can refer to the college of doctors of the medical faculty, or even to the whole faculty (Cracow). At the same time it is the standard term for the professional corporation of university-trained physicians (*doctores medicinae*) in late medieval and early modern cities. In university towns, however, the academic *collegium doctorum medicinorum* functioned mostly also as the urban college of physicians. Bordeaux was rather an exception, with three separate bodies (physicians, medical

---

in Europa tra il xiv e il xviii secolo. Atti del Convegno di Studi della Commissione Internazionale per la Storia delle Università, Siena – Bologna, 16–19 maggio 1988 (Milan, 1990), 101–18; H. de Ridder-Symoens, 'The changing face of centres of learning 1400–1700', in A.A. MacDonald and M.W. Twomey (eds), *Schooling and society. The ordering and reordering of knowledge in the Western Middle Ages* (Louvain, 2004), 115–38; W. Frijhoff, *La société néerlandaise et ses gradués, 1575–1814. Une recherche sérielle sur le statut des intellectuels à partir des registres universitaires* (Amsterdam and Maarssen, 1981), 40–1.

[5] For maps, see *Universities in the Middle Ages* (note 1), 69–74 and *Universities in early modern Europe (1500–1800)* (note 2), 90–105.

[6] N. Siraisi, *Medieval and early Renaissance medicine. An introduction to knowledge and practice* (Chicago and London, 1990), 48–77 (Medical Education); Siraisi, 'Faculty of medicine' (note 1), 360–87.

[7] There exist many monographs on local medical colleges.

professors, surgeons).[8] In Orleans, with only a law faculty, the members of the urban *collegium medicum* could enrol as *suppositi* in the university, and as such enjoy its academic privileges.[9]

Because in almost all the university cities the medical colleges were identical to or under the supervision of the medical faculty, the university claimed that only their own graduates were allowed to engage in medical practice in the city and in the neighbouring villages under city control. This claim was often extended to the provincial level. I will give only one example, for the Netherlands. In 1540 Charles V stipulated that a physician wanting to practise had to be a licentiate or doctor of an authorized university or be examined by registered doctors of Brussels or by Louvain professors.[10] But within two years the city and university of Louvain managed to require that only graduates from Louvain or other Netherlandish universities could be registered as public physicians.[11] This obligation was confirmed in the Louvain *Visitatio* of 1617, which can be considered as a kind of organic law in the Spanish Netherlands, and which lasted till the second half of the

---

[8] G. Pery, *Histoire de la faculté de médecine de Bordeaux et de l'enseignement médical dans cette ville: 1441–1888* (Paris, 1888), ch. 1 (Collège des médecins); ch. 2 (Faculté de medicine).

[9] In the historiography of the University of Orléans allusion is made to the existence of a medical faculty in the margin of the Law University. It concerns in fact the urban *collegium medicum* whose members could enrol in the University, such as the *maîtres de grammaire*: E. Bimbenet, 'Recherche sur l'origine et l'évolution de l'enseignement et de la pratique de la médecine en France, examen de deux registres concernant le collège de médecine d'Orléans', *Mémoires de la Société d'agriculture, sciences, belles lettres et art d'Orléans*, 4e s., 15 (1875), 168–235; E. Bimbenet, 'Maîtres grammairiens tenant tutelle, docteurs en médecine, docteurs régents, écoliers et suppôts de l'Université. Privilèges généraux', *Mémoires de la Société d'agriculture, sciences, belles lettres et art d'Orléans*, 4e s., 19 (1877), 141–56.

[10] *Placcaeten van Brabant*, 10 vols (Antwerp and Brussels, 1648–1768), vol. III, 261–63 (8 Oct. 1540); C. Broeckx, *Histoire du Collegium Medicum Antverpiense* (Antwerpen 1858), 10–3.

[11] The city magistrate of Louvain had complained that for many years students from the Low Countries 'pour prendre en aucune faculté et meismes en la faculté de theologie, des drois, ou de medecine le degre du doctorat ou de licence, se soyent avanchez de ce [*sic*] faire creer docteurs ou licentiez es universités situées es pays forains ... ou ils sont admis avec la multitude en payant le pris [*sic*] ad ce ordonné, et en delaissant notre université dudit Louvain ... Oultre ce que aud. moyen notredit université et ville de Louvain sont fort diminuez et fait a craindre diminueront de plus en plus, au grand detriment de la chose publique.' Emperor Charles V reacted in a positive way and declared 'que nul ... ne pourra doresenavant estre receu ne admis exercer aucun estat ou office requerant certain degre, ou obtenir benefice ou dignité ... ne soit qu'il ait prins son degre et promotion en notredit université de Louvain ou aultre université situé en noz pays, ne fust à notre expres consentement ...': F. Claeys Bouuaert, *L'ancienne Université de Louvain*, Bibliothèque de la Revue d'histoire ecclésiastique, 28 (Louvain, 1956), 96, transcription pp. 203–4.

eighteenth century.[12] It is clear that the prohibition on taking degrees outside the Netherlands had a great impact on student mobility and graduation policy.

Medical science too underwent important changes in the sixteenth century. The adage *ad fontes* ('back to the sources') went also for medicine. Hippocrates and Galen were studied in the original Greek; the medieval European and Arabic commentaries were discussed. The in-depth investigation of the classical authors cast doubt on the veracity of many former findings. In many universities professors were divided over the path to follow: Arabic or Greek medicine? This 'querelle des anciens et des modernes' raged particularly at German universities.[13] Natural philosophers also became interested in experiments, and they started to design instruments and even to build them. Consequently, the yawning gap between intellectual and manual work became less profound and thereby fruitful collaboration became possible. Furthermore, disciplines began to blend into each other. A natural philosopher needed the knowledge of several disciplines if he wanted to understand a specific field. Geography, for instance, was a mixture of mathematics, cosmography and travel accounts.

Medical Education

The new concepts regarding natural philosphy and research had effects on medical teaching, as, for instance, in the fields of surgery and clinical praxis.

The changes in the official curriculum imposed by the faculty occurred rather slowly. They went faster in another teaching circuit – not well-known to us, owing to a lack of sources – namely the so-called *privatissima* or private tuition, which escaped all inspection. The latter supplied gaps in the official and often out-of-date programme. *Privatissima* were better taught and adjusted to the individual student. This type of training, provided by chair holders or 'assistants', had to be paid for in addition to the official programme.

In the Middle Ages courses in the *medica practica* or pathologies and their treatments existed already. Until the seventeenth century they were mainly taught on a theoretical level and by a professor ('*ex cathedra*'). The curriculum was based on a fixed corpus of classical works supplemented and commented by Arab scholars.

---

12 '... ut nemo ad exercitium artis medicae admittatur, nisi qui intra Belgium promoti, vel a doctoribus nostrarum Belgicarum Universitatum, vel a cubiculariis nostris medicis examinati et approbati fuerint; sed nemo stipendia a civitatibus nostris recipiat, nisi qui in nostris Universitatibus Belgicis ad licentiam vel doctoratum promotus fuerit' (Brants, '*Visite*' (note 1), 336, art. 123).

13 G. Keil, B. Moeller and W. Trusen (eds), *Der Humanismus und die oberen Fakultäten*, Mitteilung XIV der Kommission für Humanismusforschung (Weinheim, 1987): chapters of Vivian Nutton, Gerhard Bader, Gundolf Keil and Rudolf Peitz.

The Italian medical faculties of Bologna and Padua were the first to introduce practical teaching, first anatomy and surgery. In the middle of the sixteenth century a whole range of practical courses were taught; besides surgery and anatomy, also botany and pharmacy. Thus, anatomical theatres, botanical gardens, practical training rooms were built and specialised chairs were created (Appendix 3).[14]

Bedside teaching came into use to a certain extent during the course of the sixteenth century. The professor introduced the student to his private patients or went with him to the town hospital. Many professional colleges of physicians also offered practical tuition. We have to wait till the end of the eighteenth century, at Leiden, before the first university hospital was in operation for bedside teaching.

North of the Alps, anatomical dissections were introduced only slowly, and with difficulty, in the course of the sixteenth century. Alumni from Italian universities who got medical chairs elsewhere in Europe tried to follow the good example set at their alma mater and to make their teaching more practical and adapted to the new science. This first happened in the Dutch Republic. After having declared the independence of the County of Holland in the 1570s, one of the first concerns of the authorities was the creation of a university at Leiden for the training of intellectuals and professionals in the Calvinist faith. Other provinces followed after some intervals. These Dutch universities, founded from 1575 (Leiden) onwards, followed the north-western university structure, but were not bound by the medieval traditions in teaching and research. Thus the professors, curators and other authorities dealing with higher education could introduce the medico-scientific oriented systems into the faculties of arts, insofar as these faculties could fit new disciplines and scientific methods into the straitjacket of the medieval university structure. If they could not fit, there remained only the possibility of inventing alternative forms of education. This is what happened in the northern Netherlands in the late sixteenth and seventeenth centuries. The burghers of the new Republic tried to harmonize traditional theoretical teaching and scientific research with practical application, that is to say, with applied research and experimentation. The result was that the separation between *artes liberales* and *artes mechanicae* gradually lessened and technology became as important as book knowledge.[15] Studies of those sciences that were essential for warfare (the Dutch Revolt!), commerce and navigation received the special attention of philosophers and teachers. Simon Stevin (1548–1620) and his engineering school come immediately to mind, as does the less well-known Adriaan Metius (1571–1635), professor of mathematics, who taught navigation, geodesy and fortification in Franeker around 1600. He followed

---

14 Brockliss, 'Curricula' (note 2), 609–18.

15 See e.g. W. Frijhoff, 'Medical education and early modern Dutch medical practitioners: towards a critical approach', in H. Marland and M. Pelling (eds), *The task of healing: Medicine, religion and gender in England and the Netherlands, 1450–1800* (Rotterdam, 1996), 205–20.

Stevin's example and lectured in Dutch, but his courses were more integrated into the university curriculum.[16]

In fact, the more practically oriented Netherlanders at Leiden and other Dutch universities followed the existing tradition of Italy, where engineering studies had evolved on a more scientific basis (mathematics and geometry) as early as the fifteenth century.[17] In the beginning of the sixteenth century, both inside and outside the University of Louvain (founded 1425), a similar group of scholars and technicians emerged, including Mercator, Gemma Frisius, Stevin and others. Even then the *Fiamminghi*, as the Netherlanders were called in Italy, did not hesitate to stay in Italy if their own country did not offer enough opportunities for them to follow their proper scientific calling as they saw it. Vesalius (1514–1564) left Louvain for Padua and Jozef van Goethuyse, alias Giuseppe Casabona (ca. 1515–1596) of Munsterbilzen (diocese of Liège) became the herbalist of Cosimo I in Florence and the director of the botanical garden in Pisa in 1592–1596.[18] As a result of the Dutch Revolt and the 'brain drain' to the young Republic, Leiden took over the torch of learning from Louvain and became the European centre for experimental and applied sciences.[19] Under the Leiden professor Herman Boerhaave (1668–1738), the results of the scientific revolution were applied in the medical faculties. It was the starting point of a fundamental modernisation of the medical curriculum and of teaching methods. His pupils improved medical faculties all over Europe (Vienna, Prague, Göttingen, Uppsala, Freiburg) or were founders of new medical faculties, with great success (e.g. Edinburgh 1726). This provided him with the epithet *Communis Europae Praeceptor*.[20]

---

[16] K. Van Berkel, *In het voetspoor van Stevin. Geschiedenis van de natuurwetenschap in Nederland 1580–1940* (Bonn and Amsterdam, 1985), 14–5; H.A.M. Snelders, 'Science in the Low Countries during the sixteenth century: A survey', *Janus*, 70 (1983), 213–21.

[17] A. Keller, 'Mathematical technologies and the growth of the idea of technical progress in the sixteenth century', in A.G. Debus (ed.), *Science, medicine and society in the Renaissance. Essays to honour Walter Pagel*, 2 vols (New York, 1972), 11–27; Berkel, *Voetspoor* (note 15), 17–8; G. Siraisi, *Avicenna in Renaissance Italy* (Princeton, 1987), 106–7.

[18] J.P. Goethuys, 'G. Casabona alias Jozef van Goethuyse', *Nationaal Biografisch Woordenboek*, vol. 11 (Brussels, 1985), 96–9.

[19] Berkel, *Voetspoor* (note 15), 14–5.

[20] Boerhaave is a well-researched scholar. Some titles: G.A. Lindeboom (ed.), *Boerhaave and his time*, Analecta Boerhaaviana, 6 (Leiden, 1970); G.A. Lindeboom, *Herman Boerhaave: the man and his work* (London, 1968), 360–74 and W. Frijhoff, 'Academic relations in Europe at the time of Boerhaave: A structural approach', in I.L. Bonta et al., *Hungarian-Dutch contacts in medicine since the epoch of Herman Boerhaave, Proceedings of Symposium 13 October 1994 under the auspices of The Emil Starkenstein Foundation and The Mikes Kelemen Kör* (Amsterdam, 1995), 13–28 on the imitation or adaptation of the Leiden pattern; C.J. Lawrence, 'Early Edinburgh Medicine: Theory and practice', in R.G.W. Anderson and A.D.C. Simpson (eds), *The early years of the Edinburgh medical school* (Edinburgh, 1976), 81–94; W. Kaiser, 'Theorie und Praxis in den Boerhaave-

Having sketched the evolution that occurred in the teaching of natural philosophy in general, and of medicine in particular, I would like now to turn my attention to its effects on the mobility pattern of medical students before 1800.

Mobility Patterns

For the Middle Ages, I will be brief.[21] Taking into account the state of the medical arts in the Middle Ages and the role of medical doctors in society, we can conclude that there was not a great need for university-trained physicians. Most of the healing was done by medical practitioners on the artisanal level. Although a *doctor* or *licentiatus medicinae* earned greater prestige than his practically educated counterpart, within the universities the medical faculty and its *suppositi* were considered less important and prestigious than those of the other, higher faculties of theology and law. Although a full *studium generale* consisted of four faculties, many universities north of the Alps functioned without, or only temporarily with, a medical faculty. In the thirteenth century the only famous schools of medicine were at Bologna, Montpellier and Paris. With every new university foundation in the fourteenth and fifteenth centuries university recruitment became more regionalized, so much so that in the fifteenth century external migration actually came to a halt. The statistics available for this period suggest that three-quarters of all students at the end of the Middle Ages were content to go to a regional university, usually the one nearest their home. The journeys of the remainder, especially the English, Spaniards, French and Italians, and to a lesser extent the Germans, were nearly always within their country of origin. The real itinerant scholars – those who crossed Europe – were few, most of them young men keen to continue their studies at an internationally renowned university and in disciplines not taught in their own schools.

There are two ways to know the attendance at and the popularity of the medical centres. First, we can count the matriculations in the medical faculty – if, of course, matriculation lists exist. As we know, until the late sixteenth or even seventeenth century, only the *studia generalia* in the Germanic world produced such lists. More available are the names of students who took a degree in medicine. Since they were a minority of all the enrolled students, we never will get reliable attendance figures for Italy and France, the countries with the most and the best medical centres.

Another way is prosopography. In biographical registers of medical doctors the compilers very often add the place where the physician received his education and eventually his degree. Thanks to the work of Wickersheimer and Jacquart, we have

Aere und in nachboerhaavianischen Ausbildungssystemen an deutschen Hochschulen des 18. Jahrhunderts', *Clio medica*, 21 (1988), 71–94.

[21] H. de Ridder-Symoens, 'Mobility', in Ridder-Symoens, *Universities in the Middle Ages* (note 1), ch. 9; ch. 11 (Siraisi, 'The faculty of medicine').

a lot of data for late medieval France (Appendix 4).[22] At the start of the fourteenth century 301 medical doctors were registered in France; 57.8 per cent of them had studied in Paris, 35.2 per cent in Montpellier, 2.7 per cent in other French faculties of medicine and 4.3 per cent abroad. At the end of the fifteenth century, of a total of 436 graduate physicians, the alumni of Montpellier formed only 16.3 per cent and those of Paris 47.5 per cent; other French universities now accounted for 27.6 per cent and foreign faculties for 8.5 per cent. Paris, and even more Montpellier, lost ground to Caen, Toulouse and Avignon, or to Perpignan, Cahors, Angers, Dôle, Nantes, Poitiers, Bordeaux and Bourges. The graduates of foreign (non-French) universities were nearly all foreigners (rather than Frenchmen) who, after finishing their studies, practised in France. The nearby Louvain University was the most frequented foreign *studium* (17 graduates); then came Salerno and Bologna, each with 10 graduates. Other Italian *studia* produced only a few French graduates.

The same happened in Italy. Most of the students came from the surrounding area. After having acquired a basic education in the region in arts and medicine, they went to Bologna and Padua to acquire more profound medical knowledge and to get a degree. The same happened with the ultramontane students, certainly those from the Germanic world, where medical faculties were not well equipped. The youngsters with medical ambitions had to go abroad, mostly to Italy, where medical education stood at the forefront, in comparison with the rest of Europe.[23] Of all the degrees awarded in Padua in the fifteenth century, 30 to 40 per cent were earned by ultramontane students, with an average of 5 to 10 medical graduations a year, the highest number in Europe in the fifteenth century. The university of Tübingen, for instance, only averaged one medical degree every two years between 1477 and 1532.[24]

As already mentioned, the northern Italian universities were by far the most progressive, and so the most attractive for ambitious and well-to-do medical students.[25] In the thirteenth and the first half of the fourteenth centuries Bologna was, without doubt, the most popular *studium* south of the Alps, in the first place for juridical students, in the second place for medical students. After 1350 the numbers of foreigners decreased rather drastically for more than a hundred years.

---

[22] E. Wickersheimer, D. Jacquart and G. Beaujouan, *Dictionnaire biographique des médecins en France au Moyen Age*, Ecole pratique des hautes études. 4e section: Sciences historiques et philologiques. 5: Hautes études médiévales et modernes 34–35, 3 vols (Geneva, 1979). Supplément: D. Jacquart, (Nouv. éd. sous la dir. de Guy Beaujouan) V.1–2 (Réimpr. de l'éd. de 1936); D. Jacquart, *Le milieu médical en France du 13e au 15e siècle* (Geneva, 1981), 364–5.

[23] Siraisi, 'Faculty of medicine' (note 1), 371.

[24] R. Ohl, 'The University of Padua 1405–1509: an International Community of Students and Professors', Ph. D. diss. University of Pennsylvania (1980), 59–61; Siraisi, 'Faculty of medicine' (note 1), 372–4.

[25] N. Siraisi, *Medicine and the Italian universities, 1250–1600*, Education and Society in the Middle Ages and the Renaissance 12 (Leiden, 2001)

About 1500, the Bolognese university was again in favour, but had to reckon with the competition of the Paduan *studium*, which had started a century earlier. Around 1400 the arts and medical *universitas* of Padua took over the lead, and held it till well into the seventeenth century.[26] According to a correspondent of the merchant of Prato, Francesco Datini, Padua was the most famous university in the whole of Italy (letter dated 1 June 1404).[27] But other universities were also chosen, for either geographical or political reasons. In the fifteenth century the merchants of Genoa preferred to send their sons to the nearby university of Pavia, and only in the second place to Bologna.[28]

Under the influence of ideas circulating during the Renaissance, the number of wandering students increased very quickly. The geographical mobility of students and teachers reached its peak (in absolute terms as well as proportionately) in the sixteenth century, lasting until about the 1630s. In this period of prosperity student migration was encouraged by the new humanist ideas in teaching, which helped the nobility to cope with the new cultural and intellectual demands of a fast-changing society, to which the universities also adapted themselves but slowly. Universities and university students were more aristocratic than before.

Humanism gained ground in several universities.[29] But the *iter italicum* ('Italian tour') became essential to any would-be humanist. Young and less-young Englishmen, Germans, Netherlanders, Scandinavians, Spaniards and Portuguese made an intellectual pilgrimage to the Italian universities – to Bologna and Padua, Pavia, Siena and Pisa, and in smaller numbers to Ferrara and Perugia. The university programme was wide ranging and combined sound legal or medical training with courses on classical antiquity. The growing interest in natural sciences in the sixteenth century is revealed in the choice of studies. A diploma in law or medicine meant a successful career, and the study of literature and natural science formed the 'universal man' of the Renaissance.[30]

---

26 J.H. Randall Jr., *The School of Padua and the emergence of modern science*, Saggi e Testi, 1 (Padua, 1961).

27 K. Park, *Doctors and medicine in early Renaissance Florence* (Princeton, 1985), 59 n. 37, 123.

28 J. Heers, 'L'enseignement à Gênes et la formation culturelle des hommes d'affaires en méditerranée à la fin du moyen âge', *Revue des études islamiques*, 44 (1976), 232–4.

29 A good overview is given by R. Weiss, *Italian humanism in Western Europe,* E.J. Jacobs (ed.), Italian Renaissance Studies (London, 1960), 69–93. See also C. Howard, *English travellers of the Renaissance* (London and New York, 1914), 8–10; W. Lucke, 'Deutsche Studenten in Bologna. Ein Beitrag zur Geschichte der Aufnahme des Humanismus in Deutschland', *Das Gymnasium*, 53 (1942), 43–61; W. Dotzauer, 'Deutsches *Studium* in Italien unter besonderer Berücksichtigung der Universität Bologna', *Geschichtliche Landeskunde*, 14 (1976), 102–8.

30 About the intellectual reputation of medical doctors in the Renaissance see N. Siraisi, 'The physician's task: medical reputations in humanist collective biographies', in N. Siraisi, *Medicine and the Italian universities, 1250–1600*, Education and Society in the Middle Ages and the Renaissance, 12 (Leiden, 2001), 157–83.

These multiple curriculum choices were a new phenomenon in the middle of the fifteenth century. Several disciplines were combined: law and medicine or theology and medicine, theology and law or even the three disciplines together. In the Middle Ages one went to the university to learn a profession. In the Renaissance, besides the professional choice, one followed courses in completely different disciplines out of pure interest.[31] This explains why the number of graduates in medicine surpassed the demand for practitioners in the sixteenth century. There was a group of students who wanted to practise a profession as physician but who, out of intellectual ambition, also followed classes in classical languages and literature, in philosophy, history, law or theology. Another group consists of theologians or jurists who were keen on understanding 'the Book of Nature' and were interested in the new science. They went to the medical faculty or to an arts faculty with a well-developed *quadrivium*.[32]

I will only give some striking examples, omitting the hundreds of *studiosi* who in many regions and cities were responsible for the development of a fertile intellectual and scientific climate, and who shaped the Republic of Letters.

An early example is the merchant's son Hartmann Schedel (1440–1514) from Nuremberg, who studied arts in Leipzig (1445–62) and got a degree in medicine and surgery at Padua (1466).[33] Schedel was one of the first transalpine scholars to read works in the original Greek. He also learned Italian in order to read Dante and other contemporary authors. After many wanderings he settled as a medical practitioner in Nuremberg, but he spent a large part of his time in writing (*The Nurnberg Chronicle*), editing classical texts and collecting books.[34] In the same period Thomas Linacre (c.1460–1524) from Canterbury went to Italy (1485–97) after having started his academic education in Oxford (1480–84). His peregrination led him to Bologna, Florence, Rome and Vicenza; meanwhile he applied himself to learning humanist Latin and Greek, and to the study of medicine. Linacre received his MD at Padua in 1496. In London he became the personal physician of Henry VIII and of many high nobles and humanists (such as Erasmus). He devoted his fortune to the creation of readerships in Greek medicine at Oxford and Cambridge and to the development of the London College of Physicians, founded by him in 1518. He was renowned not only as a physician, but also as a

---

31 See interesting examples in P.G. Schmidt, 'Mediziner oder Poet? Soziale Lage und Lebenspläne hessischer Humanisten', in A. Buck and T. Klaniczay (eds), *Sozialgeschichtliche Fragestellungen in der Renaissanceforschung*, Wolfenbütteler Abhandlungen zur Renaissanceforschung, 13 (Wiesbaden, 1992), 107–18.

32 Many examples in Frijhoff, *Sociéte néerlandaise* (note 4), 240–5.

33 www.ingolstadt.de/stadtmuseum/scheuerer/ausstell/schedel2.htm.

34 P. Lehman, 'Grundzüge des Humanismus Deutscher Lande zumal im Spiegel Deutscher Bibliotheken des 15. und 16. Jahrhunderts', in P. Lehman, *Erforschung des Mittelalters. Ausgewählte Abhandlungen und Aufsätze*, vol. V (Stuttgart, 1962), 487–9; www.beloit.edu/~nurember/inside/about/author.htm; www.mapforum.com/06/schedel.htm; www.ingolstadt.de/stadtmuseum/scheuerer/ausstell/schedel2.htm.

grammarian, rhetorician and philosopher.[35] His younger contemporary Renerus Snoyus (Reinier Snoy of Sonoy) (1477–1537) from Zealand, graduated MD in Bologna after studies at Louvain. Besides being court physician, Snoyus was a close friend of Erasmus. Apart from editing humanist works he was quite a prolific writer himself, dealing with history, medicine, philosophy and theology. He was also Charles V's ambassador to Scotland and Denmark.[36]

It was not uncommon for students eager to learn and in search of the best teachers to study at three, four and even eight universities.[37] An Italian doctorate in medicine or law, or a degree in medicine from Montpellier, also enhanced the holder's prestige and, even at this time, his career prospects in his native land. Andreas Gerardi Hyperius (1511–64) from Ypres in Flanders studied arts and theology in Paris and, out of personal interest, also some medicine and canon law. After that he travelled to northern Italy (Bologna), England (Cambridge) and Germany and visited the universities of Cologne, Erfurt, Leipzig and Marburg, where he finally got a chair in theology. He wrote on all kinds of topics.[38] Volkert Coyter, a student from Groningen, travelled to no less than seven universities between 1550 and 1566: Louvain, Tübingen, Montpellier (where he befriended Felix Platter), Padua, Rome, Bologna (where he got his medical degree in 1562) and finally Perugia. After his studies he lived in Germany as a Protestant physician, where he published important medical works, especially on the subject of anatomy.[39]

These are only some of the hundreds of men with analogous careers and with aspirations to belong to the Republic of Letters.[40] Students and professors circulated knowledge throughout Europe in the form of the letters, manuscripts, books, ideas,

---

35 www.britannica.com/eb/article-9048334/Thomas-Linacre; F. Maddison (ed.), *Essays on the life and work of Thomas Linacre c.1460–1524* (Oxford, 1977).

36 A. Tervoort, *The iter italicum and the Northern Netherlands. Dutch students at Italian universities and their role in the Netherlands' society (1425–1575)* (Leiden, 2005), biographies on CD-rom; C.G. van Leijenhorst, 'Reyner Snoy', in P.G. Bietenholz and T.B. Deutscher (eds), *Contemporaries of Erasmus. A biographical register of the Renaissance and Reformation*, vol. 3 (Toronto, 1987), 261–2.

37 See D. Julia, 'La pérégrination académique en France à l'époque moderne', in M. Kulczykowski (ed.), *Les Grandes Réformes des universités européennes du XVIe au XXe siècles. IIIème Session scientifique internationale, Cracovie, 15–17 mai 1980*, Zeszyty Naukowe Uniwersytetu Jagiellonskiego DCCLXI. Prace Historyczne, Z. 79 (Warsaw and Krakau, 1985), 31.

38 J.N. Paquot, *Mémoires pour servire à l'histoire littéraire des dix-sept provinces des Pays-Bas, de la Principauté de Liège et de quelques contrées voisines*, 18 vols (Louvain, 1763–70), vol. 3, 491–5: 'André Gheeraerdts, ou Andreas Gerardi Hyperius'; H. Jahr, 'Hyperius, Andreas', in *Neue Deutsche Biographie* (NDB), 10 (Berlin, 1974), 108f.; K.F. Müller, *Andreas Hyperius, ein Beitrag z.s. Charakteristik* (Kiel, 1895).

39 See for many examples in Tervoort, *Iter italicum* (note 34), 38–45; on Coyter p. 40 and biography on CD-rom.

40 Many examples in the biographical repertory of Tervoort, *Iter italicum* (note 34).

instruments, curiosities, artefacts etc.[41] It is impossible to dwell on this aspect, but it is necessary to keep this in mind when speaking of academic mobility.

Let us now come back to the Italian universities. The tables in Appendix 5 give an impression of the numbers of students and their distribution among the different universities. Till the mid-sixteenth century Padua could not compete with Bologna in numbers, certainly not with regard to the *Ultramontani*.[42] In 1506 the university of Bologna had come under the direct control of the Cardinal Legate of the Pope, who had his residence in the town. In 1562 the *Ultramontani* left the *studium* of Bologna en masse because the Papal legate had treated some of the 'heretical' students badly. Moreover, by means of the papal bull *In sacrosancta* of 1564, Pope Pius IV obliged all candidates for the doctorate in all faculties to take an oath of loyalty to the Catholic faith, the so-called *professio fidei*. For medical students the requirement of the oath was confirmed in 1566 by Pius V in the bull *Supra gregem*. However, this constraint did not change the attitude of tolerance which the civil and ecclesiastical authorities of the Republic of Venice and its *studio* had long supported.[43] They accepted Protestants as long as they remained inconspicuous and did not debate about religious matters.[44] The civil government of Venice and the university authorities went a step further.[45] After the death of Pius IV in 1565 the Venetian senate had hoped to annul the compulsory oath,

---

41 See www.circulatingknowledge.ugent.be/mission; the special issue on Circulation of Knowledge, *History of Universities,* 23, 2 (2008); example: S. Van Damme, 'Un modèle de transmission universitaire? La circulation des savoirs cartésiens en Europe', in T. Kouamé, F. Garrigues and J.-P. Vittu *(eds), Les Universités en Europe*, Homme et société, 31 (Paris, 2005), 211–25.

42 H. de Ridder-Symoens, 'Italian and Dutch universities in the sixteenth and seventeenth centuries', in C.S. Maffioli and L.C. Palm (eds), *Italian scientists in the Low Countries* (Amsterdam, 1989), 31–64; G.P. Brizzi, 'Matricole ed effettivi. Aspetti della presenza studentesca a Bologna fra Cinque e Seicento', in G.P. Brizzi and A.I. Pini (eds), *Studenti e Università degli studenti dal XII al XIX secolo*, Studi et Memorie per la Storia dell'Università di Bologna, n.s. 7 (1988), 225–9.

43 A. De Benedictis, '"Respublica stans de per se per vim contractus". Bologna, Stadt und Kirchenstaat: Politische Kultur und Recht', *Zeitschrift für Historische Forschung*, 20, 2 (1993), 153–87; A. De Benedictis, 'La fine dell'autonomia studentesca tra autorità e disciplinamento', in: Brizzi and Pini, *Studenti e Università* (note 40), 193–223; B. Brugi, 'Gli studenti tedeschi e la S. Inquisizione a Padova nella seconda metà del secolo XVI', *Atti del R. Instituto Veneto di scienze, lettere ed arti*, vol. 5 ser. 7 (1893-94), 1015-33; B. Brugi, *La scuola Padovana di diritto romano nel secolo XVI* (Padua, 1888), 22–4; A. Franceschini, *Spigolature archivistiche prime*, Dep. Prov. Ferrarese di storia patria. Atti e memorie, s. 3, 19 (Ferrara, 1975), 135–8.

44 J.J. Poelhekke, 'Nederlandse leden van de "Inclyta Natio Germanica Artistarum" te Padua 1553-1700', *Mededelingen van het Nederlands Historisch Instituut te Rome*, 3 de r., 31 (1961), 276.

45 For what follows see P. van Kessel, *Duitse studenten te Padua. De controverse Rome-Italië en het protestantisme in de tijd der Contrareformatie* (Assen, 1963), 101–2.

but it did not succeed. Therefore, both the university and the senate encouraged the students to follow the long-established but unpopular means of graduating under the authority of a Count Palatine. Emperor Sigismund (1367–1437) had given the competence to create doctors in the name of the Emperor to *comites palatini* and other papal and imperial authorities.[46] Thus, German Protestants had the possibility of avoiding the *professio fidei* by taking a less-prestigious private degree, awarded by a Venetian count palatine in his private residence. The palatine doctor's diploma could create some difficulties at home. The degree was awarded in a Catholic university which was regarded as suspect in the Protestant home country. Moreover, a private examination and an 'unofficial' diploma might cast doubt upon the scholarly quality of the newly created doctor. In view of such considerations, the student Frederick Sebiz asked the German nation of the arts faculty for a certificate stating that the doctor in question had not taken an oath of Catholicity and that the Palatine diploma had the same scholarly value as one awarded in a public graduation ceremony by the university itself. This practice was followed by other religious dissidents after him. The procedure was facilitated by the fact that several palatine counts were appointed as professors, e.g. the very popular Alramer (d. 1597), who was the promoter of many Dutch medical doctors. Further, around 1600 the private certificate was provided with the seal of the university. The last *doctor palatinus* was William Stratenus of Utrecht, who graduated as MD on 8 May 1613. This nobleman became professor at the new Utrecht university in 1636, and personal physician of the Stadholders Frederik Hendrik, Willem II and Willem III. After Stratenus' private graduation the Venetian senate no longer accepted that a degree could be awarded in the Republic of Venice by a foreign sovereign, *in casu* the German Emperor.[47] From 1616, students who wanted to avoid the public graduation ceremony in the presence of the bishop could graduate *auctoritate veneta* instead of *auctoritate imperiale*.[48] Of the 673 *promoti auctoritate veneta* listed by Weigle[49] between 1616 and 1663, two-thirds

---

46 A. Von Wretschko, 'Die Verleihung gelehrter Grade durch den Kaiser seit Karl IV', in *Festschrift Heinrich Brunner zum 70. Geburtstag dargebracht von Schülern und Verehrern* (Weimar, 1910), 689–735; F. Gall, 'Palatinatsverleihungen an italienische Universitäten und gelehrte Gesellschaften, 1530–1653', *Mitteilungen des Österreichischen Staatsarchivs*, 15 (1962), 93–113; E. Martellozzo Forin, 'Conti palatini e lauree conferite per privilegio. L'esempio padovano del sec. XV', *Annali di storia delle università italiane*, 3 (1999), 79–120.

47 Kessel, *Duitse studenten* (note 43), 101–2; P. van Kessel, 'The denominational pluriformity of the German Nations at Padua and the problem of intolerance in the 16th century', *Archiv für Reformationsgeschichte*, 75 (1984), 256–76.

48 Kessel, *Duitse studenten* (note 43), 109.

49 F. Weigle, 'Die deutschen Doktorpromotionen in Philosophie und Medizin an der Universität Padua von 1616-1663', *Quellen und Forschungen aus italienischen Archiven und Bibliotheken*, 45 (1965), 325-36.

originated from the Protestant north of Europe, including 198 (or 30 per cent) Netherlanders (125 from the north, 58 from the south, 15 unspecified).[50]

We must not confuse the graduation *auctoritate veneta* with the examination carried out by the Venetian College of Physicians (*Collegio dei medici*).[51] Padua was the most expensive Italian university for taking degrees. Medical students could escape the high costs by graduating in Venice. From the fifteenth century, the Venetian College of Physicians was allowed to examine the candidates of the *studium* of Padua, as did the *collegium doctorum medicinorum* (*Sacro Collegia dei Filosofi e Medici*) of Padua. The doctor's certificate issued by both the *collegi* testified that the degree was awarded on the basis of papal and imperial authority by the *studium generale* of Venice, located in Padua. The rivalry between the two colleges kept down the price of graduation in the long run. Over half the Venetian graduates came from within the Venetian Republic, and only a small group from outside Italy (35 of the 618 *laureati* between 1501 and 1602).[52] The number of ultramontane graduates was nevertheless disproportionately high in Padua, one third of them taking a degree at this university. The same proportion holds for students of the Low Countries. The influx of Dutch medical students in Padua occurred in the first half of the seventeenth century and represented more than 20 per cent of the total population of the German nation in that faculty. Altogether it was a constant concern for the Republic of Venice and of its alma mater to attract and retain foreign students, and more specifically the members of both the German nations. When we compare the Paduan figures with those of the other Italian universities, it is clear that they succeeded, mostly to the detriment of Padua's rival, i.e. the *studio* of Bologna (Appendix 5, Tables 3 and 4).

The most important competitor for Padua was the university of Leiden.[53] It was indisputably the largest international centre for seventeenth-century Protestants, so much so that the *Encyclopédie* of 1765 stated : 'Il semble que tous les hommes célèbres dans la République des Lettres s'y sont rendus pour la faire fleurir, depuis son établissement jusqu'à nos jours' [All the famous men of the Republic of Letters appear to have studied there and made it flourish, ever since its foundation]. The Dutch republic 'as an international center of free discussion, free printing and free learning' and the supranational network of the Republic of Letters formed an important if not essential part of student mobility.[54] The teaching of classical

---

50 These Dutch students are listed in Poelhekke, 'Nederlandse leden' (note 42).

51 For what follows see R. Palmer, *The Studio of Venice and its graduates in the sixteenth century*, Contributi alla storia dell'Università di Padova, 12 (Padua, 1983); L. Rossetti, 'I Collegi per i dottorati 'Auctoritate Veneta', in M.C. Billanovich, G. Cracco and A. Rigon (eds), *Vividarium Floridum. Studi di Storia Veneta offerti dagli allievi a Paolo Sambin* (Padua, 1986), 365–86.

52 Calculations based on the Catalogue of Graduations published by Palmer, *The Studio of Venice* (note 49), 67–192.

53 H. de Ridder-Symoens, 'Italian and Dutch universities' (note 40), 31–64.

54 Frijhoff, 'Academic relations' (note 22), 15.

and oriental philology, history, Calvinist theology, Cartesian philosophy, humanist Roman law (the Elegant School), natural science and medicine flourished there. Other Dutch universities benefited from its renown, often acting as relay stations in the *iter hollandicum* and as graduation universities.[55] In seventeenth-century Leiden and also for a short time at the small Frisian university of Franeker (founded in 1585), between one third and two-thirds of all the students were foreigners, during the heyday years of 1575–1700. In descending order they were Germans, Englishmen, Frenchmen, Scots, Swedes, Danes, Hungarians, Southern-Netherlanders, Swiss etc. A proportionally large number of them studied medicine (Appendix 6).[56]

The French medical faculties were small till the eighteenth century, with a local clientele. By 1700 there were 19 cities where local medical graduates had a monopoly on practice. Colleges of physicians and medical faculties controlled the health sector. Some of these faculties, nevertheless, did not provide any teaching; they only awarded degrees (Valence, Orange, Nantes, Bourges).[57] As we have already noted, from the beginning only Montpellier and Paris recruited on a national and even international level.[58] This does not mean, though, that foreigners avoided French medical faculties. Thanks to recent studies by Willem Frijhoff on Netherlandish *promoti* at French universities at the end of the sixteenth and in the seventeenth centuries, we get some insight into the numbers, albeit only of graduations and not of matriculations, for the universities of Angers, Avignon, Caen, Grenoble, Montpellier, Orange, Pont-à-Mousson, Reims and Valence. The universities with the highest number of Netherlandish medical students were

---

55 On graduation universities see H. de Ridder-Symoens, 'Mobility', in H. de Ridder-Symoens, *Universities in early modern Europe (1500–1800)* (note 2), 435–8.

56 Numerous figures in H.T. Colenbrander, 'De herkomst der Leidse studenten', in *Pallas Leidensis* (Leiden, 1925), 273–303; see also G.G. Simpson (ed.), *Scotland and the Low Countries, 1124–1994*, Mackie Monograph, 3 (East Linton, 1996), 122–35; G. Cohen, *Ecrivains français en Hollande dans la première moitié du XVIIe siècle*, Bibliothèque de la Revue de littérature compare, 1 (The Hague and Paris, 1921), 141–356 (Livre II: Professeurs et étudiants français à l'Université de Leyde (1575 à 1648)); O.P. Grell, 'The attraction of Leiden University for English students of medicine and theology, 1590–1642', in C.C. Barfoot and R. Todd (eds), *The Great Emporium. The Low Countries as a cultural crossroads in the Renaissance and the eighteenth century*, Studies in Literature, 10 (Amsterdam, 1992), 83–104; R.W. Innes-Smith, *English speaking students of medicine at the University of Leyden* (Edinburgh, 1932); J.K. Cameron, 'Some Scottish students and teachers at the University of Leiden in the late sixteenth and early seventeenth centuries', in G.G. Simpson (ed.), *Scotland and the Low Countries, 1124–1994* (East Linton, 1996), 122–35; K. van Strien, 'Schotse studenten in Leiden omstreeks 1700', *Jaarboekje voor Geschiedenis en Oudheidkunde van Leiden en omstreken*, 86 (1994), 133–48 (deel 1); 88 (1996), 126–48 (deel 2).

57 Brockliss, *French higher education* (note 1), 184; see also Julia, 'Pérégrination académique' (note 37), 38–40.

58 Brockliss, *French higher education* (note 1), 16–7.

Angers (130), Caen (168) and Reims (45), all three quite close to the Netherlands. In the other cities only between one and seven medical *promoti* were found.[59]

In the seventeenth century Angers was very popular among foreigners on their Grand Tour, thanks to its Académie d'équitation. Hundreds of them graduated in law or medicine.[60] Between 1601 and 1635 Frijhoff found 712 foreigners enrolled in the Académie, half of them coming from Germany, Bohemia and Poland, 30 per cent from the Netherlands, 12 per cent from the British Isles and 6 per cent from the northern countries.[61] The more regular students only aspiring to a degree, like the 130 medical doctors who graduated between 1635 and 1688, did not enrol in the Academy.

The university of Caen – much influenced by Calvinism until 1586 – was even more attractive to Dutch students, in law as well as in medicine.[62] After its reorientation towards Catholicism, reformed (i.e. Calvinist) foreigners continued to visit the Norman university in the seventeenth century, thanks to the quality of its open-minded professors, especially in the medical faculty. Jacques de Cahaignes (1548–1617) and his nephew Etienne de Cahaignes were well known in the Netherlands, having studied at Leiden and being in contact with the famous scholars of their time.[63]

Another pole of attraction for foreigners was the medical faculty of the university of Reims, founded in 1548. Till the 1680s less than 10 medical degrees per year were awarded. From then onwards their number increased, with figures between 17 and 35. Indeed, in the early eighteenth century no less than 60 per cent of its graduates in medicine were foreigners, and at the end of the eighteenth century this held for nearly 30 per cent, most of them from the British Isles – in the first half of the eighteenth century mainly English and Scots; after 1750, Irish (Appendix 7).[64] The English and Scottish Protestants attended Boerhaave's lectures in Leiden (which were revolutionary for their time) and went on to take their degree at Reims, probably on their way home. At Leiden candidates had to

59 W. Frijhoff, 'Nederlandse promoties in de geneeskunde aan Franse universiteiten (zestiende-'achttiende eeuw), *Jaarboek Centraal Bureau voor Genealogie*, 60 (2006), 75–6; see also W. Frijhoff, '"Un chemin de travers du grand tour". Gradués en Droit néerlandais et allemands à l'université de Caen au XVIe siècle, avec un inventaire chronologique', *Lias*, 34, 1 (2007), 59–68.

60 W. Frijhoff, 'Étudiants étrangers à l'Académie d'équitation d'Angers au XVIIe siècle', *Lias*, 4, 1 (1977), 13–84.

61 Frijhoff, 'Étudiants étrangers' (note 57), 20.

62 Frijhoff, 'Nederlandse promoties' (note 56), 89–102 and Frijhoff, 'Un chemin de travers' (note 56), 59–136.

63 W. Frijhoff, 'Le médecin selon Jacques Cahaignes (1548–1617). Autour de deux soutenances en médecine à Caen au début du XVIIe siècle', *Lias*, 10 (1983), 193–215.

64 P. Dubourg-Maldan, 'Histoire de la Faculté de Médecine de l'Université de Reims', *La Chronique de Champagne*, 4 (1838), 351–91; A. Ségal, 'Les liens médicaux entre Liège et Reims', *Revue médicale de Liège,* 35, 20 (15 octobre 1980), 696–7.

write a dissertation for their doctorate and the examination fees were high, whereas in Reims foreigners were given a diploma on payment of a fee which was much lower than in the Dutch university; they had to promise not to practise in France. The nine physicians who founded the faculty of medicine in Edinburgh (1726) were all alumni of Boerhaave, but only one of them was a graduate of Leiden. Three had taken their degree in Reims, one in Angers and one in Padua; and three Scots had chosen a Scottish university, Glasgow, St Andrews and Edinburgh, but many years later. The Catholic Irish appear to have studied in Paris, where in the latter half of the eighteenth century medical studies had been quite drastically brought up to date. The College of Surgery, founded in 1750, especially attracted many foreign medical students, because of its advanced theoretical and practical training.[65]

In the sixteenth and seventeenth centuries without any doubt Montpellier hosted the most international medical faculty in France. In contrast with Paris, where the medical teaching was completely under the influence of the theories of Galen and Hippocrates till the late seventeenth century,[66] notwithstanding the introduction of lectures in surgery and pharmacy into the curriculum in 1506 and 1538 respectively, in the sixteenth century Montpellier modernised its teaching more drastically by introducing courses in practical medicine (still on a theoretical basis) and by creating chairs in botany, anatomy, surgery and pharmacy. The Montpellier example was slowly taken up by other medical faculties, but it took till the eighteenth century before the whole curriculum changed more drastically.[67] In the seventeenth century it became common at Montpellier for students to accompany their masters when they visited their patients. For the rest, bachelors in medicine had to gain practical skills by working in local hospitals in Montpellier and its neighbourhood before taking their licentiate and doctorate. Only in Paris were bachelors expected to attend the faculty's weekly out-patient clinic, from 1639 onwards.[68] Montpellier attracted not only large numbers of foreigners, but

---

[65] L.W.B. Brockliss and C. Jones, *The medical world of early modern France* (Oxford, 1997), 199–200, 493–4, 517–18; D. Julia and J. Revel, 'Annexe statistique : Facultés de médecine', in D. Julia and J. Revel (eds), *Les Universités européennes du XVIe au XVIIIe siècle. Histoire sociale des populations étudiantes*, vol. 2: *France*, Recherches d'histoire et de sciences sociales – Studies in History and Social Sciences, 18 (Paris, 1989), 459–86; for the graduation universities see D. Julia and J. Revel, 'Les étudiants et leurs études', ibid., 83–6; T. Gelfand, *Professionalizing modern medicine: Paris surgeons and medical science and institutions in the 18th century*, (Westport and London, 1980); W. Frijhoff, 'L'École de Chirurgie de Paris et les Pays-Bas: analyse d'un recrutement, 1752–1791', *Lias*, 17, 2 (1990), 185–240.

[66] L.W.B. Brockliss, 'Medical teaching at the University of Paris 1600–1720', *Annals of Science*, 35 (1978), 221–51.

[67] Brockliss and Jones, *Medical world* (note 62), 94–8; general overview: Brockliss, *French higher education* (note 1), 391–440 (ch. 8: Medicine).

[68] Brockliss and Jones, *Medical world* (note 62), 167–9.

also French students in search of a modern medical education. One fifth to one third of all the medical doctoral degrees awarded in France in that period came from Montpellier.[69] The sixteenth-century university is well known to us, thanks to the vivid descriptions of the Basle students Felix (1536–1614) and Thomas Platter (1574–1628), who both went there to study medicine.[70] In the beginning of the sixteenth century (1503–1512) 36.9 per cent of the Montpellier students were foreigners, of whom one quarter came from Spain. In the last decade of that century the number of foreigners had decreased to 14 per cent, and no further Spaniards were enrolled, as a consequence of Philip II's prohibitive legislation on studying abroad. Proportionally, Montpellier had fewer graduates than students because many students went on to Avignon or Valence to get their degrees. This fact was mentioned by Felix Platter.[71] According to Felix's father, Thomas Platter the Elder (1499–1582), academic standards in French universities were so low that he advised his son to take his degree of doctor of medicine at Basle, not Montpellier, as this would be more 'honourable' for him. 'If I took my degree in France people would be sure to say that I was not up to the standards of the Basle *studium*; for everyone knew what was said of the French universities: accipimus pecuniam et mittimus stultos in Germaniam (we take their money and send them off to Germany as ignorant as they came).'[72] This did not dissuade Felix from studying in France.

The recruitment of students at Paris became more local in the early modern period. Up to 50 per cent of medical students came from the region of Paris and another 35 per cent from dioceses north of the Loire; no more than 10 per cent originated from south of the Loire and only 4 per cent were foreigners.[73] With the foundation of the Académie de Chirurgie in 1750, Paris again became attractive for professional training.

The situation in the Germanic world, Spain, the British Isles and the northern countries was not that different from the average situation in France.[74] The medical

---

69 Brockliss and Jones, *Medical world* (note 62), 199–201.

70 *Félix et Thomas Platter à Montpellier, 1552–1557, 1595–1599. Notes de voyage de deux étudiants bâlois publiées d'après les manuscrits originaux appartenant à la Bibliothèque de l'Université de Bâle* (Montpellier, 1892); S. Jennett (ed.), *Journal of a younger brother, the life of Thomas Platter as a medical student in Montpellier in the close of the sixteenth century* (London, 1963); S. Jennett (ed.), *Beloved son Felix: the Journal of Felix Platter a medical student in Montpellier in the sixteenth century* (London, 1961).

71 Julia, 'Pérégrination académique' (note 37), 30–1.

72 Quoted in Julia and Revel, 'Les étudiants et leurs études' (note 62), 39.

73 L. Brockliss, 'Patterns of attendance at the University of Paris 1400–1800', in Julia and Revel (eds), *Universités européennes* (note 62), 503 (also published in *The Historical Journal*, 21 (1978), 513–44).

74 R.G. Frank, 'Science, medicine and the Universities of early modern England: Background and sources', *History of Science*, 11 (1973), 194–216, 239–69; R.L. Kagan, *Students and society in early modern Spain* (Baltimore, [1974]).

faculties were small and ill equipped. Many of them only existed on paper, or functioned just temporarily. They educated the local or regional medical elites. For a more advanced training, as we have seen, students went to medical schools in Italy, the United Provinces, or one or two French *studia*. This pattern did not really change till the eighteenth century. Outside the Dutch Republic only Protestant institutions of ancient foundation, such as Heidelberg and Basle, dispensed multi-disciplinary teaching, with fully fledged faculties of law and medicine, many of the others teaching only arts and theology. In the Lutheran *studia* theology and law were the principal disciplines, with arts being considered as propaedeutic.[75] The medical faculties were, to a certain extent, protected by the prohibitive 'national' legislation compelling candidates for public office to have graduated at the local or regional university. For multiple reasons – which could be familial, religious, political, geographical or by chance – these smaller faculties enrolled 'foreigners' from time to time. (See an example in Appendix 8).

In the eighteenth century the landscape changed profoundly, thanks partly to the already mentioned influence of Boerhaave. The fashion of going abroad to take a degree died out in the eighteenth century. The Grand Tour was no longer looked on as the culmination of a first-class education, but rather as tourism and travel for pleasure. The idea of utility so dear to the disciples of Enlightenment began to take precedence in pedagogic thinking, also. Study abroad was still regarded as advantageous and even advisable, but only in special cases. Young intellectuals sought advanced training for a career in a carefully chosen institution and, if they failed to find one at home, went abroad for it. In short, foreign universities were used where there were no adequate facilities at home. The official religion of the *studium* was now less important, for the fashion of the times favoured severance from confessional links or, increasingly, religious tolerance. As it was necessary to submit a diploma when taking up office or applying for inscription on the rolls of a profession, it was still necessary to appear for examination at a national university (or at a foreign one if it charged less for its degree), unless the home government made difficulties for holders of foreign diplomas.[76]

Under Boerhaave, Leiden's international attendance increased spectacularly. Of the 1,919 students who attended his lectures between 1701 and 1738, about one third (659) came from the English-speaking countries, where medical training was then of indifferent quality. Comparatively few of his students (178, of whom 43 or fourth quarter were English speaking) took their degree in Leiden.[77] Under the influence of the Scottish Enlightenment, the Scottish universities flourished in the eighteenth century, Edinburgh towards the middle of the century and Glasgow at its end. As these universities did not require any profession of faith in the Church of Scotland and the programmes in their faculties of medicine –

[75] Siraisi, 'Faculty of medicine' (note 1), 360–79; Brockliss, 'Curricula' (note 2), 609–18; CRE 1 and 2; O'Malley, *History of medical education* (note 1).

[76] Ridder-Symoens, 'Mobility' (note 52).

[77] Lindeboom, *Boerhaave* (note 19).

the pride of Edinburgh and later of Glasgow – were very flexible, they had an international following of Scandinavian, Portuguese and other students (amongst them Russians), and were visited by English and Irish dissenters, and by Calvinists from the American colonies. Very few of them, however, took a degree there. In the 1780s Edinburgh's faculty of medicine had about 500 students a year, only 20 to 30 of whom took a degree there.[78]

The new universities of Halle and Göttingen were poles of attraction in the Empire, but their international audience should not be overestimated. They certainly attracted quite a large number of young people from northern and eastern Europe, western Europe being represented there almost solely by Englishmen. The reform of the Viennese *studium* in the reign of Maria Theresa made it quite widely attractive within the Habsburg Empire.[79]

Italian universities were completely out of fashion. Towards the middle of the eighteenth century the foreign nations there had to close down for lack of students. Spain never attracted foreign students. Its medical faculties remained very traditional until the eighteenth century (their written textbooks were Hippocrates, Galen and Avicenna). Only at the end of the eighteenth century were writings of the ancients supplemented with recent texts and new courses in botany, pharmacology and practical medicine.[80]

Jews at Universities

Before concluding I will mention an interesting and often-neglected group of medical students, namely the Jews. The only way Jews or converterd Jews could gain a living was to apply themselves to commerce, finance or medicine. To study medicine, they were not really free to choose a university; they had to be content with those institutions willing to accept them.[81] Happily for them, the medical faculties open to Jews and other types of dissidents were mostly the most tolerant, in religion and also in teaching and research.

In the Middle Ages Jews could register at the university of Montpellier, till their expulsion from the city and the region in 1306. In other universities only

---

[78] J.B. Morrell, 'Medicine and science in the eighteenth century', in G. Donaldson (ed.), *Four centuries of Edinburgh University life 1583–1983* (Edinburgh, 1983), 38–52; *Evidence, oral and documentary taken by the Commissioners for Visiting the Universities of Scotland*, vol. XI: *University of Glasgow* (London, 1837), 525.

[79] N. Hammerstein, 'Die deutschen Universitäten im Zeitalter der Aufklärung', *Zeitschrift für historische Forschung*, 10 (1983), 73–89.

[80] Kagan, *Students and society in early modern Spain* (note 71), 162, 197–230, 249–59.

[81] V. Colorni, 'Sull'ammissibilità degli ebrei alla laurea anteriormente al secolo XIX', *Rassegna mensile di Israel*, 16, 6–8 (1950), 202–16; H. Friedenwald, *Jews and medicine* (Baltimore, 1944).

converted Jews (*Judaei conversi*) were accepted. Jews, Marranos and Moriscos were repeatedly expelled from Spain and Portugal, notably in 1480–92 and 1609. They could not attend a university until the end of the fifteenth century, when the popes allowed Jews to register in Italian medical faculties and even to teach.[82] With the advent of Pope Paul IV (1476–1559), an orthodox Catholic proselyte and an enemy of Marranos and Jews, attendance at universities was no longer allowed. Some Italian principalities were more tolerant and disregarded the anti-Jewish decrees. Juan Roderigo de Castello Branco (1511–68), from a family of Portuguese crypto-Jews, went home after having studied at Salamanca. About 1533 he fled from his country and settled in Antwerp as a botanist and a physician. Although he had a flourishing private practice, he accepted a chair in anatomy at the university of Ferrara. Thanks to Renée de France (1510–75), wife of Duke Ercole II d'Este (1508–1559), the duchy of Ferrara was an asylum for men of letters and science and for religious dissidents.[83] In Ferrara, Roderigo changed his name to Amatus Lusitanus. Under Pope Paul IV, Amatus left for Ragusa in Dalmatia and then for Salonika (in the Ottoman Empire), where he could publicly profess Judaism.[84]

As already mentioned, the university of Padua found ways to resist the papal decrees on orthodoxy. It became the principal centre of academic training for European and North-African Jews, some of whom attended the university of Siena, which also tried to be as tolerant as possible.[85]

The expelled Iberian Jews and converted Jews sought refuge in whatever country would accept them and allow and enable them to study. In the fifteenth and sixteenth centuries they settled mainly in the great merchant cities of France

---

[82] V. Colorni, 'Ebrei in Ferrara nei secoli XIII e XIV', in *Miscellanea di Studi in onore di Dario Disegni* (Turin, 1969), 69–106.

[83] C.J. Blaisdell, 'Politics and heresy in Ferrara, 1534–1559', *Sixteenth-century Journal*, 6 (1975), 67–93; R. Bonfil, 'Ferrare: un port sûr et paisible pour la diaspora séfarade', in M. Abitbol and H. Méchoulan (eds), *Les Juifs d'Espagne: histoire d'une diaspora 1492–1992* (Liana Levi, 1998), 295–303.

[84] G.H. Tucker, 'To Louvain and Antwerp and beyond: The contrasting itineraries of Diogo Pires (Didacus Pyrrhus Lusitanus, 1577–99) and João Rodrigues de Castelo Branco (Amatus Lusitanus, 1511–68)', in L. Dequeker and W. Verbeke, *The expulsion of the Jews and their emigration to the southern Low Countries (15th-16th c.)*, Medievalia Lovaniensia, Series 1, Studia XXVI (Louvain, 1998), 83–113; D. Hashavit, 'Amatus Lusitanus discovered valves in veins and arteries', *HaLapid* (Publication of the Society for Crypto-Judaic Studies), Winter (2006); text on internet: www.cryptojews.com/Amatus%20Lusitanus.htm.

[85] J. Shatzmiller, 'Étudiants juifs à la faculté de médecine de Montpellier, dernier quart du XIVe siècle', *Jewish History*, 6 (1992), 243–55; P.C. Ioly Zorattini, 'Gli Ebrei a Venezia, Padova e Verona', in *Storia della Cultura Veneta*, 3, 1 (Vicenza, 1980), 337–576; M. Luzzati, 'Prestito ebraico e studenti ebrei all'università di Pisa (secc. XV–XVIII)', in *Studi di storia moderna e contemporanea in memoria di Nicola Carranza* (special issue of *Bollettino Storico Pisano*, 49) (1980), 23–38; J. Shatzky, 'On Jewish medical students in Padua', *Journal of the History of Medicine and Allied Sciences*, 5 (1950), 444–7.

and the Low Countries, particularly Antwerp. In the seventeenth century Holland became their place of asylum, and the Dutch universities their centres of study.[86] Basle, too, as a tolerant commercial town, accepted Jews at its university.[87] When the German *studia* opened their doors to Jews – the Protestant universities at the end of the seventeenth century and, more importantly, the Catholic universities in the eighteenth century – the process of integration flourished, with Jews even being admitted to the other faculties of arts and law.[88] Thus, the universities that accepted Jewish students are those that had already distanced themselves from the prevailing religious intolerance by accepting and even protecting students of other religious or political persuasions. These were the universities of Padua, Siena, Leiden, Franeker, Utrecht, Montpellier and even Basle, to cite only those giving courses in medicine.

Conclusion

From the fifteenth century well far into the seventeenth century almost all medical faculties were the little brothers of the higher faculties, in numbers as well as in prestige. They mainly educated the local medical elites and were responsible for the health organisation of the region or country. Only a few medical schools were at the forefront with regard to teaching and research: Bologna and Padua in northern Italy, Montpellier in France, and the universities of the Dutch Republic, with Leiden in the lead. These institutions attracted an international audience. Their graduates became professors at the local university or got leading positions as court or city physicians. Many of the Italian graduates were prominent humanists and investigators who devoted most of their time to writing and research. A medical education was also a way to get acquainted with the new natural sciences and the developments in chemistry, physics, mathematics, cosmography and so on. So even artists, jurists and theologians wanting to learn more about 'the Book of Nature' would enroll in a medical faculty and often get a degree. Under the influence of the new science and the professionalisation of health care, medical education lost more and more of its philosophical and even religious approach, and modernised drastically and, as a consequence, gained more esteem.

---

[86] Frijhoff, *Société néerlandaise* (note 4), 55–6, 237, 240; B.J. Kaplan, *Muslims in the Dutch Golden Age. Representations and realities of religious toleration* (Amsterdam, 2006) (Fourth Golden Age Lecture, 23 May 2006).

[87] G. Kisch, *Die Universitäten und die Juden. Eine historische Betrachtung zur Fünfhundertjahrfeier der Universität Basel*, Philosophie und Geschichte, 77 (Tübingen, 1961).

[88] S. Kottek, 'Sur l'ouverture progressive des universités de l'Europe centrale aux étudiants en médecine juifs au XVIIIe siècle', *Revue d'histoire de la médecine hébraïque*, 27 (1974), 113–8; M. Richarz, *Der Eintritt der Juden in die akademischen Berufe. Jüdische Studenten und Akademiker in Deutschland 1678–1848* (Tübingen, 1974).

Indeed, in the course of the early modern period, the status of medical faculties and medical doctors changed profoundly. Medical faculties in many universities lost their Cinderella position. The social status of physicians in society increased dramatically, not only as a result of the growing interest in science, but also because of the foundation of *collegia medica* which gave them complete control over the whole medical sector.

As a consequence, the study pattern of medical students changed likewise. Till the fifteenth century, physicians *in spe* were obliged to travel to the scarcely functioning medical faculties. From the end of the Middle Ages onwards students had more opportunities to study close to home, thanks to an increasing number of *studia generalia* with a medical faculty, albeit that they were sometimes compelled to gain their diploma from a more distant university.

Under the influence of Renaissance ideas and humanism, the *peregrinatio academica* received a fresh boost. The basic arts courses were mostly attended at a nearby university. For more advanced courses, youngsters sought out centres of excellence where they could combine professional quality with intellectual and cultural challenges. In that period student mobility was at its apogee. In the late seventeenth century and certainly in the eighteenth century mobility decreased considerably. The main reason was that most of the universities had started to modernise their curricula even if they were not in the forefront of innovation. Prospective physicians with local aspirations contented themselves with the most nearby medical faculty, which allowed them to start a practice. We have also to consider the fact that many local authorities required of their candidate physicians a degree awarded by the local or regional university. Furthermore, medical graduates went on a Grand Tour less frequently than law graduates, because of the high costs that the medical milieu could less easily afford.

The Enlightenment revived university life and encouraged student mobility to some extent, but such mobility was mainly within the country and confined to a few centres providing a modern education suitable for the needs of enlightened states. The direction in which students went changed drastically. France, with the exception of Paris, and Italy were now of little account. The Northern Netherlands also lost their attraction to a great extent, after Boerhaave. Students with intellectual and professional aspirations went to the new or thoroughly renovated centres, such as Göttingen and Halle, Vienna and Edinburgh. Paris remained popular, thanks to many facts: the quality of teaching, the creation of the Académie de Chirurgie, possibilities of networking and language training, facilities, cultural environment etc.

It is clear from this short review[89] that the attraction of educational institutions was manifold and changed over the course of the centuries. Looking at student numbers, we can see that the success of most medical faculties was often based on their educational reputation (for example, the modernity of the curriculum,

---

[89] For a more detailed overview see De Ridder-Symoens, 'Mobility' (notes 20 and 52).

study facilities). But the cost of tuition, and even more of graduation, local facilities, accessibility, family traditions, political and religious situations also played important roles in the choice of a *studium*. As a consequence, it would be wrong to consider medical faculties with the highest number of 'foreigners' as automatically centres of excellence. The whole context has to be taken into account, and excellence has to be defined.

The more focused chapters in this volume will provide the necessary nuances and supply more refined arguments to allow consideration of universities and their medical faculties as a centres of excellence.

Appendix I: Institutional Context – Italy

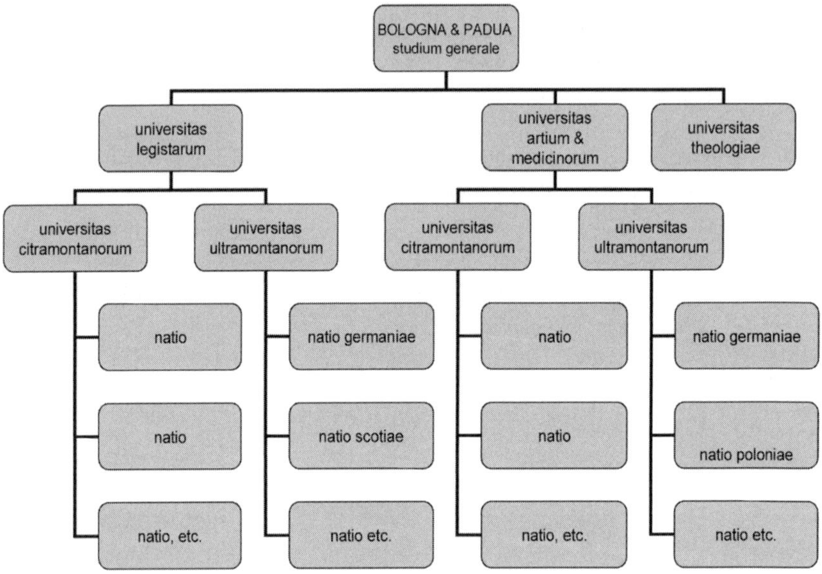

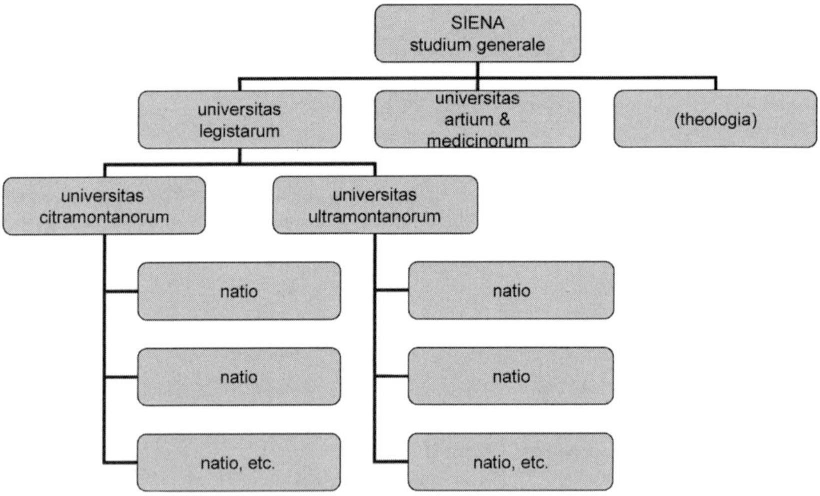

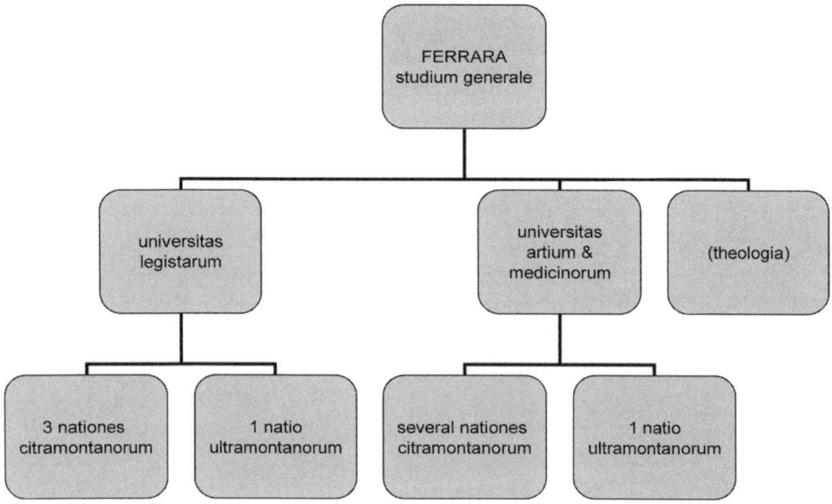
FERRARA
studium generale
universitas legistarum
universitas artium & medicinorum
(theologia)
3 nationes citramontanorum
1 natio ultramontanorum
several nationes citramontanorum
1 natio ultramontanorum

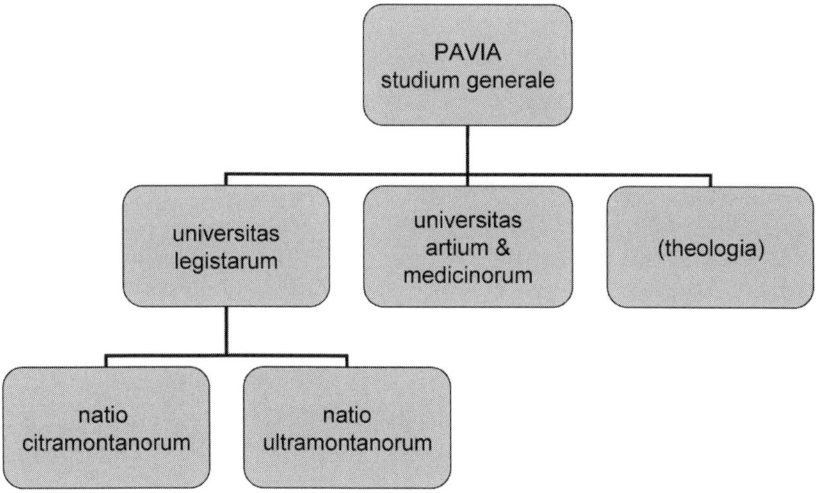
PAVIA
studium generale
universitas legistarum
universitas artium & medicinorum
(theologia)
natio citramontanorum
natio ultramontanorum

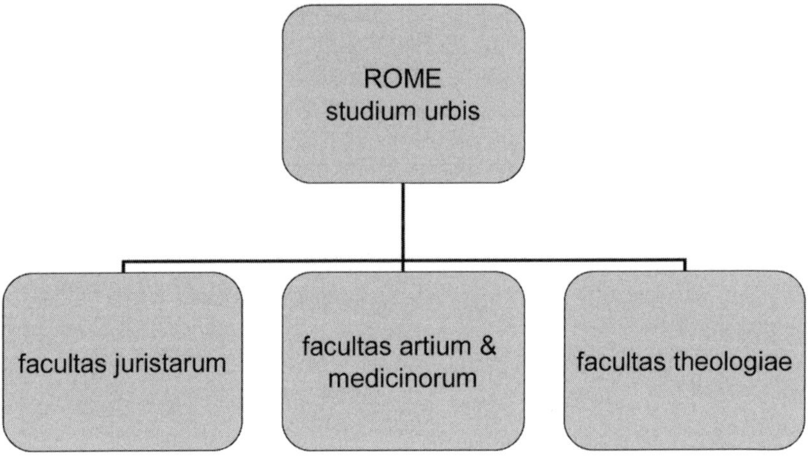
ROME
studium urbis
facultas juristarum
facultas artium &
medicinorum
facultas theologiae

Appendix II: Institutional Context – NW-Europe

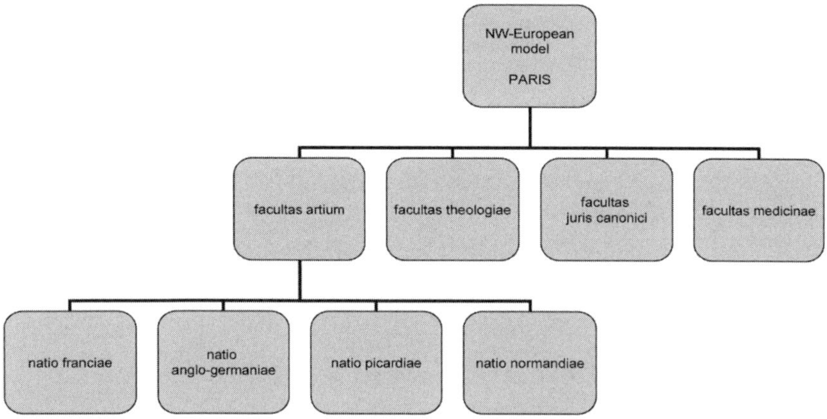

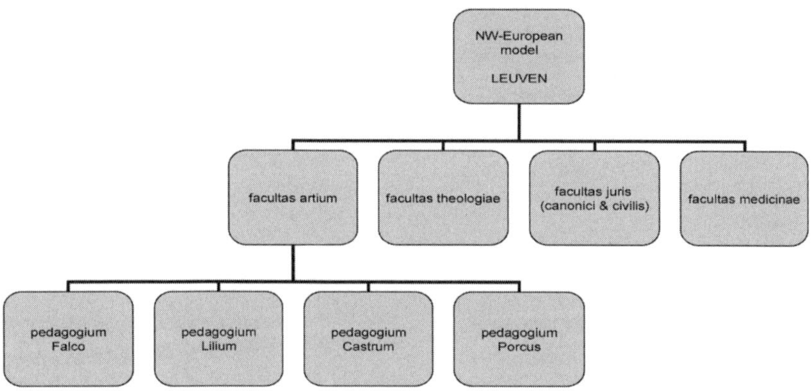

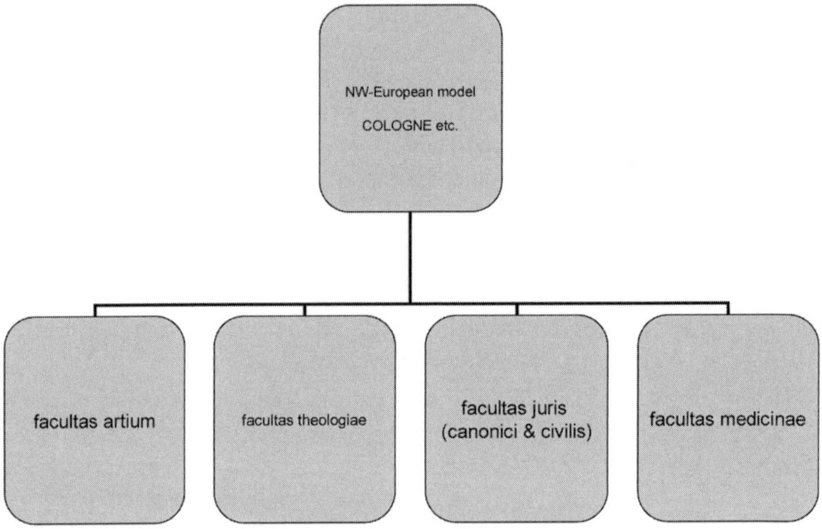
NW-European model
COLOGNE etc.
facultas artium
facultas theologiae
facultas juris
(canonici & civilis)
facultas medicinae

Appendix 3: Medical infrastructure

Botanical gardens

1545	Padua
1547	Pisa
1567–68	Bologna
1567	Valencia
1580	Leipzig
1587	Leiden
1588	Basel
1593	Montpellier
1597	Heidelberg
1600	Copenhagen
1621	Oxford
1655	Uppsala
1738	Leuven

Anatomical theatres

1595	Padua
1597	Leiden
ca. 1600	Bologna, renovated 1637–49
1604	Paris in wood
1617–20	Paris in stone
1619	Amsterdam, renovated 1691
1620s	Oxford
1640–43	Copenhagen
1663	Uppsala
1727	Halle
1744	Louvain

Clinical (bedside) teaching

1539	Padua
1636	Utrecht (not continued)
1637	Leiden
1729	Edinburgh
1749	Wenen
1689	Copenhagen
1705	Uppsala
1728	Strasbourg
1751	Göttingen

1776	Granada
1778	Würzburg
1786	Valencia

Appendix 4 Physicians in medieval France

Beginning of fourteenth century – places of study of 301 graduate physicians registered in France

Paris	57.8%
Montpellier	35.2%
Other French faculties of medicine	2.7%
Abroad	4.3%

End of fifteenth century – places of study of 436 graduate physicians registered in France

Montpellier	16.3%
Paris	47.5%
Other French universities (Caen, Toulouse, and Avignon, Perpignan, Cahors, Angers, Dole, Nantes, Poitiers, Bordeaux, Bourges)	27.6%
Foreign faculties (Louvain – 17 graduates Salerno and Bologna – 10 graduates each Other Italian studia – a few French graduates each)	8.5%

Source: Ernest Wickersheimer, Danielle Jacquart and Guy Beaujouan, *Dictionnaire biographique des médecins en France au Moyen Age*, 3 vols , Ecole pratique des hautes études. 4e section: Sciences historiques et philologiques. 5: Hautes études médiévales et modernes 34–35 (Genève: Droz, 1979). Supplément: Danielle Jacquart (Nouv. éd. sous la dir. de Guy Beaujouan) – Vol. 1–2 (Réimpr. de l'éd. de 1936).

Appendix 5 Medical students at Italian universitie

Table 1 Graduations in medicine at the University of Bologna 1480–1799

	1480–99	**1500–24**	**1525–49**	**1550–74**	**1575–99**	**1600–24**	**1625–49**	**1650–74**	**1675–99**	**1700–24**	**1725–49**	**1750–74**	**1775–99**	**1480–1799**
Total	*144*	*294*	*399*	*604*	*432*	*462*	*328*	*457*	*298*	*166*	*262*	*242*	*259*	*4347*
Citramontani														
Italy	79	132	219	351	270	300	196	204	126	79	132	173	178	**2439**
Bologna	8	24	16	51	48	80	75	83	69	58	45	29	54	**640**
Total Citra-montani	**87**	**156**	**235**	**402**	**318**	**380**	**271**	**287**	**195**	**137**	**177**	**202**	**232**	**3079**
Ultramontani														
Portugal	13	23	23	25	28	4	10		2			7	1	**136**
Spain and Colonies													2	**2**
Holy Empire	22	70	67	99	19	35	27	99	67	20	56	22	9	**612**
Southern Netherlands	5	4	12	25	24	14	7	12	8			3	2	**116**
Northern Netherlands	5	4	17	10	3	7		7			1			**54**
Poland	3	15	8	21	9	9	5	5	2		3	2	7	**89**
France	1	2	15	5	4		1	5		1				**34**
Great Britain	1	1	1		1	4	1	1						**10**
Switzerland			1	2	1	3	1	7	3	4	2	2	3	**29**

Northern countries				2	1									**3**
Southern Europe				1	1	2	1	3	1		3	1	1	**14**
Bohemia, Moravia,	1	1	5	3	6	2		20	16	2	17	2		**75**
Hungary														
Jews	1			1										**2**
Total Ultra-montani	**52**	**120**	**149**	**194**	**97**	**80**	**53**	**159**	**99**	**26**	**82**	**39**	**25**	**1176**
	36%	40%	38%	32%	22%	17%	16%	35%	35%	33%	30%	16%	10%	**28%**
Unknown	5	18	15	8	17	2	4	11	4	2	3	1	2	**92**

Source: G. Bronzino, Notitia doctorum, sive catalogus doctorum qui in collegiis philosophiae et medicinae Bononie laureati fuerunt ab anno 1480 usque ad annum 1800, Universitatis Bononiensis Monumenta VI (Milan, 1962).

Table 2 Graduations in medicine at Bologna: Citramontani

Years	Total students	Unknown	Italy	Bologna	Total Citramontani
1480–1499	144	5	79	8	**87**
1500–1524	294	18	132	24	**156**
1525–1549	399	15	219	16	**235**
1550–1574	604	8	351	51	**402**
1575–1599	432	17	270	48	**318**
1600–1624	462	2	300	80	**380**
1625–1649	328	4	196	75	**271**
1650–1674	457	11	204	83	**287**
1675–1699	298	4	126	69	**195**
1700–1724	166	2	79	58	**137**
1725–1749	262	3	132	45	**177**
1750–1774	242	1	173	29	**202**
1775–1799	259	2	178	54	**232**
1480–1799	**4347**	**92**	**2439**	**640**	**3079**

Source: Bronzini (1962).

Table 3 Graduations in medicine at Bologna: Ultramontani

Years	TTotal	Total Ultra-montani	%	Holy Empire	Southern Nether-lands	Northern Nether-lands	Portugal, Spain and Colonies	Po-land	Bohemia Moravia Hungary	France	Switzer-land	Southern Europe	Great Britain	Northern Count-ries	Jews
1480–1499	144	**52**	36%	22	5	5	13	3	1	1			1		1
1500–1524	294	**120**	40%	70	4	4	23	15	1	2			1		
1525–1549	399	**149**	38%	67	12	17	23	8	5	15	1		1		
1550–1574	604	**194**	32%	99	25	10	25	21	3	5	2	1		2	1
1575–1599	432	**97**	22%	19	24	3	28	9	6	4	1	1	1	1	
1600–1624	462	**80**	17%	35	14	7	4	9	2		3	2	4		
1625–1649	328	**53**	16%	27	7		10	5		1	1	1	1		
1650–1674	457	**159**	35%	99	12	7		5	20	5	7	3	1		
1675–1699	298	**99**	35%	67	8		2	2	16		3	1			
1700–1724	166	**26**	33%	20					2	1	4				
1725–1749	262	**82**	30%	56		1		3	17		2	3			
1750–1774	242	**39**	16%	22	3		7	2	2		2	1			
1775–1799	259	**25**	10%	9	2		3	7			3	1			
1480–1799	**4347**	**1176**	**28%**	**612**	**116**	**54**	**138**	**89**	**75**	**34**	**29**	**14**	**10**	**3**	**2**

Source: Bronzini (1962).

Table 4 Graduations in Medicine at Padua

	De Ridder-Symoens 1989	De Ridder-Symoens 1989	Rossetti 1964
Year	**Northern Netherlands**	**Southern Netherlands**	**Poland**
1450–74		2	
1475–99			
1500–24		1	
1525–49		6	
1550–74		11	
1575–99	22	8	
1600–24	55	15	47
1625–49	85	35	29
1650–74	29	18	16
1675–99	2	7	16
1700–24			7
1725–49			1
1750–74			0
1775–99			
1450–1799	**193**	**103**	**116**
1550–1799	**193**	**94**	

Sources: H. de Ridder-Symoens, 'Italian and Dutch Universities in the Sixteenth and Seventeenth Centuries', in C.S. Maffioli and L.C. Palm (eds), *Italian Scientists in the Low Countries* (Amsterdam, 1989), 31–64; Lucia Rossetti, 'Dottorati polacchi dal 1600 al 1644 nel Sacro Collegio dei filosofi e medici di Padova (dall'Archivio antico dell'Università)', in *Relazioni tra Padova a la Polonia* (Padova 1964).

Table 5 Graduations of students in medicine from Poland: Padua and Bologna 1600-1750

Years	Padua	Bologna
1600–24	47	9
1625–49	29	5
1650–74	16	5
1675–99	16	2
1700–24	7	
1725–49	1	3
1750–74	0	2
1600–1774	**116**	**26**

Sources: Rossetti (1964) and Bronzini (1962).

Table 6 Graduations of students from the Low Countries

	Medicine				**Law**		
	Padua		**Bologna**		**Padua**	**Bologna**	
Years	**NNL**	**SNL**	**NNL**	**SNL**	**SNL**	**NNL**	**SNL**
1450–74		2				7	9
1475–99			5	5	1	15	6
1500–24		1	4	4	5	8	5
1525–49		6	16	12	5	2	8
1550–74		11	8	27	11	11	42
1575–99	22	8	3	24	3		26
1600–24	55	15	7	14			4
1625–49	85	35		7			1
1650–74	29	18	9	12	1		
1675–99	2	7		8			
1700–24							
1725–49							2
1750–74			1	3			
1775–99				2			
1450–1799	**193**	**103**	**53**	**113**	**26**	**43**	**103**
1550–1799	193	94	28	92	15	11	75

Source: De Ridder-Symoens (1989).

Notes: NNL = Northern Netherlands; SNL = Southern Netherlands.

Table 7 Students from the Low Countries: matriculations and graduations (in brackets) at Italian universities

	Pisa				**Siena**		**Perugia**	
	NNL		**SNL**		**NNL**	**SNL**	**NNL**	**SNL**
	Med.	**Law**	**Med.**	**Law**				
1550–74	6(4)	6(3)	14(13)	27(12)	(13L)	(2M,24L)		
1575–99	3(2)			1	20(2L)	40(2M,9L)	3	11
1600–24			3(2)	3(2)	50(lM,3L)	32(1M)	11(2M, 1L)	13
1625–49			1		42(lL)	26(3L)	6	33(4L, 1T)
1650–74		1			18	23(1L)	2	13(2L)
1675–99					14	28	1	9
1700–24					2	5		1
1725–49								
1750–74						1(1M)		
1550–1774	9(6)	7(3)	18(15)	31(14)	146(7)	155(17)	23(3)	80(7)

Source: De Ridder-Symoens (1989)

Notes: NNL = Northern Netherlands; SNL = Southern Netherlands; L = Law; M = Medicine.

Table 8 Graduations of Austrian students 1500–1630

	Arts	**Medicine**	**Law**	**Theology**	**Total**
Bologna		2	70	2	74
Padua		31	25	4	60
Perugia	1		6	4	11
Pisa		2	12	1	15
Siena		1	30	2	35

Source: Ingrid Matschinneg, Österreicher als Universitätsbesucher in Italien (1500-1630). Regionale und soziale Herkunft - Karrieren - Prosopographie, Diss. Karl-Franzens-Universität Graz (1999).

Appendix 6 Students at Leiden 1575–1813

	Dutch Republic and Colonies		Foreigners		Total	
	Matriculations	Doctorates	Matriculations	Doctorates	Matriculations	Doctorates (% of matriculations)
1575–1600	1705	280	1020 (31.9%)	123 (30.5%)	1985	403 (12.9%)
1601–1625	3546	352	2690 (39.9%)	141 (28.6%)	3898	493 (7.3%)
1626–1650	5363	569	5713 (48%)	247 (30.3%)	5932	816 (6.9%)
1651–1675	6381	949	3559 (31.7%)	334 (26%)	7330	1283 (11.4%)
1676–1700	4533	945	3575 (37.8%)	412 (30.4%)	5478	1357 (14.3%)
1701–1725	3558	1233	3164 (38%)	353 (22.3%)	4791	1586 (19%)
1726–1750	3236	1200	2715 (36.5%)	278 (18.8%)	4436	1478 (19.9%)
1751–1775	2713	1216	1132 (21.5%)	216 (15%)	3929	1432 (27.1%)
1776–1795	2152	871	534 (14.4%)	150 (14.7%)	3023	1021 (27.5%)
1795–1813	1673	700	205 (7.5%)	139	2512	839
1575–1813	**34860**	**8315**	**24307 (36%)**	**2393 (22.3%)**	**43175**	**10708**

Source: H.T. Colenbrander, 'De herkomst der Leidse studenten', in *Pallas Leidensis* (Leiden, 1925), 273–303.

Appendix 7 Students at Reims 1547–1794

Reims 1547-1794: DMed

1547–1604	66
1604–1660	339
1660–1794	2917
1547–1794	3322

Geographical origins of the doctores medicinorum

Reims	63
Region of Reims	31
Northern France (Loire is border)	1654
Southern France (Loire is border)	244
Ireland	657
Scotland	243
England	103
Low Countries	183
German Empire	65
Switzerland	20
Sweden	17
Poland	12
America's	11
Spain & Portugal	8
Italy	6
Byzantine Greece	3
Russia	1
Africa	1
Total	3322

Source: Pierre Dubourg-Maldan, 'Histoire de la Faculté de Médecine de l'Université de Reims', *La Chronique de Champagne*, 4 (1838) 378–79.

Appendix 8 Examples of regional mobility

Medical students from Kleef and Moers 1575-1700
Komorowski 2007

	1575-1600	1601-1625	1626-1650	1651-1675	1676-1700	1575-1700	total stud.
Bologna (13e)				1		1	1
Padua (13e)		1	1	6	1	9	17
Siena (13e)							1
Leiden 1575		1	3	5	8	17	38
Franeker 1585				1	2	3	15
Groningen 1614				1		1	7
Harderwijk 1648						0	19
Utrecht 1636				1	6	7	28
Erfurt 1379						0	2
Heidelberg 1388						0	15
Basel 1460	2	3		1		6	39
Frankfurt/Oder 1498						0	2
Marburg 1527					1	1	3
Duisburg 1654				8	18	26	85
Orleans 1306						0	27
total	2	6	4	24	36	71	299

Source: M. Komorowski, 'Graduierte aus dem Herzogtum Kleve und der Grafschaft Moers 1575–1700. Eine bio-bibliographische Dokumentation', in R.C. Schwinges (ed.), *Examen, Titel, Promotionen. Akademisches und staatliches Qualifikationswesen vom 13. bis zum 21. Jahrhundert*, VGUW Band 7 (Basel, 2007), 535–74.

PART II
The *peregrinatio medica*, from the Peripheries to the Centres and Back Again

Chapter 4
Spanish Medical Students' *peregrinatio* to Italian Universities in the Renaissance[1]

Jon Arrizabalaga

Introduction

As Walter Rüegg has pointed out, '[t]he social role of the medieval university consisted primarily of training for more rational forms of the exercise of authority in church, government, and society', although what led to the foundation of universities was not 'the demand for socially applicable knowledge ... so much as the existence of certain disciplines which had shown themselves to be of value for dealing with certain social tasks'.[2]

The sons of the urban patriciate received a formalised training in the universities in theology, law (both civil and canonical), medicine and the arts that was increasingly required by the social elites who led the European cities and principalities. In fact, preachers with a solid theological training were requested to fight heresies and spread Christianity effectively against Islam and Judaism; jurists were needed to ensure that the socio-political status quo was preserved by means of civil Roman and canon law; physicians were required to attend to the health needs of an increasingly productive society; and 'artists' were summoned in order to satisfy other social needs of different and no less relevant kinds, such as administrative bureaucracy, the education of elites and the development of machines, appliances and other innovative tools for diverse purposes (architecture, engineering, etc.).[3]

In the late medieval Spanish kingdoms the university was neither a vigorous nor a plentiful institution, although, from the fourteenth century, Castilian and Aragonese monarchs promoted the foundation of several universities – Palencia

1 This chapter has been developed in the framework of the project BHA2002-00512 of the Dirección General de Investigación, Spanish Ministry of Science and Technology. I am indebted to Andrew Cunningham and Sebastià Giralt for their advice and material assistance.

2 Walter Rüegg, 'Themes', in Hilde de Ridder-Symoens (ed.), *A history of the university in Europe. Vol. 1: Universities in the Middle Ages* (Cambridge, 1994), pp. 3–34 (pp. 21, 26).

3 Jon Arrizabalaga and Lluís Cifuentes, 'La medicina: institucions, sabers, pràctiques, protagonistes', in Pere Gabriel (ed.), *Història de la cultura catalana. Vol. 1: L'esplendor medieval segles XI–XV* (Barcelona, 1999), pp. 247–70 (p. 249).

(1208), Salamanca (1218–19), Sevilla (1254–60), Valladolid (before 1300), Lérida/Lleida (1300), Perpignan (1350), Huesca (1354), Sigüenza (1489), Alcalá (1499), Valencia (1499–1502) – according to the principle of one university per kingdom, with the aim of satisfying the socio-political needs of their kingdoms and avoiding the professional elites' having to send their sons to other countries in search of a suitable training in order effectively to carry out their professional duties. The privilege by which the Aragonese King Jaume II founded the Estudi General of Lérida/Lleida in 1300 could not have been more explicit as to the purpose of the initiative, when it declared the royal will that:

> [wise] men provide among us the nourishment of every honest science, with the essential purpose that our faithful and subjects need look for foreign nations neither to investigate sciences nor to beg for them in alien regions.[4]

Students' *peregrinatio academica* was a common phenomenon in late medieval and Renaissance Europe,[5] and the founding of all these Spanish universities could not stop it. Almost 20 years ago, together with the late Luis García-Ballester and Fernando Salmón, I first approached the issue of the presence of Spanish medical students in Italian universities at the turn of the sixteenth century. We dealt then with the presence of students from the Kingdom of Aragón in four northern Italian and Tuscan universities (Siena, Pisa, Ferrara and Padua), with particular attention to the sub-group of Valencian medical students.[6] In my somewhat qualitative new approach here, the chronological term is extended to the period between the mid-fifteenth and mid-sixteenth centuries, and the universities of Bologna and Parma are also included as academic destinations of travelling Spanish medical students.

I will first characterise the major features of this academic *peregrinatio*, namely geographical origins, university destinations and itineraries. Second, I will deal with the students' backgrounds, the institutions with which they were

---

[4] '... ad id precipue curas nostras dirigimus per quod viris eisdem scientiarum quarumlibet honestarum apud nos alimenta condantur ut nec potissime nostros fideles et subditos pro investigandis scientiis naciones peregrinas expetere nec in alienis ipsos opporteat regionibus mendicare'. See Antoni Rubió i Lluch (ed.), *Documents per l'historia de la cultura catalana mig-eval* (Barcelona, Institut d'Estudis Catalans, 1908, 2 vols; facsimile reprint: Barcelona, IEC, 2000), vol. I, p. 14.

[5] Peter Denley, 'The social function of Italian Renaissance universities: prospects for research', in *Town and gown: the university in search of its origins. CRE-Information* (Geneva, quarterly published by the Standing Conference of Rectors, Presidents and Vice-Cancellors of the European Universities, 1983), pp. 48–54.

[6] Jon Arrizabalaga, Luis García Ballester and Fernando Salmón, 'A propósito de las relaciones intelectuales entre la Corona de Aragón e Italia (1470–1520): los estudiantes de medicina valencianos en los estudios generales de Siena, Pisa, Ferrara y Ferrara', *Dynamis* 9 (1989): 117–47.

associated, and the activities they undertook during their academic sojourns. Third, I will summarise some of their subsequent careers, which are indicative of the impact of medical training in Italian universities on their professional and personal biographies.

Students' Geographical Origins, Academic Destinations and Itineraries

In a stimulating historiographical article published in the early 1980s, Peter Denley drew attention to the vast quantity of documents concerning the history of Italian universities in the Middle Ages and Renaissance that have been published since the nineteenth century; and, very reasonably, among the tasks to be undertaken in this area he gave priority to making full use of this material – which was available precisely at a time when intellectual historians were becoming more aware of the need for institutional and prosopographical studies to support their claims.[7] Twenty-five years later not only do the reasons argued by Denley remain valid, but much more collected and published material is available for such work.

The data supporting the present study comes mostly from the universities of Parma, Ferrara, Padua, Bologna, Siena and Pisa. The last three seem to have been those first chosen by Spanish students in Italy; their presence at the other three was, as we will see, very limited. I am well aware that other universities, such as those of Naples (1224) and Catania (1444), because they were situated in territories belonging to the Crown of Aragón, may also have been much frequented by Spanish students. Yet they cannot be included in this study because of major heuristic difficulties.

My self-imposed chronological term is the 110 years between 1441 and 1550. While the historical sources relating to the universities of Parma, Ferrara, Padua and Bologna cover this period perfectly, those for Siena are only available for the years 1484–86, 1496–1514 and 1516–73, and those for Pisa university are restricted to the three decades between 1473 and 1503. Before analysing some specific features that characterised the *peregrinatio* of Spanish medical students to Italian universities we will look at some more general features of these universities and students' presence there.

Between 1412 and 1522 no less than 187 students from different faculties got their doctorates at Parma university.[8] Sixteen of them – scarcely 8.56 per cent – were Spaniards, all of whom got their degrees in the fifteenth century. They were

---

7 Peter Denley, 'Recent studies on Italian universities of the Middle Ages and Renaissance', *History of Universities* 1 (1981): 193–205.

8 Celestino Piana, *Ricerche su le Università di Bologna e di Parma nel secolo XV* (Florence, 1963), pp. 333–502; Celestino Piana, *Nuove ricerche su le Università di Bologna e di Parma* (Florence, 1966), pp. 505–72. On the history of the small university of Parma, see Piana, *Ricerche*, pp. 309–32; and the monographical section at the *Annali di Storia delle Università italiane*, 9 (2005), www.cisui.unibo.it/frame_annali.htm.

14 law doctorates (11 of them from the Kingdom of Aragón), 1 in theology and 1 in medicine. The latter was Joannes Bertrandi, a native of Xàtiva (a Valencian city from where Borgia family came) who had previously studied at Bologna and Siena who and got his degree in 1442.[9] His is the earliest Spanish medical doctorate that I have discovered.

The presence of Spanish students at Ferrara university was also very early, although they never frequented this university very much.[10] Indeed, of the approximately 2,700 students who got their doctorates at Ferrara between 1404 and 1555, only 30 (plus another 9 doubtful ones) were Spaniards, namely 17 (plus the 9 doubtful ones) in law, 4 in arts, 2 in theology, 3 in medicine (all in 1448) and 4 others in arts and medicine (in 1501, 1502, 1520 and 1529). Five of the seven medical doctoral students came from the Kingdom of Aragón and one from Castile. As to the origin of the seventh, it is known only that he was the son of a personal doctor to the 'King of Spain' (of Castile, presumably).

While the available records for the student population at Ferrara university remain very limited, the records concerning the *Studio* of Padua that have been published since 1969 are of monumental proportions, particularly for the acts of academic graduations.[11] Unfortunately, the presence of Spanish students at Padua was very limited during the period under review. Suffice it to say that only 53 Spanish and Portuguese students, mostly in law, are recorded in the Padua university archives for the 20-year period 1490–1510.[12] And the number of medical students was very small not only during this period (two in medicine and three in arts and medicine), but also during the whole period (1406–1550) for which I have searched through the indexes of names of the Paduan *Acta*. Indeed, between 1406 and 1460 only two medical students have been found, both of them acting as witnesses at doctorates, one in arts (1445) and another in civil law (1458).[13] And we have to wait until the last decade of the fifteenth century to run into four other Spanish medical students. One of them was a witness at a doctorate in arts and medicine (1491),[14] while the other three appear to have finished their

[9] Piana, *Ricerche*, pp. 373–4 (#46).

[10] Giuseppe Pardi, *Titoli dottorali conferiti dallo studio di Ferrara nei sec. XV e XVI* (Lucca, 1901; facsimile reprint: Bologna, 1970).

[11] *Acta Graduum Academicorum Gymnasii Patavini (1406–1806)* (Padua, 1969–) (hereafter, AGAGP).

[12] Emilia Veronese Ceseracciu, 'Spagnoli e portoghesi all'Università di Padova nel ventennio 1490–1510', *Quaderni per la Storia dell'Università di Padova* 11 (1978): 39–83.

[13] Martí de Catalunya (*Martin[us] Petri de Catilonia art. et med. scolari[s]*), witness of the arts doctorate held on 20 March 1445, and the Aragonese 'Gilbertus', who witnessed a civil law doctorate on 9 August 1458. See AGAGP, vol. I.2, p. 208 (#1913); vol. II.1, p. 166 (#525).

[14] It was the Spanish-Neapolitan *Ioannesbaptista Cathalanus de Aversa*, who witnessed an arts and medicine doctorate on 21 October 1491. See AGAGP, vol. II.5, pp.

studies at Padua. They include two students from Mallorca, namely Antoni Nadal, doctorate in arts and medicine in 1490,[15] and Gabriel Brun, who was a student of arts between 1490 and 1492 and may have got his doctorate in arts and medicine about 1500;[16] and also Tomás Tagliavia de Concha, a Neapolitan-Spanish student who got his medical doctorate in 1497.[17] Throughout the first half of the sixteenth century (1501–50) I have been able to discover only two other medical students, both during the first decade of the century, namely the Castilian Francisco Núñez, doctorate in medicine in 1506,[18] and a Joannes Spagnolus who got his medical doctorate in 1508.[19] Therefore, it was during the last decade of the fifteenth and first decade of the sixteenth centuries – and always in very limited numbers – that Spanish medical students appear to have had a somewhat noteworthy presence at Padua.

With regard to Bologna university,[20] before the 1440s there are a single medical doctorate – Martinus de Hispania (1425) – and five other medical students from the Spanish kingdoms, four of them Catalan and the fifth Valencian.[21] And for the period under review (1441–1550) we have found 56 Spanish medical doctorates at Bologna university. There are two Spanish medical doctorates – Juan de Carrillo (1442) and Fernando de Medina de Córdoba (1447) – during the 1440s, and another during the 1470s – Agustín de Campo Verde (1472) – but only from 1480 does the flow of students appear to have had more appreciable dimensions. Suffice it to say that during the seven decades between 1480 and 1550, at least 65 (7.6 per cent) of the 854 doctorates recorded in arts and/or medicine were of Spaniards.[22]

1065–6 (#1527).

15 See AGAGP, vol. II.5, pp. 983–5 (#1363–1365); Veronese Ceseracciu, 'Spagnoli', pp. 65–6.

16 See AGAGP, vol. II.5, p. 1095 (#1581); Veronese Ceseracciu, 'Spagnoli', pp. 51–2.

17 See AGAGP, vol. II.6, pp. 1358, 1366–9 (#2078, 2100, 2103, 2106).

18 See AGAGP, vol. III.1, p. 148 (#429); Veronese Ceseracciu, 'Spagnoli', p. 66.

19 See AGAGP, vol. III.1, pp. 184–6 (#528, 530, 533).

20 Our main information sources for Bologna university have been the studies and documents uncovered by Celestino Piana and Antonio Pérez Martín. See Piana, *Ricerche*, pp. 3–306; Piana, *Nuove ricerche*, pp. 1–504; Celestino Piana, *Nuovi documenti sull'Università di Bologna e sul Collegio di Spagna* (Bologna, Publicaciones del Real Colegio de España, 1976, 2 vols); Antonio Pérez Martín, *Proles Aegidiana* (Bologna, Publicaciones del Real Colegio de España, 1979, 4 vols); Pérez Martín, *Españoles en el Alma Mater Studiorum. Profesores hispanos en Bolonia (de fines del siglo XII a 1799)* (Murcia, Servicio de Publicaciones de la Universidad de Murcia, 1998).

21 Arnaldus Joannis de Catellonia, rector Universitatis scholarium medicine (1387–88); Petrus Paulus de Catelonia (1397); Dominicus Ferarii de Valentia (1405); Ioannes q. Ferari de Cathelonia (1418); Ioannes Splugas de Cathelonia (1418, 1423). See Piana, *Nuovi documenti*, vol. I, pp. 40–41, 428; vol. II, pp. 705–6, 707–8, 721, 929, 935.

22 Giovanni Bronzino, *Notitia doctorum sive catalogus doctorum qui in Collegiis Philosophiae et Medicinae Bononiae laureati fuerunt ab anno 1480 usque ad annum 1800*

At Siena university the number of Spanish doctorates during the three periods for which there is information (1484–86, 1496–1514 and 1516–79) amount to 58 out of a total of 1,375 licensed and doctoral students.[23] Only nine of them got their doctorates in either medicine or arts and medicine. Seven of them had done so by 1550, namely the Valencian Johannes Lopes de Ayora (1497), the Andalusian Didacus Santii de Antiquera (1501), the Aragonese Lupus Sancii de Orvugyno (1504), Aurelius Bartholomei de Firas from Toledo diocese (1534), Antonius Martiz de Adalia from Segovia (1548), Gabriel Vaez from Mondéjar (Toledo) (1549) and Ferdinandus de Segobia from Almodóvar del Campo (Ciudad Real) (1549).[24]

Between 1473 and 1503 Pisa university became the Florentine *Studio*, on the initiative of Lorenzo il Magnifico. During these three decades at least 1,296 students passed through its lecture rooms, 89 of whom were Spaniards, namely 22 in arts and medicine and the rest (67) in other faculties, particularly law. At least 18 Spanish students got their doctorates at Pisa, namely 5 in arts and medicine and the remaining 13 in other faculties, especially law. All the Spanish medical doctoral students came from the Kingdom of Valencia and got their degrees between 1476 and 1484.[25] I will come back later to two of them, namely Jeroni Torrella and Francesc Argilagues.

Given that most of the sources discovered from the six Italian universities under review (Ferrara, Padua, Parma, Bologna, Siena and Pisa) reflect the graduation acts, it seems appropriate to restrict our analysis to those Spanish medical students who took their doctorates at any of these and to resort, when convenient, to any additional information about other students whose graduation is not recorded. I have organised the major figures into three tables.

Table 4.1, ordered by universities and decades, summarises the major numbers for these 81 doctorates in medicine (40 of them together with arts). The Spanish medical students' *peregrinatio* to Italian universities shows variable patterns throughout the period. During the first 70 years (1441–1510) 37 students (about 45 per cent) received their doctorates, while the remaining 44 (55 per cent) did

(Milan, Giuffré, 1962), pp. 1–43; Pérez Martín, *Proles Aegidiana*, vol. I, pp. 295, 266–7, 340–41.

23 Giovanni Minnucci and Paola Giovanna Morelli, *Le lauree dello Studio senese nel XVI secolo. Regesti degli atti dal 1573 al 1579* (Siena, Edizioni Cantagalli, 1998), pp. xxiii–xxviii.

24 Giovanni Minnucci, *Le lauree dello Studio senese alla fine del secolo XV* (Milan, Giuffré, 1981), pp. 42–3; Giovanni Minnucci, *Le lauree dello Studio senese all'inizio del secolo XVI (1501–1506)* (Milan, Giuffré, 1984), pp. 23, 63–4; Giovanni Minucci and Paola Giovanna Morelli, *Le lauree dello Studio senese nel secolo XVI. Regesti degli atti dal 1516 al 1573* (Siena, Università degli Studi di Siena – La Nuova Italia, 1992), pp. 68–9, 184–5, 199, 213–14).

25 Arrizabalaga, García Ballester and Salmón, 'A propósito de las relaciones intelectuales', pp. 130–36.

so during the following four decades (1511–50). Almost 70 per cent (56 of 81) received their doctorates at Bologna university, although these graduates passed from representing about half (18 of 37) of all Spanish medical doctorates during the period 1441–1510, to comprising the majority (38 of 44) during the period 1511–50. This means that 76 per cent (19 of 25) of Spanish medical doctoral students at Italian universities other than Bologna got their degrees by 1510. Of the remaining six (24 per cent), two did so at Ferrara during the period 1511–30 and four others at Siena between 1531 and 1550, with the distribution of degrees being as follows: five at Ferrara, five at Padua, five at Pisa, three at Siena and one at Parma. During the first seven decades, Spanish medical doctorates were concentrated into two sub-periods, namely the decade 1441–1450 (3 at Ferrara and 1 at Parma, apart from 2 others at Bologna) and the four decades from 1471 to 1510 (5 at Padua, 5 at Pisa, 3 at Siena and 2 at Ferrara, apart from the remaining 16 at Bologna). The absence of Spanish medical doctorates during the 20-year period 1451–70 is striking, although it should not be ruled out that some further, undiscovered graduations could have occurred during that time from Siena, whose graduation acts for that period have been only partly preserved.

Table 4.1 Distribution of Spanish medical doctorates (1441–1550) by universities and decades

			Padua	**Pisa**	**Siena**	**Parma**	**Total**
1441–50	2	3	-	-	-	1	6
1451–60	-	-	-	-	-	-	-
1461–70	-	-	-	-	-	-	-
1471–80	2	-	-	3	-	-	5
1481–90	5	-	1	2	-	-	8
1491–1500	2	-	2	-	1	-	5
1501–10	7	2	2	-	2	-	13
1511–20	5	1	-	-	-	-	6
1521–30	7	1	-	-	-	-	8
1531–40	12	-	-	-	1	-	13
1541–50	14	-	-	-	3	-	17
Totals	**56**	**7**	**5**	**5**	**7**	**1**	**81**

Table 4.2 reflects the distribution of Spanish medical doctorates, ordered by geographical origin and decade. Of the 81, 25 came from the Kingdom of Aragón (11 from Aragón, 10 from Valencia, 3 from Mallorca and 1 from Catalonia); and 26 others came from the Kingdom of Castile (13 from Castile, 12 from Andalusia and 1 from Biscay). It is not possible to determine the origin of the remaining 31, although we can infer from the family names of 3 of them that they were Italian-Spanish. While 60 per cent of the students from Kingdom of Aragón had received their doctorates by 1510, 65 per cent of those from the Kingdom of Castile received them after that year.

Table 4.2 Distribution of Spanish medical doctorates (1441–1550) by geographical origins and decades

	Crown of Aragón	**Crown of Castile**	**Without details**	**Total**
1441–50	3	1	2	6
1451–60	-	-	-	-
1461–70	-	-	-	-
1471–80	4	1	1	6
1481–90	4	1	3	8
1491–1500	2	1	2	5
1501–10	2	5	5	12
1511–20	2	2	2	6
1521–30	-	3	5	8
1531–40	3	6	4	13
1541–50	5	6	6	17
Totals	25	26	30	81

Finally, Table 4.3 presents a chronological list of 81 Spanish medical students who received their doctorates at any of the six mentioned Italian universities during the 110 years from 1441 to 1550, with additional information about their identities and academic itineraries. From this table we can analyse the mobility patterns of Spanish students in terms of their moves to the Italian university cities where they first chose to study medicine, as well as in terms of their further *peregrinatio* to other universities before taking their doctorates. There appear to have been substantial differences between the mobility patterns of those who went directly from Spain to Bologna by virtue of their election as scholars of the Colegio de España, and of those whose first destination in Italy was one of the other five universities under review. The mobility of the latter appears to have been significantly greater than that of those students who were chosen by the ecclesiastical authorities of their native Spanish dioceses as scholars of the Bolognese Colegio de España. The prize for mobility should go to the Valencian Jacobus Álvarez, who passed through Montpellier, Lérida/Lleida, Ferrara, Bologna, Padua and Pavia before taking his doctorate at Ferrara in 1502, but the records of some students are also notable. This is particularly the case for the Aragonese Ludovicus Martinez de Camannas, who passed through Salamanca, Bologna and Vienna before getting his doctorate at Ferrara in 1520; and for two Valencians, namely Joannes Bertrandi, who studied in Bologna and Siena before taking his medical doctorate at Parma in 1442, and Gabriel Valleriola, who passed through Lérida/Lleida and Montpellier before taking his doctorate at Pisa in 1481.[26] The passing-through universities, from greater to lesser frequency, are as follows: Bologna (four times), Siena and Padua (three times), Pavia and Montpellier (twice) and Ferrara and Vienna (once); apart from three Spanish universities – Lérida/Lleida (four times) and Salamanca and Alcalá (once each), which were, incidentally, the most outstanding universities in the Kingdoms of Aragón and Castile respectively. If we turn our attention to the academic itineraries of these students beyond medicine, previous studies in arts at Salamanca (twice), Alcalá (once), Paris (once) and in theology at Bologna (once) are recorded.

26 Pardi, *Titoli dottorali*, pp. 110–11, 116–17; Piana, *Ricerche*, pp. 373–4; Armando F. Verde, *Lo Studio fiorentino, 1473–1503. Ricerche e documenti* (Florence-Pistoia, Istituto Nazionale di Studi sul Rinacimento – Memorie Dominicane – Leo S. Olschki, 1973–85, 4 vols), vol. II, pp. 678–9.

Table 4.3 Consolidated list of Spanish medical doctorates at the Italian universities of Parma, Ferrara, Padua, Bologna, Siena and Pisa (1441–1550)

Date of doctorate	**Faculty**	**Name and affiliation**	**Additional university information**
1442, 13 Feb Parma	Medicine	Joannes Bertrandi Xàtiva (dioc. Valencia)	Bologna, Siena, Parma
1442 Bologna	Medicine	Juan de Carrillo	Rector Coll. Hisp. (1442)
1447 Bologna	Medicine	Fernando de Medina Córdoba	scol. Coll. Hisp.(1442–48) lecture of medicine (1447–48)
1448, 28 Feb Ferrara	Medicine	Martín de Cataluña	Padua (1445), Ferrara lecture (extraord.) of medicine (Bologna, 1447–48)
1448, 14 March Ferrara	Medicine	Marcos Andrés de Valencia	lecture of medicine (Bologna 1448–49)
1448, 21 Nov Ferrara	Medicine	Gondisalvus de civ. Portuensi in Ispanea, f. mag.[ri] Manueli medici q. Regis Ispanee	Pavia, Ferrara father physician
1472 Bologna	Medicine	Agustín de Campo Verde Sevilla	priest lecture of medicine (1472–73)
1476, 22 Aug Pisa	Arts and medicine	Rodericus de Nodo del Vaizes Oriola (dioc. Valencia)	Lérida, Pisa
1476, 7 Oct Pisa	Arts and medicine	Jeroni Torrella Valencia Son of Ferrer Torrella, physician	Siena, Pisa

1477, 11 Aug Pisa	Arts and medicine	Francesc Argilagues Valencia	Siena, Pisa
1480, 5 Jan Bologna	Medicine	Franciscus de Trestut q. Ioannis Oliva (dioc. Valencia)	privately examined by favour of Pope Sixtus IV
1481 ,20 Nov Bologna	Medicine	Andrés Vives Alcañiz (dioc. Zaragoza)	Lérida, Bologna scol. Coll. Hisp. (1474–81) lecture of medicine (1478–79) lecture of medicine on feast days (1481–82) founder of the Collegium Vives
1481, 11 Dec Pisa	Arts and medicine	Gabriel Danielis Valleriola Valencia	Lérida, Montpellier, Pisa
1484, 15 Oct Pisa	Arts and medicine	Petrus Iacobi Alvares Oriola (dioc. Valencia)	
1487, 28 Nov Bologna	Arts and medicine	Pedro del Puerto	scol. Coll. Hisp. (1480–87) lecture of medicine (1485–86)
1487, 22 Dec Bologna	Medicine	Graciano Mejía Hispanus	scol. Coll. Hisp. (1482–88) lecture of logics (1485–86)
1488, 17 May Bologna	Arts and medicine	Juan de Fogeda Sevilla	scol. Coll. Hisp. (1483–90) lecture of medicine (1488–89)
1490, 21 Jan Padua	Medicine	Antoni Nadal Mallorca	magister in arts and student of medicine (1490)
1490, 15 Oct Bologna	Medicine	Antonius Hispanus	

1493, 2 Apr Bologna	Arts and medicine	Juan Graciano	lecture of medicine (1491–92)
1494, 30 Jan Bologna	Medicine	Bernardinus Christophorus de Almonte (Cristóbal del Monte) (dioc. Sevilla)	scol. Coll. Hisp. (1488–96)
1497, 18 Jul Padua	Medicine	Thomas Tagliavia de Concha	student of arts (1497)
1497, 7 Oct Siena	Arts and medicine	Johannes Lopes de Ayora Valencia	
c.1500, Padua	Arts and medicine	Gabriel Brun Mallorca	student of arts (1490–92)
1501, 29 Nov Ferrara	Arts and medicine	Antonius de Castera, Aragón	Padua, Ferrara
1501, 23 Dec Siena	Arts and medicine	Didacus Santii de Antiquera Antequera (dioc. Málaga)	
1502, 13 Aug Ferrara	Arts and medicine	Iacobus Alvarez Valencia	Montpellier, Lleida, Ferrara, Bologna, Padua, Pavia, Ferrara
1504, 29 Mar Bologna	Arts and medicine	Ferdinandus Tovan de Anne Ramírez	
1504, 20 Jun Siena	Arts and medicine	Lupus Sancii de Orvugyno De Albarracín (dioc. Teruel)	
1504, 8 Nov Bologna	Arts and medicine	Francisco Torres Chillón (dioc. Córdoba)	schol. Coll. Hisp. (1502–5) lecture of medicine (1503–4)

1506, 10 Jan Padua	Medicine	Franciscus Nunes Guadalafaiar (dioc. Toledo)	doctor in arts
1506, 12 Jan Bologna	Medicine	Gabriel Hispanus	lecture of rhetoric (1503–4)
1506, 12 Jan Bologna	Arts and medicine	Alfonso del Moral Trigueros, Niebla (dioc. Sevilla)	scol. Coll. Hisp. (1499–1509)
1506, 20 May Bologna	Medicine	Iacobus Hispanus	
1507, 10 Mar Bologna	Medicine	Martinus Hispanus de Cresembenis	
1508, 11 May Padua	Medicine	Joannes Spagnolus	student of medicine (1508)
1508, 15 Jan Bologna	Arts and Medicine	Diego (Jacobo, Santiago) Velázquez (dioc. Sevilla)	priest scol. Coll. Hisp. (1501–8) Rector Coll. Hisp. (1506–7) lecture of philosophy (1504–5) lecture of logics (1507–8)
1511, 26 Apr Bologna	Arts and medicine	Gonzalo Díaz de Almodóvar Almodóvar del Campo (dioc. Toledo)	scol. Coll. Hisp. (1505–11) Rector Coll. Hisp. (1511) lecture of philosophy (1509–10)
1511, 26 Apr Bologna	Arts and medicine	García Pérez de Artieda Tauste (dioc. Zaragoza)	scol. Coll. Hisp. (1505–11) lecture of philosophy (1508–09)
1513, 30 Apr Bologna	Arts and medicine	Alfonso Godínez Ciudad Real	scol. Coll. Hisp. (1504–13)

1516, 24 Oct Bologna	Medicine	Antonius Hispanus	
1520, 25 May Ferrara	Arts and medicine	Ludovicus Martinez de Camannas, f. Michaelis, Teruel	Salamanca, Bologna, Vienna, Ferrara
1520, 1 Jun Bologna	Medicine	Antonius Hispanus	lecture of philosophy (Bronzino, 18)
1521, 14 Mar Bologna	Arts and medicine	Ioannes Hispanus	
1521, 31 Aug Bologna	Medicine	Ochoa González de Buitrón Bermeo (Vizcaya)	scol. Coll. Hisp. (1515–22) lecture of medicine (1520–21)
1525, 2 Jun Bologna	Arts and medicine	Ioannes Hispanus (Juan de Villalpando?)	lecture (extraor.) of practical medicine (1528/29–1544/45)
1525, 4 Jul Bologna	Arts and medicine	Caraffa Hispanus	
1526, 22 Nov Bologna	Medicine	Petrus Thomas Hispanus	
1529, 14 May Ferrara	Arts and medicine	Lorenzo Alderete Salamanca	Salamanca (arts), Bolonia (theology), Pavia, Ferrara scol. Coll. Hisp. (1514–19)
1529, 30 Dec Bologna	Arts and medicine	Francisco Alfónsez	lecture of philosophy (1528–29)
1530, 16 Feb Bologna	medicine	Jerónimo de Colonia Burgos	scol. Coll. Hisp. (1514–23) lecture of philosophy (1517–18) doctorate in arts (1518)

1531, 12 Jan Bologna	Arts and medicine	Ludovicus Toletanus nobilis Hispanus Toledo	
1531, 3 April Bologna	Arts and medicine	Pedro Carnicer Maella (Aragón)	scol. Coll. Hisp. (1524–33) Rector Coll. Hisp. (1530–31) Rector of arts universities lecture of medicine on feast days (1530–31)
1532, 20 April Bologna	Arts and medicine	Cristóbal de Rus Quesada (dioc. Toledo)	scol. Coll. Hisp. (1526–34) Rector of arts universities lecture of medicine on feast days (1531–32)
1532, 19 June Bologna	Arts and medicine	Benito Bustamante de Paz Salamanca	Salamanca (arts), Paris (master of arts) scol. Coll. Hisp. (1529–39) lecture of medicine (1531–32) lecture of logics (1537–39)
1533, 21 Jan Bologna	Medicine	Erricus Lopes	Previous medical doctorate (Salamanca)
1533, 6 Feb Bologna	Arts and medicine	Emanuel Hispanus	
1533, 6 Mar Bologna	Arts and medicine	Melchior Giassias Hispanus	
1534, 26 Oct Siena	Arts and medicine	Aurelius Bartholomei de Firas (dioc Toledo)	
1538, 26 Jan Bologna	Arts and medicine	Álvaro Núñez del Castillo Zaragoza	scol. Coll. Hisp. (1534–43) lecture of logics (1536–37) doctorate in theology (1539) and in law both civil and canonical (1543)

1538, 11 Sep Bologna	Medicine	Petrus Lopes Hispanus	
1539, 27 Jan Bologna	Medicine	Alfonso Caballero Chillón (dioc. Córdoba)	scol. Coll. Hisp. (1537–39)
1539, 22 Feb Bologna	Medicine	Pedro Domínguez Molón Cariñena (dioc. Zaragoza)	Alcalá scol. Coll. Hisp. (1533–43) Rector of arts universities lecture of medicine on feast days (1540–41)
1540, 17 Sept Bologna	Arts and medicine	Francisco de Santa Cruz Azuaga (dioc. Córdoba)	scol. Coll. Hisp. (1536–42)
1542, 6 Jun Bologna	Medicine	Fabianus Sanchies (Sonches) Hispanus	
1543, 19 May Bologna	Arts and medicine	Antonius Spinosa Hispanus	
1544, 8 Mar Bologna	Medicine	Petrus Ximenes Valentinus Hispanus Valencia	
1545, 28 Mar Bologna	Medicine	Francisco de Artieda Zaragoza son of García de Artieda physician (Bologna, 1511)	scol. Coll. Hisp. (1543–47)
1545, 21 Apr Bologna	Medicine	Iohannes Baptista Hispanus	

1545, 10 Nov Bologna	Medicine	Andrés Laguna Segovia son of Diego Fernández de Laguna, physician	
1547, 1 Mar Bologna	Medicine	Miguel Muñoz Pedroches (dioc. Córdoba)	Alcalá (arts) scol. Coll. Hisp. (1541–48)
1548, 6 Jun Bologna	Medicine	Iacobus de Thores (Torres) Hispanus	
1548, 18–19 Jul Siena	Medicine	Antonius Martiz de Adalia Segovia	
1549, 27–28 Feb Siena	Medicine	Gabriel Vaez Mondéjar (Toledo) Son of Pedro Vaez, physician?	
1549, 16 Apr Bologna	Arts and medicine	Mateo Ramos Alcañiz	lecture of rhetoric (1548–49)
1549, 6–7 Oct Siena	Medicine	Ferdinandus de Segobia, son of Iohannes de Segobia Almodóvar del Campo (Ciudad Real)	
1550, 4 Mar Bologna	Arts and medicine	Bartolomeus Hispanus	
1550, 4 May Bologna	Arts and medicine	Bartolomeus Dominicus de Maiorica Mallorca	
1550, 20 Oct Bologna	Medicine	Lupus Garcias Bastardus Hispanus	

1550, 11 Dec Bologna	Medicine	Pedro de Estrada Córdoba	scol. Coll. Hisp. (1546–51) Rector Hispaniorum (1550)
1550, 23 Dec Bologna	Medicine	Domingo de Robres Zaragoza Son of physician	scol. Coll. Hisp. (1546–52)

Sources: Giovanni Bronzino, *Notitia doctorum sive catalogus doctorum qui in collegiis philosophiae et medicinae Bononiae laureati fuerunt ab anno 1480 usque ad annum 1800* (Milan, Giuffré, 1962); Antonio Pérez Martín, *Proles Aegidiana*, 4 vols. (Bologna, Publicaciones del Real Colegio de España, 1979).

To clarify the reasons why Spanish medical students moved so often from one university to another is beyond our ability, except in the case of migration from Siena to Pisa in the 1470s, which was motivated by the strong attraction exerted by the renewed *Studio* that Lorenzo il Magnifico opened at Pisa in 1473. The effects of this event continued for some time, such that during the period under review only seven Spanish medical students (three between 1497 and 1504 and the other four between 1534 and 1549) got their doctorates at Siena (a common destination of Spanish students until the 1470s), and all of them after 1494, when the invasion of Charles VIII's army hastened the fall of the Medicean Republic, together with the uprising of Pisa against the domination of Florence.[27] The cases of Francesc Argilagues and the brothers Jeroni and Gaspar Torrella illustrate clearly the reasons underlying this migration.[28] About 1470, these three Spaniards from Valencia had begun their medical studies at Siena university, from where Argilagues moved to Pisa during the academic year 1473–74, as did the two Torrella brothers a year later. Jeroni Torrella and Francesc Argilagues finished their medical studies in Pisa by getting their doctorates in arts and medicine in 1476 and 1477, respectively, while Gaspar Torrella only stayed at Pisa during the academic year 1474–75 and delayed his doctorate until 1483, as we will see.

Students' social background, university life and academic activities

Apart from the opportunity that the scholarship fund created by Cardinal Gil de Albornoz offered for study at Bologna, it is hard to imagine how the Spanish university students defrayed the expenses of their studies in Italy without the support of well-off families or some rich patron. In fact, the heavy economic burden on any family of defraying a student son's four- to five-year stay in Italy cannot be readily dismissed. Two examples from the second half of the fifteenth century help to evaluate this economic expense. In 1459, the medical practitioner Marco di maestro Antonio di Pistoia estimated at 30 florins per year (approximately the salary of a manual worker in Florence) the expenses required to support his son Antonio, then a medical student at Bologna.[29] In eight years (1470–78) the Valencian notary Antoni Llopis sent about 29,000 *sueldos* in Valencian currency to Italy for the living expenses and university studies of his sons Joan (theology)

---

[27] Arrizabalaga, García Ballester and Salmón, 'A propósito de las relaciones intelectuales', pp. 131, 141–2.

[28] Only Gaspar Torrella appears at the *ruolo* of the *Casa di Sapienza* of Siena. See Lodovico Zdekauer, *Lo studio di Siena nel Rinascimento* (Milan, Hoepli, 1891; facsimile Reprint: Bologna, Forni, 1977), p. 181; Arrizabalaga, García Ballester and Salmón, 'A propósito de las relaciones intelectuales', pp. 128–9.

[29] On this issue and, most generally, on the cost of university education outside the familiar residence, see Katherine Park, *Doctors and medicine in early Renaissance Florence* (Princeton, Princeton University Press, 1985), pp. 123–6, 242–4.

and Jeroni (law); an amount that obliged the notary to mobilise all his economic resources.[30]

Unfortunately, in most cases the social background of the Spanish medical doctoral students can only be presumed. We know definitely that at least six of them were the sons of physicians, namely Gondisalvus (Ferrara, 1448), whose father was magister Manuel, physician to the king of Spain (presumably Castile), Jeroni Torrella (Pisa, 1476), Andrés Laguna (Bologna, 1545), Francisco de Artieda (Bologna, 1545), Domingo de Robres (Bologna, 1550) and most probably Gabriel Vaez (Bologna, 1549).[31] We have also found among the Valencian medical students at the universities of Siena and Pisa in the late fifteenth century the family names of well-known Jewish *converso* lineages (i.e., Torrella, Santàngel, Alcanyís, Valleriola, Torregrosa and Escrivà), some of them counting many medical practitioners among their members and all of them well off.[32]

On the other hand, there are at least two rather peculiar cases of Spanish medical students, namely Erricus Lopes and Andrés Laguna. The former had previously got his medical doctorate at Salamanca, and took a second one at Bologna in 1533 because of the prestige of this Italian university, also taking advantage of his stay there as a member of Emperor Charles V's itinerant court.[33] For his part, Andrés Laguna (*c.*1511–*c.*1559) took his medical doctorate at Bologna (1545) 11 years after his medical bachelor's degree at the Sorbonne (1534), and once his professional reputation and economic resources were sufficient to overcome external resistance to his professional promotion, owing to his Jewish origins.[34]

---

30 On the cost of the studies of these two Valencian people, its itemisation and the channels through which Antoni Llopis got the money to his sons, see José M. Cruselles Gómez, *La familia de Antoni Lopiç, notario de la ciudad de Valencia (1433–1493). Promoción social de un profesional de la escritura* (Universitat de València, M.Ph. Dissertation, 1985), pp. 230–44 and appendix (pp. 3–9); and José M. Cruselles Gómez, *Els notaris de la ciutat de València. Activitat professional I comportament social a la primera meitat del segle XV* (Barcelona, Fundació Noguera, 1998), pp. 71, 252, 264–5, 285, 362–5.

31 Pardi, *Titoli dottorali*, pp. 22–3; González Manjarrés, Miguel Ángel, *Andrés Laguna y el humanismo médico* (Salamanca, Junta de Castilla y León, 2000), pp. 40–41; Pérez Martín, *Proles Aegidiana*, vol. II, pp. 525–6, 791–3, 830–31; Antonio Hernández Morejón, *Historia bibliográfica de la medicina española*, (Madrid, Imp. de la Vda. De Jordán – Imp. de la Calle de San Vicente, 1842–52, 7 vols; facsimile reprint: New York–London, Johnson Reprint Corporation, 1967), vol. III, pp. 257–8; Anastasio Chinchilla, *Anales históricos de la medicina en general y biográfico-bibliográficos de la española en particular* (Valencia, Imp. López y Cía – Imp. Mateu y Cervera, 1841–46, 4 vols; facsim. reprint: New York-London, Johnson Reprint Corporation, 1967), vol. II, pp. 116–18.

32 Arrizabalaga, García Ballester and Salmón, 'A propósito de las relaciones intelectuales', p. 145.

33 'Hic erat in curia Cesaris etiam doctor Salamanche sed voluit Bononiae quoque laureari ob famam nostri Studii' (Bronzino, *Notitia*, p. 24).

34 Jon Arrizabalaga, 'The world of Iberian converso practitioners, from Lluís Alcanyís to Isaac Cardoso', in Víctor Navarro Brotons and William Eamon (eds), *Más allá de la*

Hilde de Ridder-Symoens has emphasised that the multiple curriculum was a new phenomenon at European universities from the mid-fifteenth century onwards, meaning that some medical doctoral students were spurred on to study medicine not by any primary concern to become medical practitioners, but by their intellectual ambition.[35] This feature can be illustrated by some of the Spanish doctoral students at the Italian universities under review, such as Benito Bustamante de Paz, who was bachelor in theology and had been professor of philosophy at Salamanca university before he entered the Colegio de España in 1529 as a medical student at Bologna university, where he got his doctorate in 1532, and subsequently lectured in the mornings on logic for two academic years (1537–38 and 1538–39). The same could be suggested about Álvaro Núñez del Castillo, who (at Bologna the whole time) took doctorates in theology (1539) and in civil and canonical law (1543) after his doctorates in arts and medicine (both in 1538).[36]

To the economic burdens arising from such long academic sojourns should be added the obligation of paying *in advance* the whole cost of lodging for four or five years and the extra expenses of the graduation ceremony. The outlay in advance was, for example, one of the conditions imposed by the Casa di Sapienza, the most celebrated college (*collegium*) at Siena university. Founded in 1404 for the purpose of allowing poor local students to pursue university studies, the Casa di Sapienza soon moved away from its initial aims and became the lodging place of most well-off ultramontane students who came to Siena, lured there – as to other Italian universities – by the prestige of its *Studio*.[37] Siena municipality, which directly controlled the Casa di Sapienza and selected the students accepted there, knew how to use this college as a means of obtaining diplomatic advantages and of forging good political relations with other European powers, both inside and outside Italy.[38] In addition to its contribution to the flourishing of Siena university throughout the fifteenth century, because of its innovative character within the

Leyenda Negra: España y la Revolución Científica / Beyond the Black Legend: Spain and the Scientific Revolution, Valencia, IHCDLP (Universitat de València-CSIC), 2007, pp. 307–22 (pp. 315–16).

[35] See Hilde de Ridder-Symoens' essay in this volume. The same could be suggested about Álvaro Núñez del Castillo, who – always at Bologna – took the doctorates in theology (1539) and civil and canon law (1543) after his doctorates in arts and medicine (1538). See Pérez Martín, *Proles Aegidiana*, vol. II, pp. 681–3, 728–30.

[36] Pérez Martín, *Proles Aegidiana*, vol. II, pp. 681–3.

[37] Zdekauer, *Lo Studio*, pp. 31–5; Giuliano Catoni, 'Genesi e ordinamento della Sapienza di Siena', *Studi Senesi (III Serie 22)* 85(2) 1973: 155–98; Peter Denley, *The University of Siena, 1357–1557* (University of Oxford, PhD dissertation, 1981); Peter Denley, *Commune and Studio in late medieval and renaissance Siena* (Bologna, CLUEB, 2006).

[38] Giuliano Catoni, 'Il Comune di Siena e l'amministrazione della Sapienza nel secolo XV'. In: Centro Italiano di Studi di Storia e d'Arte (ed.), *Nono Convegno Internazionale: Università e società ei secoli XIII-XVI (Pistoia, 20–25 settembre 1979)* (Pistoia, C.I.S.S.A, 1982) pp. 121–9 (p. 123); Peter Denley, 'The social function', pp. 52–4.

college movement, the Casa di Sapienza also served as an inspirational model for other similar institutions that were founded in other parts of Italy.[39]

Even the expenses of the graduation ceremonies were not insignificant. During the fifteenth century, the *Studio* of Ferrara, for example, charged each graduate student a fee of no less than 70 ducats.[40] Thus, little wonder at the frequency with which students about to graduate formally petitioned the university authorities for exemption from payment of these fees. A typical case is that of Gaspar Torrella, who, along with his brother Jeroni, studied medicine at Siena and Pisa. While the latter got his doctorate at Pisa in 1476, Gaspar only did so seven years later. Apparently the reason for this delay was the high cost of the academic fees, which he had been unable to pay earlier, as he argued in his petition addressed to Pope Sixtus IV in order to receive his doctorate from any university. By virtue of this petition, which Gaspar Torrella sent from the Roman court of Cardinal Rodrigo de Borja, he got his medical doctorate at Rome in April 1483. A member of his examining board was the Aragonese Andrés Vives, who had received his medical doctorate at Bologna two years before (1481) and, like Torrella, was a cleric.[41] Vives' status as 'Knight of Saint Peter' and 'Count palatine' may explain how Torrella could receive his degree outside any university, since these noblemen had the power to confer doctorates in the name of the Holy Roman Emperor from the time of Sigismund (1433–37) until the early seventeenth century.[42]

To Torrella's case those of two Spanish medical students at Padua can be also added. The case of Antoni Nadal, a master of arts from Mallorca, is particularly striking. In 1490 he successfully pleaded poverty, due to losses in a shipwreck, in order to obtain exemption from paying 12 ducats of his medical doctorate fees to the Paduan College of Doctors in Arts and Medicine, after this institution had recognised his 'very learned' condition and the many years he had studied at Padua

---

39 Peter Denley, 'Academic rivalry and interchange: the universities of Siena and Florence', in Peter Denley and Caroline Elam (eds), *Florence and Italy. Renaissance studies in honour of Nicolai Rubinstein* (London, Westfield College–University of London, 1988), pp. 201–3.

40 In the fifteenth century the *Studio* of Ferrara, for example, charged no less than 70 ducats to each graduate. See Girolamo Secco-Suardo, 'Lo Studio di Ferrara a tutto il secolo XV', *Atti e memorie della Deputazione Ferrarese di Storia Patria* 6 (1894): 25–294 (pp. 192–6).

41 Jon Arrizabalaga, 'Medicina universitaria y *morbus gallicus* en la Italia de finales del siglo XV: el arquiatra pontificio Gaspar Torrella (*c.* 1452 – *c.* 1520)', *Asclepio* 40/1 (1988): 3–38 (p. 9); Pérez Martín, *Proles Aegidiana*, vol. I, pp. 373–5.

42 See Hilde de Ridder-Symoens' essay in this volume. On Vives' titles, see Pérez Martín, *Proles Aegidiana*, vol. I, p. 373; Juan Ramón Royo García, 'Fundaciones piadosas de un humanista aragonés, el alcañizano Andrés Vives (c. 1450–1528)', in Agustín Hevia Ballina (ed.), *Memoria Ecclesiae XI. Beneficencia y hospitalidad en los archivos de la iglesia santoral hispano-mozárabe en las diócesis de España* (Oviedo, Asociación de Archiveros de la Iglesia en España, 1997), pp. 129–39 (p. 130).

(*qui iam tot annis in hac civitate nostra studuit et est doctissimus*).[43] On the other hand, there is Tomás Tagliavia de Concha, a Spanish-Neapolitan and *familiar* to the King of Naples, to whom in 1497 the bishop of Padua gave the grace to obtain his medical doctorate for free after he had claimed economic insolvency and proved his status as a student at Padua university for many years (*qui pluribus annis studuit in hoc Gymnasio et pauper est*).[44]

While the Casa di Sapienza was the flagshsip institution for the lodging of foreign students in Siena (among them, Spaniards), in Bologna, from its foundation in 1369, according to the will of Cardinal Gil de Albornoz, the Colegio de España was established for lodging Spanish students at the university.[45] According to its 1377 statutes, of the 30 places it granted, 18 were intended for students of canon law, 8 for theological students and 4 for students of medicine (eventually suppressed from 1627). In the absence of candidates in any of these faculties, the respective grants could be given to students in any other. Candidates for scholarships of the Colegio de España were presented by the different dioceses of the Kingdom of Castile, Zaragoza being the only diocese of the Kingdom of Aragón with legal authority to propose candidates. Cardinal Gil de Albornoz' aim was that the Colegio de España should lodge poor students: the 1377 statutes prescribed that candidates' rents should never exceed 50 florins per year. This rule lost validity over time and was formally omitted from the new statutes of 1644. From the last decades of the fifteenth century, candidates were required, apparently with great meticulousness, to have 'purity of blood'.[46]

It is possible that some of the 28 Spanish medical doctoral students who were linked to the Bolognese Colegio de España during the period under review (1441–1550) were brilliant students from poor families. Yet it is hard to go beyond the formulation of this hypothesis. It is known, however, that at least four of them, namely Agustín de Campo Verde (doct. 1472), Andrés Vives (doct. 1481), Diego Velázquez (doct. 1508) and Lorenzo Alderete (doct. 1529), were already clergymen when they entered the Colegio de España; and two more, Francisco de Artieda (doct. 1545) and Domingo de Robres (doct. 1550), were sons of physicians, as already mentioned above. Incidentally, García Pérez de Artieda, the

---

43 AGAGP, vol. II.5, p. 983 (#1363): "Pauper quidam scholaris sed doctissimus mag. Antonius de Maiorica vellet sibi de speciali gratia concedi quod se conventuare possit in med. ... Humiliter exposuit extremam paupertatem suam et miserimum casum naufragii quorumdam bonorum que a patre suo sibi mittebantur; ex quo supplicabat sibi gratias fieri in med. Pro ducatis duodecim, quia impossibile sibi erat posse plures reperire ob eius paupertatem." See also Veronese Ceseracciu, 'Spagnoli', pp. 65–6.

44 AGAGP, vol. II.6, pp. 1366–7 (#2100).

45 On the *Colegio de España* see Berthe M. Marti, *The Spanish College at Bologna in the fourteenth century. Edition and translation of its statutes with introduction and notes* (Philadelphia, University of Pennsylvania Press, 1966); Piana, *Nuovi documenti*, vol. I, pp. 62–153; vol. II, pp. 933–5; Pérez Martín, *Proles Aegidiana*.

46 Pérez Martín, *Proles Aegidiana*, vol. I, pp. 15–113.

father of the former, had also got his doctorate at Bologna in 1511.[47] The average duration of the sojourns of these 28 Spanish medical scholars was 7 years, varying from a minimum of 2 to a maximum of 10 years. All of them eventually got their doctorates at Bologna university, except Lorenzo Alderete, who was – for reasons that are unclear – obliged to renounce to his scholar's rights in return for 48 golden ducats on the condition that he should study for two years at a university other than Bologna,[48] and who eventually got his doctorate at Ferrara in 1529, after passing through Pavia university. Residents could remain in the Colegio de España for up to eight years, but they had to leave as soon as they got their doctorates. Hence the petition that Graciano Mejía made on the day prior to his doctorate, to be authorised to continue living there for an undetermined length of time,[49] and the authorisation that Andrés Vives received to extend his residence there until Easter 1482, almost six months after taking his doctorate.[50] When in charge of any lectureship at Bologna university, they could extend their stay for up to three more years after their doctorate; this may have been the reason for those stays that exceeded the authorised limits with no apparent justification. Five of these Spanish medical doctoral students were also rectors of the Colegio de España: Juan de Carrillo (1442), Diego Velázquez (1506–7), Gonzalo Díaz de Almodóvar (1511), Pedro Carnicer Aragonés (1530–31) and Pedro Estrada (1550).[51]

The 'festive lectureships' were a way for students to participate in university life. They were an honour that was given to the most brilliant students in any faculty, and included a financial reward. We know, for example, that the Valencian Francesc Argilagues was appointed to occupy the festive lectureship during the penultimate year (1475–76) of his medical studies at Pisa, where the doctorate was usually taken the following year, and that he received 64 Florentine pounds for this lectureship in September 1476.[52] At Bologna, however, most 'festive lectureships' – e.g. those held by Pedro Carnicer (doct. 1531) in 1530–31, Cristóbal de Rus (doct. 1532) in 1531–32 and Pedro Domínguez Molón (doct. 1539) in 1540–41 – were kept for those students who were rectors of the universities, as a means of assigning them a salary,[53] while outstanding students were given the so-called 'university lectureships' (*lecturae universitatis*).[54] This is the case with the lectureships

---

[47] Pérez Martín, *Proles Aegidiana*, vol. I, pp. 340–41, 373–5; vol. II, pp. 505–7, 590–1, 791–3, 830–31.

[48] Pérez Martín, *Proles Aegidiana*, vol. II, pp. 590–91.

[49] Piana, *Nuovi documenti*, vol. I, pp. 151–2.

[50] Piana, *Nuovi documenti*, vol. I, 150–51.

[51] Pérez Martín, *Proles Aegidiana*, vol. I, p. 265; vol. II, pp. 505–7, 530–31, 659–61, 828–30.

[52] Verde, *Lo studio fiorentino*, vol. III.1, pp. 269, 342. On the meaning of the 'festive lectureships' at the Studio of Pisa, see ibid., vol. II, pp. 613–14.

[53] Pérez Martín, *Españoles en el Alma Mater Studiorum*, pp. 16, 103–4; Pérez Martín, *Proles Aegidiana*, vol. II, pp. 659–61, 674–6, 721–3.

[54] Pérez Martín, *Españoles en el Alma Mater Studiorum*, pp. 16–17.

of medicine held by Fernando de Medina (doct. 1447) in 1447–48, Martín de Cataluña (doct. 1448) in 1447–48, Marcos Andrés de Valencia (doct. 1448) in 1448–49, Agustín de Campo Verde (doct. 1472) in 1472–73, Andrés Vives (doct. 1481) in 1478–79, Pedro del Puerto (doct. 1487) in 1485–86, Juan de Fogeda (doct. 1488) in 1488–89, Juan Graciano (doct. 1493) in 1491–92, Francisco Torres (doct. 1504) in 1503–4, Ochoa González de Buitrón (doct. 1521) in 1520–21 and Benito Bustamante de Paz (doct. 1532) in 1531–32;[55] as well as with the lectureships of logics held by Graciano Mejía (doct. 1487) in 1485–86, Diego Velázquez (doct. 1508) in 1507–8 and Álvaro Nuñez del Castillo (doct. 1538) in 1536–37; the lectureships of rhetoric held by Gabriel Hispanus (doct.1506) in 1503–4 and Mateo Ramos (doct. 1549) in 1548–49; and the lectureships of philosophy held by Diego Velázquez (doct. 1508) in 1503–4, García Pérez de Artieda (doct. 1511) in 1508–9, Gonzalo Diaz de Almodóvar (doct. 1511) in 1509–10, Jerónimo de Colonia (arts doct 1518; med. doct. 1530) in 1517–18 and Francisco Alfónsez (doct. 1529) in 1528–29.[56] It is, however, more difficult to define the meaning of the logic lectureship that was assigned to Benito Bustamante de Paz (doct. 1532) in 1537–39, or that of the philosophy lectureship held by Antonio Hispano (doct. 1520) sometime during his studies.[57]

A final relevant chapter among the activities undertaken by these Spanish medical students and newly graduated doctors relates to the copying of medical manuscripts. This activity could provide medical students in their final years with some income to meet their expenses, and was also a means of support for those who chose to stay in Italy rather than to return home after having finished their studies. The case of Francesc Argilagues is very typical in this respect. He got his doctorate in arts and medicine at Pisa in August 1477. His credentials for taking the degree were endorsed by three of his professors, namely Alessandro Sermoneta (ordinary lecturer in theoretical medicine), Pierleone da Spoleto (ordinary lecturer in practical medicine) and Giovanni da Venezia (lecturer in logic). Between 1476 and 1479, in different Tuscan cities (Pisa, Siena, Florence and Pistoia) Argilagues copied most of the 18 medical writings that he later (1483) had bound into a single volume. An autograph codex (Vatican Library, Rossiano, ms. 672) contains 10 works by or attributed to Arnau de Vilanova, 2 by Pierleone da Spoleto, Arnau's Latin translation of Abu Salt's *De medicinis simplicibus*, an antidotarium from

[55] Pérez Martín, *Proles Aegidiana*, vol. I, 266–7, 340–41, 373–5, 397, 414–15; vol. II, pp. 509–11, 601–2, 681–3; Pérez Martín, *Españoles en el Alma Mater Studiorum*, p. 93; Bronzino, *Notitia*, p. 4.

[56] Pérez Martín, *Proles Aegidiana*, vol. I, pp. 405–6; vol. II, pp. 505–7, 507–8, 525–6, 530–31, 591–3, 728–30; Pérez Martín, *Españoles en el Alma Mater Studiorum*, pp. 100, 103, 104; Bronzino, *Notitia*, p. 18.

[57] Pérez Martín, *Proles Aegidiana*, vol. II, pp. 681–3; Bronzino, *Notitia*, p. 18.

the Salernitan tradition, 1 work by Stephanus Arlandi and 3 others of unknown authorship.[58]

It is not easy to answer the question of why Argilagues copied these 18 medical works. However, some useful speculations can be made concerning the two writings by Pierleone da Spoleto – *Consilium de ardore urine* and *De urinis*[59] – the copying of which he completed at Florence in January 1478, because they provide us with partial answers to this enigma, which could also be applied to the remaining works in the codex. It is possible that Argilagues copied them because of his personal regard for Pierleone, who, in addition to being his professor and a promoter of his doctorate, was court physician to Lorenzo il Magnifico and an outstanding member of Marsiglio Ficino's neo-Platonist circle. On the other hand, Argilagues' regard for Arnau's medical works could have been instigated by Pierleone, as the latter had copied works by Arnau and Ramon Llull during his time as a student in Paris.[60] But this copying initiative, which caused Argilagues to move from Pisa to Florence, could also have come about by order, with Argilagues also keeping a copy for himself. And this order could have come from Alessandro Sermoneta – who was well known as an employer of ultramontane students for this kind of copying task – and the newly qualified doctor may have accepted with the dual purpose of getting his finances into shape and retaining the confidence of his protector.[61] Furthermore, Argilagues could also have copied all or part of these manuscripts as an employee of the famous Florentine librarian Vespasiano de Bisticci (1421–88). That they were on good terms is suggested by the fact that in July 1476, when Argilagues was still a student, he had designated De Bisticci and another Florentine trader as his attorneys before the Pisa Studio in order to negotiate the payment of the amount assigned to the festive lectureship of he had been in charge during the previous academic year.[62] In fact, Vespasiano da Bisticci had a *scriptorium* in Florence and a wide network of private copyists – no fewer than 45 scribes – all of them dedicated to preparing manuscript codexes of

---

58 Jon Arrizabalaga, 'De la copie a l'édition: Francesc Argilagues et les manuscrits médicaux aux premiers temps de l'imprimerie (fin XVe–debut XVIe siècle)', *Médiévales. Langue Textes Histoire* 52/1 (2007): 119–34 (pp. 122–6).

59 Vatican Library, Rossiano 672, f. 116v: 'Amen. Florencie scripta sunt 1478 Ianuarii 18. Franciscus Argilagues'. This codex includes two works by Pierleone da Spoleto, namely the *Consilium de ardore urine* (ff. 74r–83v) and *De urinis* (ff. 84r–116v).

60 On Pierleone da Spoleto's interest for Arnau de Vilanova, see Luis García-Ballester and Eustaquio Sánchez-Salor (eds), *Arnaldi de Villanova Opera Medica Omnia. XV. Commentum supra tractatum Galieni de malicia complexionis diverse* (Barcelona, Universitat de Barcelona, 1985), p. 142.

61 See Zdekauer, *Lo Studio*, pp. 91–3; Tiziana Pesenti, *Professori e promotori di medicina nello studio di Padova dal 1405 al 1509: Repertorio bio-bibliografico* (Trieste, Lint, 1984), pp. 196–8.

62 Verde, *Lo studio fiorentino*, vol. III.1, p. 269.

any work the Medicis and other well-off Florentine citizens requested.[63] It also cannot be ruled out that Argilagues copied Pierleone's writings for the purpose of preparing a printed edition – though they remained unpublished until 1514.[64] He could even have copied Arnau's writings in connection with his preparation of the second edition of the *Opera Arnaldi de Villanova* (Venice, 19 January 1505), as this new printed edition has some peculiarities in comparison with the *editio princeps* (Lyon, 1504) that indicate the intervention of an unidentified person in the editorial process. I will return to this issue when I refer to Argilagues' professional activities as an editor of medical writings for the early printing press.

Further professional careers of travelling students

Tracing the professional careers of the Spanish students who received their medical doctorates at the six Italian universities under review between the mid-fifteenth and mid-sixteenth centuries is possible in only a limited number of cases. But the information available about some of them clearly illustrates the profound impact of their Italian medical education on their professional and personal biographies. Here, as a thread of my exposition, I will follow certain distinct areas of professional practice, namely public positions in the area of health and sanitary administration, princely courts, universities and the editing of medical texts for the printing press.

Whether we gain more detailed results or not from further prosopographical research, it is known that after having taken his medical doctorate at Padua in January 1490 (with exemption from fees because he lost his goods in a shipwreck), Antoni Nadal returned to his native Mallorca, where he was designated as the physician in charge of the *Morberia* or *Llatzeret*. This institution, which had been established in Palma de Mallorca during the second half of the fifteenth century, took care of the public health of the island by controlling maritime traffic. Its officers inspected the ships before they docked at the city harbour and, if necessary, subjected their crews and goods to quarantine.[65] In the early sixteenth century he was succeeded in this position by Guillem Caldentei, another Mallorcan physician who got his doctorate before 1496 and had received all or part of his medical

63 On the figure and activities of Vespasiano da Bisticci, see Giuseppe M. Cagni, *Vespasiano da Bisticci e il suo epistolario* (Roma, Edizioni Storia e Letteratura, 1969), particularly pp. 46–85; Rudolf Hirsch, *Printing, selling and reading, 1450–1550* (Wiesbaden, Otto Harrassowitz, 2nd edition, 1974), p. 14.

64 Pesenti, *Professori*, p. 129.

65 Antonio Contreras Mas, 'La primera obra mallorquina impresa', *Medicina Balear* 10/2 (1995): 95–9.

training at Pavia, where, as we will see, he also worked for a while as a medical editor for the printing press.[66]

Still more striking, however, are the further professional links of these itinerant Spanish medical doctoral students to princely courts – beginning with the Roman one, where, soon after their medical studies, Andrés Vives (*c.*1450–1528)[67] and Gaspar Torrella (*c.*1452–*c.*1520)[68] were established as *familiares* to Cardinal Rodrigo de Borja. Both of them were clergymen with numerous ecclesiastical benefices that increased as time elapsed, and their careers converged at Rome from late 1482 or early 1483. When Cardinal Borja was elected as the new pope, Alexander VI (1492–1503), Torrella and Vives shared with Pere Pintor and Alejandro de Espinosa the positions of papal doctors. After Alexander VI's death, Torrella continued in the service of Julius II (1503–13), and Vives later served popes Leon X (1513–21) and Clement VII (1523–34), as well as Archduke Ferdinand of Austria. To their medical careers both added ecclesiastical ones at the papal court: Torrella was domestic prelate to Alexander VI and Julius II and he was bishop of Santa Giusta, Sardinia (from 1494), as well as being the librarian of the Vatican Library (1498–1500); while Vives held, among other positions, those of pontifical writer (1493–95), apostolic protonotary (1495–1503), Knight of Saint Peter and Count Palatine. Torrella was the author of six scientific writings, all of them printed at Rome between 1497 and 1507. They include an astrological prognosis and five medical works: two on the 'French disease' (both addressed to Caesar Borgia) are among the earliest ones about this new disease; one *consilium* about another new disease that was popularly known as *modorrilla*; a treatise on plague; and a *regimen sanitatis* addressed to Julius II.

Vives and Torrella were still young when they were appointed as papal doctors, but the Hellenist physician Andrés Laguna (*c.*1511–*c.*1559) had to wait until the last decade of his life to achieve his professional ambitions by being appointed court physician to Pope Julius III (1550–55), after a lifetime of travelling throughout different European countries (Spain, England, Low Countries, Germany, Italy and France) in search of protection from very powerful patrons, such as the Emperor Charles V and Pope Paul III. In any event, only his prestige and money, gathered thanks to his distinguished clientele and to the numerous books he published

[66] Jon Arrizabalaga, 'En los inicios de una nueva ocupación: médicos de la Corona de Aragón y la edición científica en la primera imprenta italiana', *Medicina & Historia* 4th series 4 (2004): 1–15 (pp. 6–8).

[67] On Andrés Vives, see Gaetano Marini, *Degli archiatri pontifici* (Roma, Pagliarini, 1784, 2 vols), vol. I, pp. 248–50; Piana, *Ricerche*, pp. 148–50, 169; Piana, *Nuove ricerche*, pp. 378, 383; Piana, *Nouvi documenti*, pp. 138, 150–51, 172–4; Pérez Martín, *Proles Aegidiana*, vol. I, pp. 373–5.

[68] On Torrella, see Arrizabalaga, 'Gaspar Torrella', in W.F. Bynum and Helen Bynum (eds), *Dictionary of medical biography* (Westport, CT–London, Greenwood Press, 2007, 5 vols), vol. V, pp. 1230–31; and the bibliography referred to there.

throughout his life, allowed him eventually to overcome, far away from his native Castile, the stigma of his Jewish *converso* lineage.[69]

Linked to other princely courts were, in addition to Pedro Carnicer Aragonés (proto-physician to Emperor Ferdinand I (1556–64), the brother of Philip II[70]), Jeroni Torrella and Juan de Fogeda. Torrella (*c.*1450–*post* 1508) was physician to Juana de Aragón (1455–1517) – a sister of Ferdinand the Catholic who married King Ferrante I of Naples (1423–94) – first in Naples (1477–99) and then in Valencia (1499–1504). Later he went into the service of Ferdinand the Catholic at the royal court of Valladolid. At the end of 1496 he finished a treatise on astrological images that he dedicated to Ferdinand the Catholic and published in about 1500.[71] Of Juan de Fogeda[72] we know that he studied arts and medicine at the university of Bologna, where he got his doctorate in 1488. His lectureship in medicine during the academic year 1488–89 and his role as the bursar of the Colegio de España in the following year (1489–90) may have allowed him to extend his connection to this institution, which he had entered in 1483. Then he may have returned to Spain, where in the mid-1490s he was bound to Juan Téllez Girón (*c.*1456–1528), the Count of Ureña – a Castilian nobleman who had been one of the most significant opponents of Isabel la Católica's party during the Castilian civil war in the mid-1470s. Early in 1496 at Seville, he completed writing a medical tract dedicated to his master which should be considered the earliest printed medical work on the French disease from the Kingdom of Castile.[73]

Some of the Spanish medical doctoral graduates in Italian universities devoted themselves to university life. In addition to Jeroni Torrella, who was professor of medicine at the newly founded Estudi general of Valencia between 1505 and 1508, this is also the case of Lorenzo Alderete and Benito Bustamante de Paz. Alderete (*c.*1500–57) spent all of his professional career at Salamanca university, where he occupied first (1530) the *catedrilla* ('little chair') of Avicenna (endowed with 10,000 *maravedíes* per year) and then (1548) the first chair (*cátedra de prima*) of Avicenna, which he kept until his death. Alderete's Italian medical education was doubtless behind his steady campaign for the creation of the chair of anatomy at Salamanca university, as well as his responsibilities there during the 1550s as commissioner to promote the building of an anatomical theatre and as a member of the commission to reform the statutes of its medical faculty (1552). Alderete

---

69

70 On Laguna, see Arrizabalaga, 'Andrés Laguna', in W.F. Bynum and Helen Bynum (eds), *Dictionary of medical biography* (Westport, CT–London, Greenwood Press, 2007, 5 vols), vol. III, pp. 761–2; and the bibliography referred to there.

71 Pérez Martín, *Proles Aegidiana*, vol. II, pp. 659–61.

72 On Jeroni Torrella, see Nicolas Weill-Parot, *Jérôme Torrella (Hieronymus Torrella). Opus praeclarum de imaginibus astrologicis* (Florence, SISMEL-Edizioni del Galluzzo, 2008), pp. 11–16; and the bibliography referred to there.

73 See Piana, *Nuove ricerche*, p. 384; Piana, *Nuovi documenti*, vol. I, pp. 110–12; Pérez Martín, *Proles Aegidiana*, vol. I, pp. 414–15.

was the author of at least three medical writings, namely *De pleuresi*, *De febribus pestilentialibus* and *In fen 2ª primi Avicennae expositio*.[74] Of Bustamante de Paz we know that he had been professor of philosophy at Salamanca university and that later he lectured on logic in the mornings at Bologna university for two academic years (1537–38 and 1538–39), after his medical studies at this Italian university (1529–32).[75]

The editing of medical texts for the printing press is the fourth and last professional position that was occupied by some of our Spanish medical doctoral graduates in the Italian universities; in this case, as early as the two last decades of the fifteenth century. Once more, the biography of Francesc Argilagues is very revealing. Apparently, from 1483 until his last days, Argilagues lived in Venice, where he combined medical practice with the editorial preparation of medical works for the flourishing local printing press. Argilagues' editorial work, undertaken precisely at the time when this new occupation was rising in Europe, was devoted to the Venetian editions of the *Articella* – a sort of textbook of university medicine that was very popular in the late Middle Ages and Renaissance – which were printed in 1483 and 1487, as well as to three editions (Venice 1483 and 1496; Pavia 1490) of the *Conciliator* by the scholastic master Pietro d'Abano (1250-*c.*1315).[76]

That Argilagues' professional profile was not exceptional for the period is confirmed by the editorial activities of Guillem Caldentei (*fl.*1496), a physician and clergyman from Mallorca. After having studied arts and medicine at Pavia university – the most outstanding university in the Dukedom of Milan – where he may have taken his doctorate by 1496, Caldentei took care of the commentary by the scholastic master Ugo (Benzi) da Siena (*c.*1370–1439) on Galen's *Tegni*, which was first printed in Pavia in early 1496.[77] Caldentei – who, in contrast to Argilagues, returned to his native land in 1502 – dedicated this edition to 'his excellent patron' Ambrogio Varese da Rosate (1437–1522), a physician, medical professor at Pavia university, astronomer and advisor to the Duke of Milan, whose

[74] Juan de Fogeda, *Tractatus de pustulis que sahaphati nominantur* [Salamanca, the printer of Nebrija's *Gramática*, *c.* 1496]. On this work, see Jon Arrizabalaga, 'Tha changing identity of the French Pox in early Renaissance Castile', in Florence Eliza Glaze and Brian K. Nance (eds), *Between text and patient: The medical enterprise in medieval and early modern Europe* (Florence, SISMEL-Edizioni del Galluzzo, 2010 [forthcoming]).

[75] On Lorenzo Alderete, see Guadalupe Albi Romero, *Lorenzo Alderete y el avicenismo en la Universidad de Salamanca* (Valladolid, Universidad de Valladolid, Seminario de Historia de la Medicina, 2003); Guadalupe Albi Romero and Juan Riera Palmero, 'Galenismo y humanismo salmantino. Lorenzo Alderete', *Llull*, 22/43 (1999): 209–19.

[76] Pérez Martín, *Proles Aegidiana*, vol. II, pp. 681–3.

[77]

patronage of medical studies was notable in late fifteenth- and early sixteenth-century Pavia.[78]

I cannot end this section without adding a piece of information concerning the probable editorial activities also undertaken in Italy by Gabriel Brun, another Spanish medical student from Mallorca, who received his doctorate in about 1500 at Padua, where, in mid-November 1501, being seriously sick (he died soon after), he made his will. Among his testamentary dispositions, he left 'the bed he had in the house of the master printer Aldo [Manuzio]' to his maid Zana, and 25 ducats that, according to his words, Aldo owed him, to a brother-in-law of his with whom he lived in Padua, to cover the expenses of his funeral. Brun also left a copy of the printed Greek edition of Aristotle's *Ethics* (Venice, Aldo Manuzio, June 1498), to a close friend, apparently an arts student who would take his degree at Padua in September 1502. All these facts strongly suggest that Brun had been working at Aldo Manuzio's printing press, that his job demanded that he have a place to sleep in Venice, and that his connection to Aldo was sufficiently close for him to be permitted to stay overnight at Aldo's house or workshop.[79]

Conclusion

From the beginnings of the university movement, the *peregrinatio academica* of university students to undertake their studies beyond the borders of the Spanish kingdoms was a reality that the foundation of a great number of universities in these kingdoms during the late Middle Ages could not stop but, on the contrary, may have encouraged. With regard to medical studies, during the thirteenth and fourteenth centuries Montpellier university appears to have been the destination of first choice for the few Spanish students – from the Crown of Aragón especially – who dared to undertake studies outside their native kingdom. Throughout the fifteenth century, however, the pole of attraction for these itinerant medical students gradually shifted to the Italian universities. In order to explain this feature, which was particularly notable during the second half of the fifteenth and first half of the sixteenth centuries, we have to look for political reasons (e.g., the Kingdom of Aragón's dominion over the Kingdom of Naples, consolidation of the Spanish presence in Italy and the pontificates of the two Borja popes, namely Calixte III and Alexander VI), as well as for socio-professional ones (the prestige of the

---

[78] On Francesc Argilagues, see Jon Arrizabalaga, Luis García Ballester and José Luis Gil Aristu, 'Del manuscrito al primitivo impreso: la labor editora de Francesc Argilagues (fl. c.1470–1508) en el Renacimiento médico italiano', *Asclepio* 43/1 (1991): 3–49; Arrizabalaga, 'De la copie a l'édition'.

[79] Ugo da Siena, *Expositio in libros Tegni Galieni* (Pavia, Antonio Carchano, 29 Feb. 1496). On Caldentei and his editorial activities in Italy, see Arrizabalaga, 'En los inicios de una nueva ocupación', pp. 6–8.

Italian universities, in contrast with the weakness of medical studies in the Spanish kingdoms and the increasing demand for health practitioners in the latter).

In the patterns of Spanish medical students' academic itinerancy there are substantial differences between those who went directly from Spain to Bologna – by virtue of having been accepted as scholars at the Colegio de España – and those students whose first Italian destination was any of the other five universities under review. The inter-university mobility of the latter appears to have been greater than that of those who were elected as scholars of the Colegio de España by the ecclesiastical authorities of their native Spanish dioceses.

The fact of the disappearance after 1510 of Spanish medical doctoral students in the Italian universities other than Bologna reinforces the impression that the latter consolidated itself as the Italian university of preference for Spanish medical students and, presumably, for those of other faculties too. We cannot entirely rule out the possibility that some other Italian universities (e.g., Naples, Catania, Rome and even Pavia) whose graduation acts we have not been able to consult continued to play some role as destinations for Spanish medical students. Yet we also cannot underestimate the dissuasive effect that the increasing availability of medical studies at the old or new Iberian universities might have had on the *peregrinatio* to Italian and other university cities of Europe.

Apart from the opportunity to study at Bologna that the scholarships of the Colegio de España offered, it is very difficult to explain what moved these Spanish students to go to such different Italian cities to undertake a university medical education. Certainly, paying for their sons' studies in Italy was only available to well-off families, whose heads also needed to appreciate the economic, socio-political and/or cultural profitability of such an investment for the future professionals and their families. Yet, behind this critical career move, in not a few cases there may also have been powerful negative reasons. The repression unleashed by the Tribunal of the Inquisition among the Jewish *converso* sections of the Valencian patriciate from 1480, in addition to causing the migration of professionals, may have also made it advisable for these sons of well-off families to study in places outside the strained local atmosphere, and definitely beyond the reach of the Holy Office.

Then, as now, the new professional perspectives open to the itinerant students – to those who returned to their native places after having finished their studies, as well as to the minority who chose to settle professionally in Italy or in other regions of Europe – were related to the quality of the education they received at their university destinations, as much as to the social networks they were able to establish with their student companions, many of whom were the offspring of the elites of Spain, Italy and the rest of Europe, and with their professors and tutors. Doubtless, institutions such as the Casa di Sapienza of Siena or the Colegio de España of Bologna may have played an essential role in this respect as places for making contacts, establishing acquaintances and forging friendships that would facilitate the future professionals' recruitment by European elites. The frequency with which these Spanish medical students who got their doctorates at Italian universities throughout the fifteenth and sixteenth centuries were recruited by the elites can be illustrated by the outstanding professional careers of a small but significant group of them who had public responsibilities in the fields of health and sanitary administration, practised medicine at important princely courts (both civil and ecclesiastical) of Christendom, devoted themselves to university life and/or worked as editors for the medical printing press.

Last but not least, I cannot end this essay without briefly referring to the historical question of Philip II's 1559 prohibition on his subjects' attending or teaching at any university outside the territories under the Spanish monarchy, and its eventual consequences for Spain's intellectual communication with the rest of Europe.[80] Certainly, this feature should be put into the wider context of the increasing confessionalisation from the mid-sixteenth century onwards, on both sides of the religious divide between Roman Catholic and Protestant, that led to a progressive closing of most universities to those students and lecturers who did not share the local religious faith,[81] and contributed to the abandonment of student pilgrimages beyond the borders of their native countries – which had been going on for reasons other than religious. Yet, as I have already mentioned, Bologna appears to have been the only exception after 1510 to the factual disappearance of Spanish medical doctorates from the Italian universities under review. Thus, the effect of the legal restraint that was promulgated 50 years later might not have been so great on the numbers of Spanish students who stopped attending foreign universities (at least, the Italian ones) during the immediately following decades as it was long-lasting on new generations of travelling students, dissuading them from crossing the borders of Catholic Europe. Not even Bologna appears to have been entirely immune to the decline of medical students at Italian universities. Indeed, Table 4.4 shows that the numbers of medical doctorates continued to increase throughout the sixteenth century (94 of the 124 doctorates for the period 1441–1700), but substantially decreased during the first half of the seventeenth century (15), to be reduced to 1 doctorate for the whole second half of that century (in 1685). The suppression of grants for places for medical students at the Bolognese Colegio de España in 1627 might have accentuated this decline but did not provoke a collapse: while six students took their doctorates between 1601 and 1620, the

80 On Ambrogio Varese da Rosate, see Mario Cosenza, *Biographical and Bibliographical Dictionary of the Italian Humanists, 1300–1800* (Boston, G.K. May & Co., 1962–67, 5 vols), vol. I, pp. 160–61; vol. V, p. 401; Alfonso Corradi, *Memorie e documenti per la Storia dell'Università di Pavia* (Pavia, Tip. Successori Bizzoni, 1877–78, 3 parts), part I, p. 120; Bartolomeo Corte, *Notizie istoriche intorno ai medici scrittori milanesi* (Milan, Pandolfo Malatesta, 1718), pp. 37–42; Filipo Argelati, *Bibliotheca scriptorum Mediolanensis* (Milan, in aedibus Palatinis, 1745, 2 vols; facsimile reprint: Farnborough, Gregg Press Ltd., 1965–66), vol. II.1, cols. 1572–1575.

81 Veronese Ceseracciu, 'Spagnoli', pp. 51–2.

remaining nine for the period 1601–50 did so between 1638 and 1641.[82] As to the other universities under review, in their published records for the period after 1550 I have only come across two Spanish medical doctorates at Siena in 1561 and 1575.[83]

Table 4.4 Distribution of Spanish medical doctorates at Bologna (1440–1700)

	Numbers (absolute)	Percentages
1441–1500	11	8.9
1501–1550	45	36.3
1551–1600	52	41.9
1601–1650	15	12.1
1651–1700	1	0.8
Totals	**124**	**100**

*Bronzi*no, *Notitia doctorum*, 141–5.

*Minucc*i and Morelli, *Le lauree* (1992), pp. 292–3; Minucci and Morelli, *Le lauree* (1998), pp. 38–9.

---

82 José Mª López Piñero, *Ciencia y técnica en la sociedad española de los siglos XVI y XVII* (Barcelona, Labor, 1979), pp. 140–8.

83 See Hilde de Ridder-Symoens's essay in this volume as well as her chapter 'Mobility', in Hilde de Ridder-Symoens (ed.), *A history of the university in Europe. Vol. II: Universities in early modern Europe (1500–1800)* (Cambridge, Cambridge University Press, 1996), pp. 416–48 (at pp. 424–6).

Chapter 5

On Portuguese Medical Students and Masters Travelling Abroad: An Overview from the Early Modern Period to the Enlightenment

Mário Sérgio Farelo

It is well known that the Iberian *peregrinatio academica* was a major movement within the Peninsula, and a much lesser one outside it.[1] Subject to the intervention of the political powers, especially royal power,[2] the Iberian universities were considered mostly as centres of learning for royal court officials. This does not mean that many royal – and even municipal – officials were not educated abroad. This remains an open question. In fact, while we have a fair knowledge, acquired since the late 1980s,[3] of the educational curricula of royal bureaucrats, the same cannot be said of the careers of medieval and early modern Portuguese scholars in the kingdom, which are still in need of systematic attention in terms of a biographical or prosopographical treatment.

This is also the case for those Portuguese who studied medicine during the period, since we lack a comprehensive study that could expand the general overview that we have. Studying this historiographical panorama is nowadays a backwater of the medieval and early modern history of universities, following on from their very visible state during the 1990s. That very valuable period, when the history of universities was viewed as a fashionable subject, was mainly

1 Hilde de Ridder-Symoens, 'Mobility', in Walther Rüegg (ed.) *A history of the university in Europe*, vol. II: *The universities of the modern era (1500–1800)* (Portuguese edition, Lisbon, 2002, pp. 410–11).

2 Mariano Peset, 'Modelos y Estatutos de las Universidades Españolas y Portuguesas (Siglos XIII–XVIIII)', in Andrea Romano (ed.) *Dall'Università degli studenti all'Università Degli Studi* (Messina, 1991), p. 95.

3 Armando Luís de Carvalho Homem, 'État, institutions, société politique sous Jean 1er et Edouard 1er', *Arquivos do Centro Cultural Português*, XXVI (1989), pp. 35–48; idem, *O Desembargo Régio (1320–1433)* (Oporto, 1990); idem, 'L'État portugais et ses serviteurs (1320–1433)', *Journal des savants*, July–December 1987, pp. 181–203; idem, 'Les Officiers Royaux (XIIIe–XVe Siècles): Une élite politique?', *Anais – Série História. Universidade Autónoma de Lisboa*, II (1995), pp. 23–7.

used, among Portuguese historians, to publish sources and synthetic essays on the institution and its components at different periods of its existence.[4] With a few exceptions,[5] less attention was given to the biographical details of Portuguese physicians educated at universities within Portugal and outside, a situation that is only now being addressed.[6]

Even with all these difficulties, it is still possible to provide a sketch of the situation for the period of the sixteenth to the eighteenth centuries. Some of the issues under discussion derive from the earlier period. In that sense, we need a general overview of the 'medieval heritage' of the phenomenon, and we need to explain why Lisbon-Coimbra was not a centre of excellence for medical studies at the time and why it could therefore not prevent the Portuguese educational pilgrimage abroad.

At the only Portuguese university 'no one who had ever studied there had learned anything; and when someone talks about a man who studied in Coimbra, he is held in a much lower regard than someone who studied in Salamanca or in some other obscure place'.[7] This opinion, put forward by an Italian at the end of the sixteenth century, indicates the low prestige of higher education in Portugal. This is normally attributed to the deficient teaching structure in place between the Middle Ages and the beginning of the modern age.[8] To start with, the poor reputation of the Portuguese university is ascribed to its lack of geographical

---

[4] For an overview of the subject, see Saul António Gomes, 'Escolares e Universidade na Coimbra Medieval', in *Estudos em homenagem a João Francisco Marques*, vol. I (Oporto, 2001), pp. 511–12.

[5] Like the paper of Saul António Gomes referred to in the previous footnote.

[6] The University of Lisbon is organising a team project to produce biographies of masters and students who attended it up to 1536. This last project is included in the commemorations of the centenary of that institution, expected in 2011. Furthermore, the Centre of History of the same university welcomed a project subsidised by Portugal's Foundation for Science and Technology entitled *Historical Dictionary on Portuguese Sephardim: a prosopography of men of culture and science*, which has the objective of creating a who's who of every Portuguese Jewish scientist in modern times.

[7] António Henrique de Oliveira Marques, 'Uma descrição de Portugal em 1578–1580', *Nova História*, 1 (June 1984), p. 119, quoted by Armando Luís de Carvalho Homem, Luís Miguel Duarte and Eugénia Pereira da Mota, 'Percursos na burocracia régia (séculos XIII–XV)', in Francisco Bethencourt and Diogo Ramada Curto (eds) *Actas do Colóquio 'A Memória da Nação'* (Lisbon, 1991), p. 421.

[8] For the state of the art, see António Resende de Oliveira, 'As Instituições de Ensino', in Joel Serrão and A.H. de Oliveira Marques (dirs.) *Nova História de Portugal*, vol. III: Maria Helena da Cruz Coelho and Armando Luís de Carvalho Homem (eds) *Portugal em definição de Fronteiras (1096–1325). Do Condado portucalense à Crise do Séc. XIV* (Lisbon, 1996), pp. 635–59; idem, 'A mobilidade dos universitários', in *História da Universidade em Portugal*, vol. I/1: *1290–1536* (Coimbra, 1997), pp. 339–56; Sebastião Tavares de Pinto, 'A mobilidade dos universitários', in *História da Universidade em Portugal*, vol. I/2: *1537–1771* (Coimbra, 1996), pp. 989–1014.

and institutional stability,[9] which was partly responsible for the engaging of bad teachers, which in turn forced some students, according to the People in the Cortes of Lisbon in 1371, to seek their higher education abroad.[10]

On the other hand, it is well known that the Iberian universities specialised in the teaching of law. Thus, in the case of the Portuguese university, one might assume that the study of medicine held a secondary place. One indicator that this was the case may be the surviving curricula, although lack of information does not allow an extensive view of the details of this issue.[11] The same can be said of the number and remuneration of the teachers of medicine. By the fourteenth century, the university was functioning with only one regent in medicine, who received a mere 200 pounds per year, one third of the stipend of a *magister regens* in law.[12] Add to this the fact that the bachelors graduated by the Portuguese university were required to possess the degree in arts plus eight years of study in medicine – while in other universities, like Salamanca, the same degree was acquired after three years of arts and another three of medicine[13] – which meant a reduction in the importance of that science in the medieval Portuguese university and an inevitable search for new opportunities of higher learning elsewhere.

Another possible factor that may have influenced the academic pilgrimage movement was the prevalent royal ideology, which tended to restrain it. Some

---

9 The University during the Middle Ages was located in two different towns: in Lisbon during 1290–1308, 1338–54 and 1377–1537, and in Coimbra from 1308 to 1338 and from 1354 to 1377.

10 In the words of the king, 'the university has not the number and the quality of teachers it should have, thus many of our land are going abroad to learn, [a situation] that is not in our [that of the king's] service and honor'. *Cortes Portuguesas. Reinado de D. Fernando I (1367–1383)*, A.H. de Oliveira Marques (org.) vol. I (Lisbon, 1982), p. 49; Artur Moreira de Sá, *Chartularium Universitatis Portugalensis*, vol. I (Lisbon, 1966), p. 297; Salvador Dias Arnaut, 'A Medicina', in *História da Universidade de Coimbra*, vol. I/1 (Coimbra, 1996), pp. 289, 292–3. The issue of the *peregrinatio academica* surfaced again in the *Cortes* of 1440, in which the People stated that the students of the Portuguese *studium generale* graduated abroad (*Cortes* (1982), p. 299).

11 According to José Mattoso, the central work in the medicine course was at the time the *Regimen Sanitatis* of Salerno, although it had already been replaced in Montpellier by Avicenna's *Canon* or Dioscorides's *De material medica*. José Mattoso, 'A Universidade portuguesa e as universidades europeias', in *História da Universidade de Coimbra*, vol. I/1 (Coimbra, 1996), p. 297.

12 See Arnaut (1996), p. 287. Many other authors frequently mention these facts.

13 Joaquim Veríssimo Serrão, *Portugueses no Estudo de Salamanca*, vol. I: *1250–1550* (Coimbra, 1962), p. 119. This allowed for the medical students in Coimbra to obtain the respective baccalaureate in Salamanca, as mentioned by Fr. Diogo de Murça to King John III in a letter dated 12 August 1550 (see, for instance, A. Marcos de Dios, 'A transferência de escolares entre Salamanca e Coimbra', in *Universidade(s). História. Memória. Perspectivas. Actas do Congresso 'História da Universidade' (No 7º Centenário da sua Fundação). 5 a 9 de Março de 1990*, vol. 3 (Coimbra, 1991), p. 158).

measures were taken that were designed to promote the education abroad of some scholars,[14] but these must be seen in specific contexts, such as the need for highly trained lawyers for the king's service, or for theologians and preachers for Christianisation during the discoveries of the New World. The hostility towards the *peregrinatio academica* led, in part, to the creation of an academic structure in line with foreign practices. One very important step, in this sense, was the transfer of the university to Coimbra in 1537, where it was henceforth established around newly specialised colleges,[15] with academic degrees the subject of privileges.[16]

Further, this thinking manifested itself in a legislative form. For example, in 1532 the university board decided to favour the integration of masters, licentiates and bachelors who had graduated abroad.[17] Equally relevant was the law promulgated by royal authority in 1564, by which the bachelors in medicine attending Salamanca could be admitted at Coimbra.[18] However, this positive legislation had a coercive counterpart, expressed in the prohibition of Portuguese scholars from obtaining the desired degrees abroad,[19] again mainly in Salamanca.[20] This legal set-up particularly affected medical studies, as bachelors in the discipline

[14] Like the award of scholarships in Paris during the second quarter of the sixteenth century, as seen below.

[15] Pinto (1996), p. 1001.

[16] Pinto (1996), p. 1001. For an overview of the medical studies at Coïmbra's university in this period, see Fernando Taveira da Fonseca, 'A Medicina', in *História da Universidade em Portugal*, vol. I/1 (Coimbra, 1996), pp. 835–74.

[17] Joaquim Veríssimo Serrão, *Les Portugais à l'Université de Montpellier (XIIe–XVIIe siècles)* (Paris, 1971), pp. 86–7.

[18] Serrão (1971), p. 87; Marcos de Díos (1991), p. 158.

[19] We have testimonies for the fifteenth century, pertaining to the *Cortes* of Évora in 1481, where the king agreed to end the funding of students living abroad. The same policy would be applied later on by John III, according to a law published in 1541 (António Domingues de Sousa Costa, 'Estudos superiores e universitários em Portugal no reinado de D. João II', *Biblos*, LXIII (1987), p. 257; Manuela Mendonça, *D. João II. Um Percurso Humano e Político nas Origens da Modernidade em Portugal* (Lisbon, 1991), p. 222; eadem., 'Portugueses na Universidade de Siena. Contribuição para a sua história', in José María Soto Rábanos (ed.) *Pensamiento medieval hispano: homenaje a Horacio Santiago-Otero*, vol. I (Madrid, 1998), p. 836; Mário Brandão, *Documentos de D. João III*, vol. II (Coimbra, 1941), pp. 67–8; Serrão (1971), p. 87; Marcos de Díos (1991), p. 158), even if the latter produced a visible effect only two decades later (A.H. de Oliveira Marques, 'As Realidades Culturais', in Joel Serrão and A.H. de Oliveira Marques (dir.) *Nova História de Portugal*, vol. V: João José Alves Dias (ed.) *Portugal. Do Renascimento à Crise Dinástica* (Lisbon, 1998), p. 475). In the following decade, more precisely in 1575, King Sebastian ordered that every Portuguese attending the universities of Salamanca and Alcalá must return to Coimbra within one year (Serrão (1971), p. 87).

[20] Pinto (1996), p. 997.

who wished to practise in the Portuguese kingdom had first to obtain confirmation of the degrees they had received abroad.[21]

Until the end of the fifteenth century, the pattern of the Portuguese academic pilgrimage for medical studies closely resembled that of the other university disciplines, in that attendance was mainly at southern centres of learning. To observe a more significant movement of Portuguese students of medicine abroad, one has to turn to the French Midi, where the *causa discendi* drew the Portuguese to Montpellier from the thirteenth century, or even before, according to the thesis proposed by Iona McCleery.[22] With the proximity of the papacy at Avignon during the fourteenth century, the southern French universities became the main centres of learning for the Portuguese, although the 25 students found listed at Montpellier and the 8 scholars found at Toulouse[23] for the whole of that period would appear to be fewer than the actual total.

In the fifteenth century, the increasing importance of other centres of learning in the curricula of Portuguese scholars seems to have reduced the recruitment of Portuguese students to France. This was probably the main reason for the almost complete disappearance of Portuguese physicians from Paris, since only one student has been detected during the whole century.[24] In addition, Joaquim Veríssimo Serrão has only found one Portuguese student at Toulouse during the same period, which he ascribes to that centre of learning's being an intellectual backwater from the end of the fourteenth century up to 1450.[25] Similar reasons may well lie behind Portuguese medical students' rejection of Montpellier during the same period.[26]

---

21 As stated by the Ordonnance of the *Físico-mor* in 1515 (Serrão (1971), p. 5). According to this author, this law was responsible for the almost total absence of Portuguese medical students from Castille (Serrão (1962), p. 118).

22 Iona McCleery, 'Opportunities for teaching and studying medicine in medieval Portugal before the foundation of the University of Lisbon (1290)', *Dynamis*, 20 (2000), pp. 309–13, 315, 326.

23 Oliveira (1996), p. 346.

24 Roland l'Escripvain, *magister regens* in Paris, also known as a physician of the Duke of Bedford and later of the Dukes of Burgundy, interested in physiognomy and astrology. Thérèse Charmasson, 'L'établissement d'un almanach médical pour l'année 1437', *Comptes-rendus du 99e Congrès national des sociétés savantes, Besançon, 1974. Section des sciences*, fasc. V (Paris, 1976), pp. 217–34; eadem, 'Roland l'Écrivain, médecin des ducs de Bourgogne', in *Actes du 101e Congrès national des sociétés savantes, Lille, 1976, Section Sciences*, fasc. III (Paris, 1976), pp. 21–32; eadem, 'L'*Arithmétique* de Roland l'Éscrivain et le *Quadripartitum numerorum* de Jean de Murs', *Revue d'Histoire des Sciences*, vol. 31, 2 (1978), p. 171–6; eadem, *Recherches sur une technique divinatoire: la géomancie dans l'Occident médiévale* (Paris-Genève, 1980), pp. 177–93.

25 Joaquim Veríssimo Serrão, *Les Portugais à l'Université de Toulouse (XIIIe–XVIIe siècle)* (Paris, 1970), pp. 41–2.

26 Serrão (1971), p. 62.

The passage of Portuguese scholars through the universities of Belgium and Germany seems to have begun with the Great Schism and the closure of the Clementine universities to students from states loyal to the Roman pope.[27] That is certainly why a Portuguese presence – mostly ecclesiastics – has been detected in the University of Cologne between 1396 and 1416, though there were only a few until the middle of the fifteenth century.[28] The same can be said in the case of the University of Leuven (Louvain), where, from the fifteenth to the seventeenth centuries, at least 33 Portuguese scholars have been found.[29]

As we saw at the beginning, the Portuguese educational pilgrimage seems to have been mostly an Iberian affair. Thus it is not difficult to show that the most popular Iberian university for the Portuguese (besides Lisbon-Coimbra during the Middle Ages) was undoubtedly Salamanca.[30] There had been Portuguese participation in the founding of Salamanca in the middle of the thirteenth century,[31] but it was only two centuries later, when past political difficulties between the two kingdoms had been surmounted, that the choice of Salamanca became truly popular.[32] Nonetheless, the Portuguese student population in medicine remained small, as medical learning in Portugal became increasingly parochial.

The Early Modern Period

The end of the fifteenth century marks an important turning point in our subject. By then, the traditional recognition of the liberties and special status of the Moorish

27 António Domingos de Sousa Costa, *Monumenta Portugalie Vaticana*, vol. III/1 (Braga, 1982), p. 137, note 50.

28 Farelo (1999), p. 67, note 244, from the consultation of the *Die Matrikel der Universität Köln*, Hermann Keussen, ed., 2nd edn, vol. I, (Bonn, 1928) (Reprint Dusseldorf, 1979).

29 María Jesús Rodero Rodero, *Estructura social y población de las universidades en el Sacro Imperio-Nación Alemana en los siglos XV, XVI y XVII y los estudiantes hispano-lusos en ellas según los libros de matrícula*, Licence Dissertation (Salamanca, 1983); Ángel Marcos de Díos, 'Estudiantes de la archidiócesis de Évora en la universidad de Salamanca (1580–1640)', *A Cidade de Évora*, vol. 33, 59 (Jan.–Dez. 1976), p. 84. We did not have access to the conclusions of Thomas Cole's research about the Portuguese students at the University of Leuven, under the direction of Prof. Hilde de Ridder-Symoens.

30 Serrão (1962).

31 José Antunes, 'Portugueses no processo histórico da fundação da Universidade de Salamanca', *Revista de História das Ideias*, 12 (1990), pp. 19–53.

32 We know that close to a thousand Portuguese passed through the University of Salamanca before 1550 (Marcos de Dios (1991), p. 156). Between 1526 and 1547 alone 745 have been detected (Pinto (1996), p. 996). By reading the register books ('Books of the cloisters'), Armando de Jesus Marques has identified a total of 30 Portuguese for the period from 1464 to 1481 (Armando Marques, 'Portugueses nos 'claustros salmantinos' do séc. XV', *Revista Portuguesa de Filosofia*, vol. 19, 2 (1963), p. 6).

and Jewish minorities in the kingdom had been replaced by fear of religious persecution, following the Jewish Expulsion (or better said, General Conversion) of 1496–97.[33] This is important, because the Jews had played a pre-eminent role in the medical professions since the Middle Ages.[34] As a result, there were created simultaneously a group of newly converted Christians, generally called *cristãos-novos*, who maintained their educational activities in the Portuguese kingdom,[35] and other groups of Sephardic Jews, who formed the first wave of Portuguese Jewish communities across Europe. Later on, some of these *nations*, like that of Bayonne,[36] helped to integrate those who were forced into exile as a result of the strengthening of measures against the Jews in 1534 and the establishment of the Inquisition two years later.[37] In fact, these communities helped to form the backbone of the structure around which those physicians could gather, meet other people and develop important scientific careers,[38] as in the case of two of the most important doctors of the period, Garcia da Orta and Amatus Lusitanus, who would have astonishing careers across Europe.[39]

These exiles made possible the development of a cultural interchange between Portuguese physicians and their European counterparts, from the rare encounters

---

[33] This is a subject for which there is a large bibliography. The latest study is by François Soyer, *The persecution of the Jews and Muslims of Portugal. King Manuel I and the end of religious tolerance (1496–7)* (New York, 2007).

[34] It does not seem incorrect to suggest that many urban doctors in medieval and early modern Portugal may have been Jews or newly converted Jews, if we take into account the numerous royal letters of authorisation of practice delivered to members of that minority between 1481 and 1495 (Costa (1987), p. 255). Alfredo Rastreiro notes that in the sixteenth century almost every Portuguese physician was a Sephardi (Alfredo Rastreiro, *Medicina Judaica Lusitana. Século XVI* (Coimbra, 2000), p. 11).

[35] We must not forget that the measures taken by King Manuel I in terms of forced baptisms and marriages, between the Edict of Expulsion of 1496 and the establishment of the Inquisition in 1536, allowed for the appearance of Jews in the universities, a situation somewhat peculiar in the European scene.

[36] Gerard Nahon, 'The Portuguese Jewish nation of Saint-Esprit-Les-Bayonne: The American dimension', in Paolo Bernardini and Norman Fiering (eds) *The Jews and the expansion of Europe to the West, 1450 to 1800* (New York, 2001), p. 255.

[37] It is normally assumed that the persecution of Judaisers did not start with the General Conversion of 1496–97, but only with the establishment of the Inquisition 40 years later. Mirian Bodian, *Hebrews of the Portuguese nation. Conversos and community in early modern Amsterdam* (Bloomington and Indianapolis, 1997), p. 12.

[38] These were the cases of Luís Nunes and Amato Lusitano. Serrão (1962), p. 243; Pinto (1996), pp. 998, 1005.

[39] Maximiliano de Lemos, *Amato Lusitano. A sua vida e a sua obra* (Porto, 1907); I.S. Révah, 'La famille de Garcia de Orta', *Revista da Universidade de Coimbra*, 19 (1960), pp. 407–20.

from the fifteenth century until the 1520s.[40] From that time on, the rapid spread abroad of these physicians and students of medicine changed the geography of the Portuguese *peregrinatio medica* drastically. The medieval situation thus remained in only a few places, like England, for example. There, the occasional Portuguese students followed the same type of recruitment, chose the same curricula and attended the same universities as before.[41]

The new reality was very different. Even if the traditional universities continued to attract Portuguese medical students, the expulsions of Jewish physicians expanded not only the number but also the range of institutions attended. Obviously, these physicians chose communities where their work and even their lives could evolve without persecution by royal, municipal and papal authorities, as was the case in various places in France, Italy or in the distant Turkish Salonica[42] and, later, in the Low Countries. The founding of such communities was especially frequent in France and Italy during the second half of the sixteenth century, mainly in the French littoral cities such as Bordeaux, Bayonne, Marseilles and Montpellier, and in northern Italy.[43] This made the establishment of Portuguese doctors in French cities other than the traditional university cities more frequent, especially after Henri II's privilege of 1550, which allowed every Portuguese merchant and New Christian to benefit from all of the privileges afforded to French citizens.[44] For instance, Avignon was served by a family of Portuguese doctors consisting of Manuel Ribeiro, his sons Miguel and Lopo, and Henrique, son of Lopo.[45]

This situation also changed the patterns of mobility, making them more flexible, following the humanist ideal of attending various centres of learning. This meant that there was no single path of progression in the course of studies pursued, although France seems to have become a place of some interest to those who had studied in Portugal or Spain. As in the case of Manuel Alves, a student could graduate at Lerida before pursuing a teaching career at Salamanca and

---

40 António Rosa Mendes, 'A Vida Cultural', in José Mattoso (ed.) *História de Portugal*, vol. III: *No Alvorecer da Modernidade (1480–1620)* (Lisbon, 1993), p. 380 quoted by Adalgisa Botelho da Costa, *O reportório dos tempos de André do Avelar e a Astrologia em Portugal no Século XVI*, MA in Science dissertation (S. Paulo, 2001), p. 39.

41 Luís de Matos, *Les Portugais en France au XVIe siècle. Étude et documents* (Coimbra, 1952), p. 154.

42 The reason for choosing Ottoman cities like this one was the religious tolerance provided there by their authorities. Aristea D. Kanellaki, *Os Judeus de origem portuguesa em Salónica no século XVI*, MA dissertation (Lisbon, 2002), p. 27.

43 Gerard Nahon, *Les nations Juives Portugaises du Sud-Ouest de la France (1684–1791). Documents* (Paris, 1981).

44 Nahon (2001), p. 255.

45 Matos (1952), p. 154–5. For other examples see Augusto da Silva Carvalho, *Notícias sobre alguns médicos Judeus do Alentejo*, offprint of *Jornal da Sociedade das Sciências Médicas de Lisboa* (Lisbon, 1930), pp. 3–20.

Toulouse.[46] This last university could also be the final stopping point for a scholar after passing through Bordeaux, Rome and Montpellier, as occurred later on with Francisco Sanches.[47]

Even so, these examples cannot disguise the fact that the French universities were not necessarily the destination of choice for those desiring an eminent medical career outside Portugal. It is true that during the first half of the sixteenth century Paris – now together with the college of Guyenne at Bordeaux[48] – continued to be an important centre of learning for Portuguese scholars, as is shown by the many dozens who are listed in the works of Luís de Matos and José Terra.[49] But looking closely, one can actually see a decline in the numbers of those studying medicine there.[50] In fact, the ranks of these *parisienses* were filled by royal grant holders, almost exclusively students of theology, in view of the desperate need for ecclesiastics to preach in the New World. With a decrease in the importance of these scholarships around the middle of the sixteenth century, the same happened to the Portuguese scholarly presence there. Taking into consideration the political problems during that century and the primacy of Salamanca after 1580, we can safely assume the disappearance of the Portuguese from the Seine's university in the last decades of the century.[51]

The same can also be said of the attendance at the southern French universities, in particular at the renowned University of Montpellier, where only 23 Portuguese scholars have been found during this time.[52] It is interesting to know that not all the Portuguese there were students, since a few medical *magistri* can be found at Toulouse, like Manuel Alves and Álvaro Peres.[53] Certainly, their presence was coincidental and centres of learning like Montpellier and Toulouse were no longer on the main European route of education for the Portuguese. In addition, we should not forget that the Portuguese scholars had to deal with orthodox Catholic universities, as was the case with Toulouse,[54] as well with the instability brought about by the latent war between Spain and France (1525–1558), together with religious problems (1560–62). Assimilation with the Spanish scholars, and thus

---

46 Pinto (1996), p. 1003–4; Serrão (1970), pp. 132–40.

47 Pinto (1996), p. 1004; Serrão (1970), pp. 140–53.

48 Ernest Gaullier, *Histoire du Collège de Guyenne: d'après un grand nombre de documents inédits* (Paris, 1874).

49 Luís de Matos, *Les Portugais à l'Université de Paris entre 1500 et 1550* (Coimbra, 1950); José F. da Silva Terra, 'Nouveaux documents sur les Portugais à l'Université de Paris (XVIe siècle)', *Arquivos do Centro Cultural Português*, V (1972), pp. 190–260.

50 Matos (1950), pp. 12, 27, 52, 53, 54, 58, 74, 82, 86, 173.

51 Ibid., p. 10; Pinto (1996), p. 1003.

52 Serrão (1971), p. 84. Only three Portuguese scholars have been identified in Montpellier during 1580–1640. Pinto (1996), p. 1006.

53 Serrão (1971), pp. 121–3; Serrão (1970), pp. 140–52; Pinto (1996), pp. 1003–4, 1006.

54 Serrão (1970), pp. 96–7.

hostile treatment by the French population, were all that was needed to force the Portuguese into exile.[55]

Many of them passed on to Italy. Part of its attraction derived from the prestige that Italian education enjoyed in Portugal, as seen in the actions of Portuguese royalty to attract learned Italians to the royal court. Similarly, from the fifteenth century universities like Rome, Pisa, Siena and Parma seem to have received a fair number of Portuguese students in medicine who reproduced, *mutatis mutandis*, the itineraries of the scholars in law.[56]

This flow continued during the sixteenth century, generally increased by Jewish and newly converted students and physicians, who were welcomed by the Portuguese communities recently founded in some northern Italian cities. For instance, they encountered favourable conditions in the tolerant ambiance provided by the Venetian authorities, who permitted hundreds of Jews to attend and to graduate from the University of Padua,[57] at that time considered the best university in Europe for medical education.[58]

In fact, these conditions made possible a high degree of mobility, a sort of tour of the centres of learning located there, like Bologna, Padua, Pisa, Venice, Ferrara and Florence. This can be illustrated by the routes followed by physicians such as Filipe Rodrigues de Montalto[59] or Rodrigo da Fonseca. The latter started as a professor of philosophy, logic and medicine at Pisa from 1575 to 1615, when he became professor at Padua.[60] The city of Ferrara is another good example of the point we are trying to make. Having a university that was recognised as a reference point in medical studies, the city attracted many Portuguese Jews during the

55 Serrão (1971), pp. 81–4, 92–3; Serrão (1970), p. 59.

56 Mendonça (1998), p. 831–60. The Portuguese *peregrinatio academica* to Italy in the fifteenth century was a very important theme in the work of (among others) António Domingues de Sousa Costa, O.F.M., *Portugueses no Colégio de S. Clemente e Universidade de Bolonha durante o século XV* (Bolonha, 1990) 2 vols.

57 The fact that the Venetian authorities exercised their domination over the university has been stressed by David R. Rudeman, 'Medicine and scientific thought. The world of Tobias Cohen', in Robert Charles David and Benjamin Ravid (eds) *The Jews in early modern Venice* (Baltimore/London, 2001), p. 191. The Jewish attendance at this university was studied by Shaul G. Massry, Miroslaw Smogorzewski, Elizur Hazani and Shaul M. Shasha, 'Jewish medicine and the University of Padua: contribution of the Padua graduate Toviah Cohen to nephrology', *American Journal of Nephrology*, vol. 19, 2 (1999), pp. 213–21. For other considerations of Padua's attraction for medical students, see the chapter by Cinthia Klestinec in this volume.

58 David B. Ruderman, 'Padua and the formation of a Jewish medical community in Italy', in David B. Ruderman (ed.) *Jewish thought and scientific discovery in early modern Europe* (New Haven–London, 1995), p. 105.

59 Peter van Rooden, 'A Dutch adaptation of Elias Montalto's *Tractado sobre o principio do Capítulo 53 de Jesaias*. Text, Introduction and Commentary', *Lias*, 16 (1989), p. 2.

60 Pinto (1996), p. 1005.

first half of the sixteenth century. This community was sufficiently influential to recommend to the Duke of Ferrara the name of Amatus Lusitanus, who eventually occupied medical chairs in Ferrara University from 1540 to 1547,[61] before leaving for another important place that admitted Portuguese Jews, Ancona.[62] During this time, Amatus interacted with other Portuguese men of science, like the physician Duarte Gomes (David Zaboca), three times accused of Judaism in Venice, and the astronomer Francisco Mendes Vezinho (Esdras Vezinho), son of Yosef Vezinho, Jewish physician of the Portuguese monarch John II[63] and the first person to determine the latitude in the southern hemisphere.[64] The same kind of arguments could explain the number of Portuguese physicians lecturing at Pisa, as is shown by the cases of Rodrigo da Fonseca, Gabriel da Fonseca, Sebastião Ferreira Lopes and Estêvão Rodrigues de Castro,[65] or of João Lopes at Florence.[66] In the south of the country, the centrality of Rome made it a destination of choice for those able

---

[61] Pier Cesare Ioly Zorattini, 'Sephardic settlement in Ferrara under the House of Este', in Yedida K. Stillman and George K. Zucker (eds) *New horizons in Sephardic studies* (Albany, 1993), p. 6–8. About the 'Portuguese Nation' there, see Aron di Leone Leoni, 'Due personaggi della "Nation Portughesa" di Ferrara: Un martire e un avventuriero', *La Rassegna Mensile di Israel*, vol. LVII, 3 (1991), pp. 407–48.

[62] For the Portuguese Jewish presence in this city, see Bernard Dov Cooperman, 'Portuguese Conversos in Ancona: Jewish political activity in early modern Italy', in Bernard Dov Cooperman (ed.) *In Iberia and beyond: Hispanic Jews between cultures* (Newark, 1998), pp. 297–352; H. Rosenberg, 'Alcuni documenti riguardanti i marrani portughesi in Ancona', *La Rassegna Mensile di Israel*, X (1935), pp. 306–23; Viviana Bonazzoli, 'Ebei italiani, portoghesi, levantini sulla piazza commercial di Ancona entorno alla matà del Cinquecento', in Gaetano Cozzi (ed.) *Gli ebrei a Venezia, secoli XIV–XVIII* (Milan, 1987), pp. 727–70; Aron di Leone Leoni, 'Per una Storia della Nazione Portoghese ad Ancona ed a Pesaro', in Pier Cesare Ioly Zorattini (ed.) *Miscellanea di Studi sul Marranesimo* (Firenze 2000), pp. 27–97.

[63] Zorattini (1993), pp. 6–8.

[64] Filipe Duarte Santos, 'Portugal na Historia da Ciências', in *História e Desenvolvimento da Ciência em Portugal. I Colóquio – até ao século XX*, vol. I (Lisbon, 1986), pp. 292–302.

[65] Giacinto Manuppella, 'Os lentes portugueses na Universidade de Pisa (ligeiros apontamentos para o futuro historiador)', in Estêvão Rodrigues de Castro, *Obras Poéticas [...]* (Coimbra, 1967); Pinto (1996), pp. 1006, 1008; Giuliana Volpi Rosselli, 'I portoghesi nell'Ateneo Pisano in epoca medicea (1543–1737)' and Barbara Marangoni, 'Un medico portoghese nello studio di Pisa – Rodrigo Fonseca', in *Toscana e Portogallo. Miscellanea storica nel 650º aniversario dello Studio Generale di Pisa. Studi del Departimento di scienze della politica dell'universita di Pisa* (Pisa, 1994), pp. 117–32, 209–21; Bruno Martins Boto Leite, *Les enseignants de médecine Portugais à l'Université de Pise (XVIe-XVIIe siècles)* (paper presented at the 40th International Congress on the History of Medicine, 26–30 August 2006 in Budapest).

[66] Costa (1987), p. 298; Costa (1990), p. 824.

to gain access via the papal court, helped by the increasing importance of medical studies there as a result of the will of Paul III.[67]

From another perspective, one must bear in mind that the decision on which university to choose depended not only on the prestige of the school, the curricula offered, the presence of one's countrymen and the existence of trade routes,[68] but also on the distance. This factor can actually be taken as one of the reasons why the Portuguese *peregrinatio academica* was mainly peninsular, and not extra-peninsular. We all know that the international pilgrimage normally involved relatively long stays, which demanded economic resources available only to a few. In that sense, having a prestigious centre of learning so close to the Portuguese kingdom as was Salamanca undoubtedly changed the scholarly flow from the moment that political relations between Portugal and Castile (later Spain)[69] improved. As a result, it was not long before Torme's university became a true 'cultural *vivarium*' for the Portuguese,[70] and their main centre of learning. In consequence, it is not surprising that by the beginning of the sixteenth century one of the university counsellors was always Portuguese.[71] As far as medicine was concerned, 47 Portuguese studied there during the year 1526–27, according to the data uncovered by Joaquim Veríssimo Serrão.[72] On average, the Portuguese medical students represented around 21 per cent of the total local student population between 1550 and 1572.[73] Similar figures are presented by Mercedes Grangel, who has identified at least 616 Portuguese medical students during the period 1500–61.[74] Many of these may have developed their studies under the guidance of one or other of their countrymen who were

[67] Filippo Mafia Renazzi, *Storia dell'Universit`a degli Studi di Roma, detta comunemente La Sapienza*, (Roma, 1804), p. 107.

[68] Mário Farelo, 'Les Portugais à l'Université de Paris au Moyen Âge. Aussi une question d'acheminements de ressources', *Memini. Travaux et documents publiés para la Société des études médiévales du Québec*, 5 (2001), pp. 101–29.

[69] For political relations between the two kingdoms in the fifteenth century, see Julieta Maria Aires de Almeida Araújo, *Portugal e Castela (1431–1475): ritmos de uma paz vigilante*, PhD dissertation (Lisbon, 2003).

[70] Joaquim Veríssimo Serrão, *História de Portugal*, 4th edn, vol. I (Lisbon, 1990), p. 230; vol. II, p. 381; Serrão (1962), pp. 36–48; Marques (1963), pp. 167–86; Américo da Costa Ramalho, 'O Humanismo (depois de 1537)', in *História da Universidade em Portugal*, vol. I/2 (Coimbra, 1996), p. 697.

[71] Armando Marques, 'Conselheiros portugueses na Universidade de Salamanca (1505–1506)', *Anais da Academia Portuguesa de História*, 2nd series, 25 (1979), p. 400.

[72] Serrão (1962), p. 118.

[73] These averages were calculated from the data compiled in Marco de Díos (1991), p. 162.

[74] Mercedes Grangel, 'Salamanca y la formación de médicos portugueses en el siglo XVI', *Medicina na Beira Interior. Da Pré-História ao Século XXI – Cadernos de Cultura*, 14 (November 2000), p. 9.

teaching there, such as the physicians Luís Nunes, Gonçalo Fernandes, Agostinho Lopes, Manuel Alves or Ambrósio Nunes.[75]

We can safely say that these numbers grew during the Dual Monarchy (1580–1640), with the return of thousands of Portuguese *conversos* to Spain. We must not forget that the opening of the border between the now 'united' kingdoms had immediate repercussions, since Portuguese medical students gained much easier access to the university. Also, their presence in Salamanca made them unaccountable for any crimes that they might have committed in Portugal. In view of this, around ten thousand Portuguese students improved their education in Torme's university during this time, according to statistics furnished by Ángel Marcos de Dios.[76] Students of medicine represented a significant proportion of this number.[77]

There are factors that enable us to see the direction and importance of the studies pursued and of the degrees obtained in Salamanca. The transfer of the Portuguese university to Coimbra in 1537 was one such. King John III decided to reform this institution, which had been in a very precarious situation, by taking it out of Lisbon. At the same time, the monarch recognised a shortage of teaching personnel, a problem settled by recourse to Portuguese and foreign scholars from Bordeaux, Paris and Salamanca.[78] The chairs of medicine thus were soon filled by professors arriving from Salamanca. In 1539, after obtaining his doctorate, Tomás Rodrigues da Veiga came to Coimbra, eventually becoming a *magister regens* of that institution for the next four decades.[79] Two years later, the University of Coimbra received another bachelor in medicine from Salamanca, António Barbosa, also a bachelor in arts and philosophy, who was given the chair of *Tercia*.[80]

The same may have occurred in other peninsular centres of learning. As one might suspect, the existing data for other Spanish universities, such as Valladolid and Alcalá de Henares, show the declining importance of those places for Portuguese students. In the case of Alcalá, only 12 students have been identified in the 19 years

[75] Pinto (1996), p. 1005; Rastreiro (2000), pp. 24–5.

[76] Marco de Díos (1991), p. 159; Serrão (1962), pp. 92–3; Pinto (1996), p. 1003. During the period 1580–1640, that university hosted on average 500 new Portuguese students each year.

[77] Ángel Marcos de Dios gives us eloquent data about the importance of this matter. While in 1579–80, 1597–98 and 1607–8 they correspond respectively to 26, 39 and 36 per cent of the total Portuguese population, from 1612–1640 to 1640 they always represent around 44 per cent. A peak of 64 per cent can be detected in 1633–34. Marco de Díos (1991), p. 162.

[78] Pinto (1996), p. 991.

[79] Professor of *Vesperas* from 1539 to 1557, he remained in the chair of *Prime* between 1557 and 1579. Pinto (1996), pp. 992, 999.

[80] Pinto (1996), p. 993.

from 1561 to 1580.[81] Even so, the period 1580–1640 saw increasingly favourable conditions for such moves. This can be confirmed by the 86 Portuguese students discovered in Valladolid for that period by Isabel Maria Drummond Braga[82], and the more than 50 scholars in the case of Alcalá, most of them specialising in the study of arts and theology.[83] The medical students in Valladolid during that time accounted for 18.6 per cent of the 86 scholars referred to earlier.[84] The Portuguese were also very rare in Lleida,[85] a fact confirmed by Marisa Costa, who has identified them at only two distinct times, 1446 and 1515.[86] Lack of research prevents us from drawing any conclusions about the Portuguese presence in the other peninsular universities of Palencia, Lerida, Perpignan, Huesca, Barcelona, Saragossa, Palma de Majorca, Sigüenza[87] and Valencia. Finally, we should bear in mind that the training of physicians could take place in other Castilian institutions outside the faculties of medicine. The best-known of them remain the hospitals of the Guadalupe monastery, which served as training centres for Portuguese physicians during the sixteenth century.[88]

The Low Countries provided a welcoming centre for Portuguese fleeing the Inquisition. Benefiting from a climate of religious toleration, physicians like Luís Nunes and Amatus Lusitanus could come to Antwerp[89] and breathe the air of

[81] Joaquim Veríssimo Serrão, 'Contributo para o estudo dos portugueses na Universidade de Alcalá (1509–1640)', *Revista Portuguesa de História*, 17 (1978), p. 39; Pinto (1996), p. 1003. We must add that, as mentioned by the author, his research was done only on the records of St Anthony College and not on all of the available university documentation.

[82] Isabel Maria Ribeiro Mendes [Drummond Braga], 'Estudantes bragantinos na Universidade de Valladolid (1567–1640)', *Brigantia*, vol. 9, 3–4 (1989), p. 50; Pinto (1996), p. 1003.

[83] Serrão (1978), p. 49; Marco de Díos (1991), p. 323; Pinto (1996), p. 1006.

[84] Mendes [Drumond Braga] (1989), p. 50.

[85] Artur Moreira de Sá, *Chartularium Universitatis Portugalensis*, vol. XI (Lisbon, 1993), p. 353, note 1, mentioned by Marisa Costa, 'O elemento estrangeiro em cidades catalãs. Portugueses em Lleida nos finais da Idade Média', in *XVII Congrés d'Història de la Corona de Aragó. Barcelona-Lleida, 7–12 de setembre del 2000*, vol. II (Barcelona, 2003), p. 119.

[86] Costa (2003), pp. 113, 116.

[87] Maria Benedicta Aires de Almeida Araújo, 'Os médicos portugueses e a inquisição de Évora', in *Universidade(s). História. Memória. Perspectivas. Actas do Congresso 'História da Universidade' (No 7° Centenário da sua Fundação). 5 a 9 de Março de 1990*, vol. 4 (Coimbra, 1991), p. 273.

[88] Isabel Maria Ribeiro Mendes Drumond Braga, *Península Ibérica: um Espaço, dois Reinos (Interrelações na Época de Carlos V)* (Lisbon, 2001), pp. 534–5; eadem and João Carlos Oliveira, 'A Saúde', in Joel Serrão and A.H. de Oliveira Marques (dir.) *Nova História de Portugal*, vol. V: João José Alves Dias (ed.) *Portugal. Do Renascimento à Crise Dinástica* (Lisbon, 1998), p. 646.

[89] Ridder-Symoens (2002), pp. 415–16.

freedom before going on to the more prestigious French and Italian universities for their medical education. Later, the attraction of the Dutch cities proved significant. It actually grew towards the end of the sixteenth century, with the increasing importance of the Portuguese community in Amsterdam.

Towards the Enlightenment

Even if the seventeenth century remains the least well known in terms of the history of sciences in Portugal,[90] we can safely say that the University of Coimbra continued to receive students. For instance, between 1573 and 1624 the annual average of matriculations in medical studies was about 63 students.[91] This is actually a fair number by Portuguese standards. Even so, the fact that it was a faculty with a conservative curriculum, still attached to a theoretical form of medical teaching rather than a more practical one,[92] helped to maintain the exodus of Portuguese students and physicians to foreign institutions.

This was especially the case with the Jewish practitioners of medicine, who passed through difficult times in Portugal. On the one hand, they had to deal with the increasing repression by the Holy Office after 1620.[93] Being generally persecuted for their Judaising tendencies, Jewish medical practitioners also found themselves the object of the 'corporative' response of Old Christians, who, by means of introducing themselves into the Inquisition as consultants, started to systematically denounce their Jewish 'colleagues'.[94] In time, the Crown actually contributed to this new segregation. By a decree of November 1568, King Sebastian instituted 30 scholarships for Old Christians to study medicine. Later, Philip I augmented their value and added other grants, for those belonging to the same group who wished to follow pharmacy. Finally, in 1671, the monarch decided to

---

[90] Henrique Leitão, 'Review of Luís Miguel Carolino, *Ciência, Astrologia e Sociedade. A Teoria da Influência Celeste em Portugal (1593–1755)* (Lisboa: Fundação Calouste Gulbenkian, Fundação para a Ciência e a Tecnologia, 2003). 431 pp.', *Journal of the history of science and technology*, vol. 1 (summer 2007).

[91] This average was calculated by me from the data mentioned in Mendes (1993), p. 499.

[92] About the medical teaching at Coimbra, see Fernando Taveira da Fonseca, 'A Medicina', in *História da Universidade em Portugal*, vol. I/2 (Coimbra, 1996), pp. 835–73.

[93] Bodian (1997), p. 12.

[94] Timothy Walker, 'Physicians and surgeons in the service of the Inquisition: The nexus of religion and conventional medical training in Enlightenment-era Portugal', in Ole Peter Grell and Andrew Cunningham (eds) *Medicine and religion in Enlightenment Europe* (Aldershot, 2007), p. 30; Harold J. Cook, *Matters of exchange: Commerce, medicine, and science in the Dutch Golden Age* (New Haven–London, 2007), p. 211.

close the University of Coimbra to 'New Christians' altogether and to direct them to commercial activities.[95]

This new reality brought a new perspective to the *peregrinatio*, one much closer to the idea of Enlightenment. No longer would the New Christians preoccupy themselves simply with obtaining a degree. Conceptually speaking, they became those *estrangeirados*, 'foreigners' who, through their social and professional networks with European intellectual circles,[96] provided a theoretical basis for medical reform in their home country.[97] Engaged on the Grand Tour,[98] they looked for news of scientific advances in England, the Netherlands, France, Italy and the German states, thus showing more and more how backward the Portuguese were scientifically.[99]

The most important of these *estrangeirados* were unquestionably António Ribeiro Sanches and Jacob Castro Sarmento. The first defended the theories of Boerhaave and Harvey, and his *Método para Aprender a Estudar Medicina* (1763) [*Method for learning how to study medicine*] inspired the reform of the faculty of medicine of the University of Coimbra, thus at last providing Portuguese medicine with a scientific basis.[100] The latter fled the kingdom in 1721, upon persecution by the Inquisition, and established himself in England, where he pursued a scientific career, leading to a teaching position at the University of Aberdeen. Like António Sanches, he promoted the modernisation of scientific studies in Portugal through the translation of Francis Bacon's work *Novum Organum*. At the same time, he was the first to spread Newtonian ideas in Portugal.[101]

---

95 José Antonio Saraiva, *The Marrano factory: the Portuguese Inquisition and its new Christians 1536–1765* (Leiden, 2001), p. 152. Therefore only old Christians were admitted at Coimbra , clean of Jewish or Muslim blood or that of slaves or men considered by the Inquisition to be guilty (Araújo (1990), p. 275).

96 Ana Simões, Ana Carneiro e Maria Paula Diogo, 'Constructing knowledge: eighteenth century Portugal and the new sciences', *Archimedes*, 2 (1999), p. 20.

97 Walker (2007), p. 46.

98 In a article in Hebrew that we could not obtain, Reuven Faindolg discusses the exile of 70 Portuguese Jewish physicians obliged to flee Portugal in the seventeenth century: Reuven Faingold, 'Flight from the Valley of Death – Converso physicians leaving Portugal in the early 17th century', *Peamim*, 68 (summer 1996), pp. 105–38.

99 Ana Simões, Ana Carneiro, Maria Paula Diogo, 'Travels of learning. Introductory remarks', in Ana Simões, Ana Carneiro, Maria Paula Diogo (eds) *Travels of learning. Towards a geography of science in Europe* (Dordrecht, 2003), p. 1; and eaedem, 'Building the Republic of Letters. The scientific travels of Portuguese naturalist Correia da Serra (1751–1823)', *Revue de la Maison Française d'Oxford*, vol. I, 2 (2003).

100 Simões, Carneiro and Diogo (1999), p. 1.

101 Joaquim de Carvalho, *Jacob de Castro Sarmento et l'introduction des conceptions de Newton em Portugal* (Lisbon, 1935); Timothy Coates, 'Timothy D. Walker, *Doctors, folk medicine and the Inquisition. The repression of magical healing in Portugal during the Enlightenment* (Brill: Leiden.Boston, 2005)', *e-JPH*, vol. 5, 1 (Summer 2007).

Naturally, all of these changes transformed the geography of the teaching of medicine. The Spanish domination over Portugal until 1640 favoured the life of the Portuguese Jews in the Spanish kingdom and their presence in its universities, mainly in Salamanca. Portuguese independence after that date led to the end of the massive exodus to Torme's university. As an example, by 1650–51, only 11 new Portuguese students had matriculated in Salamanca.[102] The same can be observed in other countries, following the end of the persecution of the Jews.[103] As a result, Portuguese scholars became very rare in the French Midi. In Montpellier, only two Portuguese medical students have been found between 1600 and 1640, while five attended the University of Toulouse in the period 1570 to 1660, according to data provided by the classic studies of Joaquim Veríssimo Serrão.[104]

Eventually this resulted in a preference for the Dutch Low Countries, especially Amsterdam,[105] and later for cities such Hamburg[106] and London.[107] The Portuguese Jews in the first of these cities formed a noticeable community, with an elite of well-educated persons that thrived upon real religious toleration.[108] The cultural environment was obviously bound to attract people such as Isaac Orosio de

---

[102] Marco de Díos (1991), p. 159.

[103] As an example, the traditional protection offered by the dukedom in Ferrara ended towards the end of the century, with its return to the Church. Zorattini (1993), p. 9.

[104] Serrão (1971), pp. 129–32; Serrão (1970), p. 129.

[105] For the Portuguese Jewish presence in Amsterdam, see Yosef Kaplan, *From Christianity to Judaism: The story of Isaac Orobio de Castro* (Oxford, 1989); idem, 'The Portuguese community of Amsterdam in the 17th century. Between tradition and change', in A. Haim (ed.) *Society and community* (Jerusalem, 1991), pp. 141–71; Bodian (1997); Daniel M. Swetschinski, *Reluctant cosmopolitans: The Portuguese Jews of seventeenth-century Amsterdam* (London, 2000); Shana Loise Stuart, *The Portuguese Jewish community in seventeenth-century Amsterdam: Images of commemoration and documentation (Volumes I and II)*, PhD dissertation (Kansas, 1992) and the articles presented in Chaya Brasz and Yosef Kaplan (eds) *Dutch Jews as perceived by themselves and by others. Proceedings of the Eighth International Symposium on the History of the Jews in the Netherlands* (Leiden, 2000).

[106] Dean Phillip Bell, *Jewish identity in early modern Germany: Memory, power and community* (Aldershot, 2007), pp. 39, 91–2. Famous Portuguese Jewish physicians such as Rodrigo de Castro, founder of gynaecology, and his sons Henrique Rodrigues (Samuel Cohen) and Samuel da Silva, all lived there (Cecil Roth, *História dos Marranos. Os Judeus Secretos da Península Ibérica.* Translated by José Saraiva and edited by Herman P. Salomon (Barcelos, 2001), pp. 155–6).

[107] Evelyne Oliel-Grausz, 'A study in intercommunal relations in the Sephardi diaspora: London and Amsterdam in the eighteenth century', in *Dutch Jews as perceived by themselves and by others...* (Leiden, 2000), p. 41; Aron Leoni *The Hebrew Portuguese nations in Antwerp and London at the time of Charles V and Henry VIII. New documents and interpretations* (New Jersey, 2004).

[108] Yosef Kaplan, '*Gente política:* the Portuguese Jews of Amsterdam vis-à-vis Dutch society', in *Dutch Jews as perceived by themselves and by others...* (Leiden, 2000), p. 22.

Castro. After passing through France he arrived in Amsterdam, where he defended Jewish ideals and the Jewish way of life.[109] The educational situation was also favourable factor, since it was common in Dutch universities to attend for only a few days, the time needed to present a thesis prepared in advance and to meet all the necessary bureaucratic requirements for obtaining a degree. This was the case with the 11 Jewish students belonging to the Portuguese and Spanish communities of Amsterdam who received the degree of MD from Leiden University between 1655 and 1686.[110]

Establishing where these individuals found employment is only one of the ways of studying this aspect of the *peregrinatio medica* during this period. The available bibliography enables us to introduce another question concerning this matter: their occupations following their medical studies.

The Careers of Physicians Who Studied Abroad

It is not easy to propose a synthesis of information about this cohort, since our knowledge of these individuals is mostly restricted to evidence of their having attended university.[111] It is also difficult to draw a social portrait of the group, since strategies for social and family promotion varied from one individual to another[112] and can be reconstructed, with great difficulty, in only a few cases.

The prestige acquired through prominent teaching careers could open the way to more profitable offices. In first place, clearly, came service to the king as a royal physician,[113] as in the examples provided by the biographies of Jerónimo de Miranda, Próspero Dias, Manuel Afonso or Manuel Fernandes de Moura.[114] We should add that this service was not exclusively to the Portuguese Crown,

[109] Kaplan (1989).

[110] Yosef Kaplan, 'An alternative path to modernity', in Yosef Kaplan (ed.) *An alternative path to modernity. The Sephardi diaspora in western Europe* (Leiden, 2000), p. 14.

[111] Obviously the specific studies of scholars, such as those of Joaquim Veríssimo Serrão, are very important for this characterisation because they gather, from a large range of sources, all the biographical data available at the time about the individual. Unfortunately, the biographies concern a limited numbers of scholars, generally those with important humanistic careers or with a known scholarly production.

[112] Although in some cases it is possible to assume that the study and practice of medicine was a 'family affair'. Pinto (1996), p. 1000; Serrão (1971), pp. 118–19; Matos (1952), pp. 154–5.

[113] The importance of Jewish physicians at the royal court began in the reign of King John I (Domingos Maurício, 'Judeus Portugueses', *Verbo – Inciclopédia Luso-Brasileira de Cultura*, vol. 11 (Lisbon, 1971), p. 838. For a general overview, Reuven Faingold, 'Judeus nas Cortes Reais Portuguesas' (electronic edition: www.reuvenfaingold.com/artigos/12.pdf).

[114] Pinto (1996), p. 998, 1001; Serrão (1971), pp. 73–4, 128, 130–3.

since teaching abroad provided excellent opportunities for serving other royal families,[115] or even the pope.[116]

But for the majority of these scholars – for whom personal service to the Crown was completely unattainable – a degree in medicine allowed them to assume the profession of physician in a wide range of institutions. Among the most significant, for their size and importance, were the hospitals established throughout the Portuguese kingdom from the beginning of the sixteenth century.[117] The presence of some of these *estrangeirados* in the most important of them all, the hospital of All Saints in Lisbon, is thus not surprising.[118] A similar career was also possible outside the kingdom, as is evidenced by the presence of Portuguese doctors working at Toulouse's Hotel-Dieu[119] or practising their skills in the hospitals of the monastery of Guadalupe.[120]

The municipalities were other institutions which frequently called on the services of physicians, as in the town of Elvas in 1498.[121] But probably most common of all was private practice in the urban centres, since it was in these places that a large proportion of the population was concentrated. A city like Lisbon had from 40 to 60 physicians working within its limits around the middle of the sixteenth century.[122] The same occurred abroad, with Manuel Alvares, who worked around Toulouse, while Ambrósio Nunes did the same at Seville and Francisco da Silva at Bordeaux.[123] Curiously, however, not every physician practised in the big cities, as is shown by the cases of Francisco Rodrigues, Francisco Lopes and Francisco Alvares, who practised respectively in Vila da Foz do Lima, in the north, and Crato and Vidigueira, both located in southern Portugal.[124] Finally, is

---

115 Luís Nunes was one of the physicians of Catarina of Medicis. Pinto (1996), p. 998.

116 Amato Lusitano practised medicine in Ancona, Rome, Pesaro and Salonica, becoming one of Pope Jules III's physicians (Maximiliano de Lemos, 'Amato Lusitano em Ferrara', *A Medicina Contemporânea*, vol. 24, 37 (1906), pp. 294–6; 38 (1906), pp. 299–301, among many other studies.

117 On this matter, see Isabel M.R. Mendes Drumond Braga, *Assistência, Saúde Pública e Prática Médica em Portugal. Séculos XV–XIX* (Lisbon, 2001).

118 Pinto (1996), p. 1001.

119 Pinto (1996), p. 1004; Serrão (1970), pp. 140–55.

120 Luís de Pina, *As relações de Portugal com a escola de medicina de Nossa Senhora de Guadalupe* (Lisbon, 1935).

121 In one of their chapters of the Cortes of Lisbon, their procurators said that the town always had to pay a physician and a grammar master. Costa (1987), p. 255.

122 These numbers are supplied from testimonies of the time. Cristóvão Rodrigues de Oliveira mentions the presence of 57 physicians, 60 surgeons and 46 apothecaries. João Brandão's testimony, around the same date, puts forward the number of 40 physicians. Cristóvão Rodrigues de Oliveira, *Lisboa em 1551. Sumário* (Lisbon, 1987), pp. 94, 129.

123 Pinto (1996), pp. 1003–4, 1006 ; Serrão (1971), pp. 134–6.

124 Serrão (1971), pp. 106–7, 128–9.

not impossible that a few physicians educated abroad chose to follow medical careers in the Portuguese Empire.

The statistics referred to above for the number of physicians working in Lisbon raise the problem of their education. Were they all graduates from the Portuguese university, or from a foreign centre of learning? Had they actually graduated? Of course we do not have a definite answer to that question. From other examples,[125] one can assume that educated physicians were never sufficient in number to satisfy the needs of the kingdom. In fact, from the fourteenth century onwards it is possible to observe the royal preoccupation with the elimination of charlatans and with obliging physicians, surgeons and apothecaries to submit to a mandatory examination prior to starting practice.[126] Excluded by the enormous cost of a university education, these men were primarily practitioners without any specialist education. Learning by observing and repeating the practice of more experienced physicians, they were as far removed as could be from the learned and graduate royal physician who was appointed to examine them.[127]

Excluded from the university institutions of their own country, at least some of them had profitable careers after passing through foreign medical faculties. The case of Abraão Zacuto Lusitano is a perfect case in point. After studying

[125] Jon Arrizabalaga, 'The ideal medical practitioner in Counter-Reformation Castile: The perception of the *converso* physician Henrique Jorge Henriques (c. 1555–1622)', in Samuel S. Kottel and Luís García-Ballester (eds) *Medicine and medical ethics in medieval and early modern Spain. An intercultural approach* (Jerusalem, 1996), pp. 61–91.

[126] The scholars would not have needed this authorisation since they had their diplomas by which they could confirm their studies. The first mention of this obligation dates from 1338, when these exams seem to have taken place in Lisbon before the royal physicians Masters Alfonso and Gonçalo, after which a royal charter of proof was presented. Existing during the reign of Alphonse IV, the same practice was followed in the time of John I and his son Edward, even if none of these charters is registered in the royal chanceries up to the time of the latter. These measures were in place until the beginning of the sixteenth century, when the king's physicians and surgeons were responsible. All of these facts were studied by Iria Gonçalves, who gathered 296 of these charters dated between 1434 and 1495 (Iria Gonçalves, 'Físicos e cirurgiões Quatrocentistas. As cartas de exame', *Do Tempo e da História*, 1 (1965), pp. 69–112; Serrão (1962), p. 117).

[127] For instance, in the case of the two masters referred in to 1338, only for Master Alfonso do we have enough information about his biography. Graduated in arts, medicine and theology by the University of Paris, he was very close to Alphonse IV, who, after Alfonso had been his physician and secretary, gave him the bishoprics of Guarda and Évora (António Domingues de Sousa Costa, 'Mestre Afonso Dinis, médico e secretário de D. Afonso IV, Professor na Universidade de Paris', *Itinerarium*, vol. III, 15 (May–June 1957), pp. 370–417; 16–17 (July–August 1957), pp. 510–607; José F. Meirinhos, 'Afonso de Dinis de Lisboa: percurso de um filósofo, médico, teólogo, tradutor e eclesiástico do século XIV', *Península. Revista de Estudos Ibéricos*, 4 (2007), pp. 47–64; Mário Farelo, 'Ao serviço da Coroa no século XIV. O Percurso de uma família de Lisboa, os "Nogueiras"', *Lisboa Medieval. Os rostos da Cidade* (Lisbon, 2007), pp. 150–51.

philosophy in Coimbra and medicine at Sigüenza, he practised in Lisbon for a while.[128] Despite the legislation against them,[129] the Jews were numerous in Salamanca during the Dual Monarchy. According to the information available, none of them was excluded on the grounds of the 'limpieza de sangue', and they formed around 70 per cent of the total of Portuguese medical students there.[130]

This overview raises more questions than there are answers. The decision to seek a better medical education outside the schools of Portugal was based on a mixture of ambition and necessity. The geography of the universities attended shows that distance or prestige could play a decisive role when it came time to choosing a centre of learning. As shown by the Jewish case, political circumstances and family/social relations were also factors to be borne in mind when discussing the reasons for such a move.

This is not the place to determine whether ambition or necessity was the driving force, nor have we sufficient data to do so. In fact, this overview reflects the great amount of work still needing to be done: research on the matriculation records of northern and central European universities, so profoundly ignored by Portuguese historians, as well as prosopographical research to determine the education of individuals and the paths they took, using Portuguese and foreign sources of information. Only then can we go beyond general ideas based on poor data or on the prevalence of better-known cases, and characterise with certainty the various flows of Portuguese students across Europe, and see to what extent they may have differed according to the students' religions.

Despite all of this, one fact seems firm. Faithful to the humanistic ideals of culture and education, Portuguese medical students did not hesitate to follow prestigious physicians, some of them their own countrymen. In the end, it was a small price to pay for a degree that could pave the way to an eminent teaching career or to introduction into royal courts and important charitable institutions.

---

[128] Araújo (1990), p. 273.

[129] Grangel (2000), p. 4.

[130] Joaquim Candeias Silva, 'Estudantes do distrito de Castelo Branco na Universidade de Salamanca (1580–1640)', *Medicina na Beira Interior. Da Pré-História ao Século XX – Cadernos de Cultura*, 11 (November 1997), p. 64.

Chapter 6

Pieter van Foreest and the Acquisition and Travelling of Medical Knowledge in the Sixteenth Century

Catrien Santing

The epitaph of Pieter van Foreest (1521–97) ran: *Hippocrates batavus si fuit ille fuit* – 'if there had been a Batavian Hippocrates, it was him'. The line indicates how, at the end of his life, Van Foreest's fame had acquired an overwhelming status, although he did not aspire to an academic career and had only started to publish late in life. Even his travelling had not been exceptionally extensive for his generation of medical doctors. As far as is known, he did all his long-distance travelling before 1546, during the first 25 years of his life. After his marriage in Alkmaar, in September 1546, to Eva van Teylingen, the daughter of his home town's mayor, his radius of action shrank considerably: from Alkmaar he moved to Delft, where he practised as an official town physician for almost 40 years. From Delft he occasionally took trips to Alkmaar, Amsterdam, Haarlem, the Hague, Rotterdam and Leiden, which in those days were all very doable distances.[1]

Nonetheless, his student itinerary via Louvain towards Bologna, Padua, Rome and finally Paris can be appraised as fairly typical, as well as crucial for his development into a famous medical doctor and author, as will be demonstrated in the first half of this chapter. One might argue that while, in his youth, Van Foreest travelled and acquired medical knowledge by passing and sojourning at the centres of medical excellence of his day, during his professional years he concentrated on

[1] On Van Foreest there are several publications in Dutch which contain more or less the same information. See, firstly, Henriette A. Bosman-Jelgersma (ed.), *Pieter van Foreest. De Hollandse Hippocrates* (Krommenie, 1996) and eadem, *Petrus Forestus Medicus* (n.p., n.d.). Also H.L. Houtzager (ed.), *Pieter van Foreest. Een Hollands medicus in de zestiende eeuw* (Amsterdam, 1989). A biography was published by Bosman-Jelgersma, *Pieter van Foreest*, as above, pp. 9–17. On the medical context see H. Beukers, 'Theoretische achtergrond'; Anthonie Luyendijk-Elshout, 'Een humanistisch arts te midden van zijn tijdgenoten', in Bosman-Jelgersma, *Pieter van Foreest*, pp. 49–57, and H.L. Houtzager, 'Opleiding in Frankrijk en verblijf in Italië', in eadem, pp. 81–6. Two German-language dissertations have been published on his medical works: R. Burri, *Die Delfter Pest von 1557 nach den Beobachtungen von Petrus Forestus* (Zürich, 1982), and I.W. Müller, *Iatromechanische Theorie und ärztliche Praxis im Vergleich zur galenistischen Medizin: Friedrich Hoffmann – Pieter van Foreest, Jan van Heurne* (Stuttgart, 1991).

the collection and exploitation of medical knowledge to be demonstrated in his writings. This implies that during this time he mainly made do with travelling medical expertise. Both types, the knowledge that travelling medical students and doctors acquired, as well as itinerant medical knowledge sought by writing letters to colleagues and the exchange of books, are reflected in his written oeuvre.

Throughout his life he conducted a busy correspondence with friends, colleagues, patrons and authorities, which for the professional-medical part mainly originated from his – or his friends' – student days. In cases of doubt, Van Foreest did not hesitate to consult colleagues, if necessary through the help of others. In 1563, for instance, the wife of Willem Cripius, the Delft burgomaster, had a miscarriage and he was unable to stop the resulting bleeding. Via the court of Prince William of Orange, then resident at Delft, he knew the Brussels councillor Viglius van Aytta, who advised him to submit the problem to an old acquaintance of them both, the Louvain medical professor and astronomer Cornelius Gemma Frisius (1535–78). So the case history was sent to Louvain, whereupon Gemma advised by written word to purge with sienna and rhubarb. Later on, the correspondence was incorporated in Van Foreest's vast collection of case histories, *Observationes et curationes medicinales*.[2] This series of books might be hailed as an embodiment of sixteenth-century travelling medical knowledge, and in the following will be perused as such. This series of works, together with the unpublished dialogue against itinerant healers entitled *Van der Empiriken*, make up the focus of the second half of this chapter. They will be analysed to show Van Foreest's medical network, for his books functioned as a medium for the circulation of professional information in what might be called the '*res publica medica*' of the second half of the sixteenth century. At that time its centre of gravity was shifting from south to north, although the Italian contacts remained very important and a lot of information moved back and forth.

Towards the end of his life Van Foreest sent a letter to a colleague, the Leiden medical professor Johannes Heurnius (1543–1601), in which he looked back on his long career. In this letter he congratulated himself on having published so many books that had brought such great benefit to society. Even better was the fact that the most eminent physicians of his time – he mentions specifically the Paduan professor Hieronymus Mercurialis (1530–1606) and the German Joachim Camerarius (1566–1643) – had sent him their reactions.[3] Heurnius held his older friend in the same high esteem. In his answer, the town of Alkmaar is congratulated for having hired the best physician of that time. This praise, Heurnius says, was not just his own personal opinion, but sung by all civilized countries alike: Italy,

---

[2] Gerard van der Waa, 'De medische praktijkvoering van Forestus', in Bosman-Jelgersma, *Petrus Forestus*, pp. 46–7. *Observationes*, Lib. 28, obs. 64.

[3] Letter inserted in *Observationes*, Libri 24–25, also Chris L. Heesakkers, 'Petrus Forestus in gedichten en brieven. Een overzicht van het materiaal en editie van zijn correspondentie met Johannes Heurnius', in Bosman-Jelgersma, *Petrus Forestus Medicus*, pp. 129–244, esp. 173.

Germany, France and England.[4] Apparently, Pieter van Foreest's expert medical knowledge had travelled all over Europe.

Van Foreest's Itinerary

Pieter van Foreest was born in 1521 in Alkmaar, which at that time was a rich commercial centre in the north of the county of Holland. Seventy-six years later, he passed away there too. This exemplifies the circle of life of sixteenth-century professionals from northern Europe. They travelled south, usually in the company of fellow townsmen or other persons from the same area, to return home and make a career on the basis of the knowledge, outlook and professional network acquired elsewhere.[5] In case of Van Foreest, close ties within his extended family also stimulated the successful course of his career. The circumstances of his birth were favourable, for he sprang from a very prolific patrician family which fostered its connections with the governmental elite of Holland. His father, Jorden van Foreest, served as mayor of Alkmaar.[6]

Young Pieter attended the local Latin school under the well-known humanistic pedagogue Petrus Nannius (1500–57), who happened to be a maternal uncle. The two of them may have travelled south together, because in 1537 uncle Nannius was appointed at the Louvain college of St Hieronymus and soon transferred as a professor of Latin to the prestigious Collegium Trilingue.[7] The medical profession seems to have run in the family, although allegedly Van Foreest's father had wanted him to read law, at that time a more prestigious discipline. Only after the mediation of uncle Nannius did he get permission to concentrate on the study that, in his own words, 'in dignity, excellence, utility and indispensability surpassed all other disciplines'.[8] In his *Brief over de scheurbuik* [*Letter on scurvy*] (1590), addressed to his nephews Adam and Jorden van Foreest, both at the time medical students at Padua, he boasted that the Van Foreest family had already known four academically trained medical doctors.[9] His namesake Pieter had been

---

[4] Ibid., p. 77. On the medical work of Van Foreest and Heurnius, see Müller, *Iatromechanische Theorie.*

[5] Willem Frijhoff, 'Graduation and careers', in H. De Ridder-Symoens, *A History of the University in Europe* (Cambridge, 1996) vol. 2, pp. 355–415.

[6] For a survey of his life see Henriette A. Bosman-Jelgersma, 'De levensloop van Pieter van Foreest', in eadem, *Pieter van Foreest*, pp. 9–16. On the Van Foreest family see H.A. van Foreest, *Het oude geslacht Van Foreest, 1250–1570* (Assen, 1950).

[7] Emiel Lamberts and Jan Roegiers, *De universiteit te Leuven, 1425–1985* (Louvain, 1988) p. 72.

[8] Remark about his choice in Dedication to the town of Delft in *Observationes*, Libri 1–2. Also Heesakkers, 'Petrus Forestus', p. 129

[9] Ibid., p. 135. For a modern edition of this treatise, see M.A. van Andel, 'Petrus Forestus *De scorbuto malo conoscendo et curando*', *Opuscula selecta Neerlandicorum de*

town physician of Dordrecht, while one Dirk van Foreest (ca. 1485–1535), after having qualified in medicine in Louvain and Italy, landed up, via Constantinople, in Poland. Through holding the position of personal physician to the archbishop of Vilnius, he earned the epithet 'the Polish doctor'. This does not mean that family contacts came to an end. For once in a while this doctor travelled home, as Pieter van Foreest recalled a visit of his kinsman to Alkmaar, during which he encouraged the then young schoolboy to pursue a medical career. Finally, there were his own brothers Jacob and Jan. The first graduated in 1565 in Ferrara, having studied medicine in Louvain and Padua.[10]

Turning 15 or 16, Van Foreest left the local Latin school and started at the Louvain *artes* faculty or at one of the propaedeutic *paedagogia* of that same town.[11] At that time, for students from the west and south of the present-day Netherlands, it was normal to begin their university studies in Louvain, while those from the north and east also might opt for Cologne. Because of its blossoming humanistic fame during the course of the sixteenth century Louvain, however, outshone Cologne to the extent that the majority of students went to the southern Netherlands.[12] Due to his comprehensive training in Alkmaar, Van Foreest did not need much time for the arts, as his approximately three years at Louvain were also used to make a start with medicine. He matriculated in the medical faculty in April 1539. Nevertheless, his medical studies cannot have been very extensive, for in 1540 he was back home in Alkmaar to prepare for his voyage south.

Due to sour comments by Andreas Vesalius and their interpretation in secondary literature, sixteenth-century medical education at Louvain university acquired a somewhat dubious reputation.[13] Van Foreest's years in Louvain, however, may have been quite interesting from a medico-professional point of view. Not only was Vesalius again temporarily present at that time, but his accomplice in performing illegal dissections, Reinerus Gemma Frisius (1508–55), also had his

---

arte medica (Amsterdam, 1935) vol. 13, pp. 17–93.

[10] Youth Jurjen N.M. Vis, 'Alkmaarse jaren 1528–1528', in Bosman-Jelgersma, *Pieter van Foreest*, pp. 71–81. Biographies of the family members who studied in Italy are to be found in A.L. Tervoort, *The Iter Italicum and the Northern Netherlands. Dutch students at Italian universities and their role in the Netherlands' society* (1426–1575) (Leiden, 2005), biographies on CD-ROM.

[11] A. Schillings, *Matricule de l'université de Louvain* (Brussels, 1961), vol. 4, p. 191. This is only Van Foreest's matriculation in medicine from 1539. The matriculation was together with three other youngsters from Alkmaar and two from the nearby town, Den Helder. On the *paedagogia* and their preparatory tasks, see Willem Frijhoff, 'Patterns', in H. de Ridder-Symoens, *A History of the University in Europe* (Cambridge, 1996) vol., 2, pp. 43–110, esp. 47–57.

[12] Tervoort, *Iter Italicum*, pp. 27–8, 30. See for surveys of student mobility Hilde de Ridder-Symoens, 'Mobility', in eadem, *A History of the University in Europe* (Cambridge, 1992) vol. 1, pp. 280–304 and eadem, 'Mobility', in ibid. vol. 2, pp. 416–48

[13] C.D. O'Malley, *Andreas Vesalius of Brussels, 1514–1564* (Berkeley, 1964) pp. 32–4 and 62–72.

domicile in the town. The two of them together constructed an articulated skeleton by stealing bones hanging from the gibbet, which they left at the home of their friend and fellow student Gisbertus Carbo. The latter, by the way, would become town physician of Louvain. Of course, one cannot help wondering whether Van Foreest admired the skeleton during his stay. After his sojourn in Paris Vesalius had returned to Louvain in August 1536 to study with Johannes Heems of Alementières, alias Armentarius. Under the authority of this medical professor, in February 1537 Vesalius defended his baccalaureate thesis, *Paraphrase on the Ninth Book of Rhazes*. Contact with both his professor and the town administration must have been very good, as Vesalius obtained permission to conduct a public dissection for his fellow students. It had been 18 years since the city had witnessed such a performance. Again, it is very tempting to conclude that Van Foreest was in attendance, although later he claimed to have mastered in Louvain only theoretical medicine, learning its practical equivalent in Italy.[14]

Thanks to Vesalius' visit, and maybe due to open-minded academics such as Armentarius, Carbo and Gemma, all much praised by Vesalius, the town turned into a short-lived, albeit still rather bleak, centre of medical excellence. For all that, it is quite understandable that Van Foreest studied medicine in Louvain only very briefly. On the whole, Vesalius' criticism of Louvain medical studies seems to have been justified, for in 1541 the two official *ordinarii medicinae*, Leonardus Willemaers and Arnoldus Noot, were fired due to negligence and incompetence. Both Vesalius and Van Foreest had already studied under their substitute, Jeremias de Drijvere of Brakel, alias Jeremias Thriverius Brachelius (1504–44). The latter is still known for his famous dispute with Vesalius on bloodletting. Thriverius had defended the practice, following the methods of the Arab physicians, which were ridiculed by his pupil in public and in very harsh words. This youthful criticism developed into the sarcasm to be found in Vesalius' *Six tables* [*Tabulae sex*] and in his *Venesection Letter*.[15] From his *Observationes*, it is clear that Van Foreest knew this controversy very well, again because he may have witnessed the beginning of

---

[14] Pieter van Foreest, *Van der Empiriken, Lantloeperen ende valscher Medicijns bedroch. Unpublished Manuscript*, Regional Archive Alkmaar, Inv. van Foreest nr 33, f. 318. Partial transcription by Henriette A. Bosman-Jelgersma, 'Handschrift tegen kwakzalverij en onbevoegde geneeskunde', in eadem, *Petrus Forestus Medicus*, pp. 257–90 and eadem, 'Van die tweede species Therapeutices', in idem, *Petrus Forestus Medicus*, pp. 299–326. On this see Vivian Nutton, 'Idle old trots, cobblers and costardmongers. Pieter van Foreest on quackery', in Bosman-Jelgersma, *Petrus Forestus Medicus*, pp. 245–58. Dedication to the town of Delft in *Observationes*, Libri 1–2, also in Heesakkers, 'Gedichten en brieven', p. 129. On the medical faculty in Louvain, see Lamberts and Roegiers, *Universiteit van Leuven*, pp. 77–85, and Omer Steeno en Maurits Biesbrouck, 'Gisbert Coolen alias Gisbertus Carbo, een Leuvense vriend van Andreas Vesalius', in Luc Misotten (ed.), *Omtrent Vesalius* (Louvain, 2007), pp. 21–40.

[15] Hieremias Thriverius, *De missione sanguinis in pleuritide* (Louvain, 1532). On this, Francine de Nave and M. de Schepper (eds), *De Geneeskunde in de Zuidelijke Nederlanden (1475–1660). Tentoonstelling Museum Plantijn/Moretus, 1 september /25 november 1990*

the dispute, but of course also because he had read the antagonists' publications. Nevertheless, he was cautious about taking sides, as sometimes he defends Galen and at other times Avicenna.[16]

In those days ambitious young men broadened their outlook by attending more than one university. They started their *artes* studies close to home and then quite often travelled further afield to continue their studies in one of the higher faculties. From the end of the fifteenth century onwards, the so-called *peregrinatio academia* acquired a different character. Humanism advocated studious travelling not only for mastering knowledge that was not available at home, but also for intellectual and ethical self-development. Later in his life Van Foreest looked back very fondly on his Italian and French time as a period in which he had enjoyed many 'wonderlicke dingen'– marvellous phenomena.[17] The 'man of the world' attitude, indispensable for a profitable career at home, was thought to be attained via visiting famous men, places and natural phenomena. For a man with a patrician background, such as Van Foreest, and an aspiring medical doctor, Italy was the obvious goal. Like many of his countrymen, Van Foreest chose to stay in Bologna, which was from the fifteenth century onwards the most popular place to continue for medical students who had started in Louvain. Only after 1550 did Padua gradually take over in popularity. The numbers of former Louvainians at other universities are very low.[18]

In Bologna the most famous physicians of the time, Berengario da Carpi, Benedetto Vettori, Luca Ghini and others became his teachers.[19] Taking the medical faculty of Bologna as his base, Van Foreest also travelled to Venice and Padua. In Padua he further developed his expertise with Giambattista da Monte (1488–1551), one of the first medical professors to lecture from the bedside of his hospital patients.[20] He also clearly spent some time there with Vesalius (Figure

(Antwerp, 1990), nr 53, pp. 180–81. In general, O'Malley, *Vesalius*, pp. 65–8 and Lamberts and Roegiers, *Universiteit Leuven*, p. 80.

16 Harm Beukers, 'Theoretische achtergrond', pp. 25–6.

17 *Van der Empiriken*, f. 318. On the *peregrinatio* of Dutch students, see Tervoort, *Iter Italicum*, esp. ch. 2, pp. 25–142.

18 Ibid., *Iter Italicum*, pp. 8–39 and map 2.3.1, p. 381.

19 A survey of medical developments in the sixteenth century can be found in A. Wear, R. French and I.M. Lonie (eds), *The Medical Renaissance of the sixteenth century* (Cambridge, 1985). For Italian medical faculties, see Paul F. Grendler, *The universities of the Italian Renaissance* (Baltimore, 2002) pp. 314–52.

20 Giuseppe Cerveto, *Di Giambattista da Monte e della medicina italiana nel secolo XVI* (Verona, 1839), pp. 47–8 and 53; Jerome J. Bylebyl, 'The school of Padua. Humanistic medicine in the sixteenth century', in Charles Webster, *Health, medicine and mortality in the sixteenth century* (Cambridge, 1979), pp. 335–70, esp. and Bylebyl, 'Teaching *Methodus medendi* in the Renaissance', in Richard J. Durling and Fridolf Kudlien, (eds) *Galen's Method of Healing* (Leiden, 1991), pp. 157–89, esp. pp. 183–5. Also Grendler, *Italian Universities*, pp. 341–2 and Nancy G. Siraisi, *Avicenna in Renaissance Italy* (Princeton, 1987), pp. 248–54, who discusses Da Monte's commentary on Avicenna.

6.1), who at that time was busy preparing his 1543 *Seven books on the fabric of the human body* [*De humani corporis fabrica libri septem*].[21] Apart from performing public dissections as lessons for surgical trainees and midwives in the context of his job as a Delft town physician, Van Foreest never became much of an anatomist. His interests remained thoroughly clinical. The *Observationes* demonstrate that he used anatomy primarily to prove the accuracy of his diagnosis in retrospective. The Van Foreest family, however, cherished the story of their ancestor's friendship with Vesalius. There exists (Figure 1) a nineteenth-century rendering of the visit, done for Sir – the family had certainly been upwardly mobile – Cornelis van Foreest. The watercolour goes back to Pieter Van Foreest's *Against irregular healers* [*Van der Emperiken*], an unpublished colloquy which remained for centuries in manuscript in the possession of the family. In this work Pieter van Foreest mentions his visit to Vesalius, who, he does not forget to underscore, received his countrymen very nicely and friendlily, although he was very busy opening up corpses and anatomising them. In later life contact between the two doctors must have been sparse. The *Observationes* contain just one consultation by Vesalius, one that is, tellingly, not on anatomy. It concerns an advice dating from 1556 over an unstoppable bleeding of the nose of the then Louvain student Augustinus van Teylingen, probably a nephew of Van Foreest´s wife. The *consilium* by Vesalius was sent to Van Foreest in the form of a written clinical lesson. The patient recovered, although it was found that the use of his legs remained defective. Nevertheless, his physician claims, the patient continued his studies in France and Italy.[22] This assertion is true, as Van Teylingen matriculated in 1562 in Padua, graduated in 1565 in law at Siena and finished off his education in 1565 in Orléans.[23] Despite the shared background with Vesalius, Van Foreest's anatomical knowledge must have been mainly acquired under the Bolognese anatomist Berengario da Carpi (1470–1550), whom in his *Observationes* he calls a 'chirurgus expertissimus'. Da Carpi was an accurate observer and the author of a well-known handbook in the field and in those days even more famous than Vesalius.[24]

---

[21] O'Malley, *Andreas Vesalius*, 20–21 and R.Van Hee (ed.), *Ziek of gezond ten tijde van Keizer Karel. Vesalius en de gezondheidszorg in de 16de eeuw* (Ghent, 2000), pp. 29–56.

[22] O'Malley, *Vesalius*, pp. 266–7. Henriette A. Bosman-Jelgersma, 'Hoe Pieter van Foreest de geleerde Petrus Forestus werd', in Houtzager, *Pieter van Foreest*, pp. 22–3. *Observationes*, Lib. 10, obs. 97.

[23] Tervoort, *Iter Italicum*, biography nr. 58 on CD-ROM.

[24] Berengario da Carpi, *Isagogae breues et exactissimae in anatomiam humani corporis* (Bologna, 1530). For developments in anatomy see Roger French, 'Berengario da Carpi and the use of commentary in anatomical teaching', in Wear, *Medical Renaissance*, pp. 42–74.

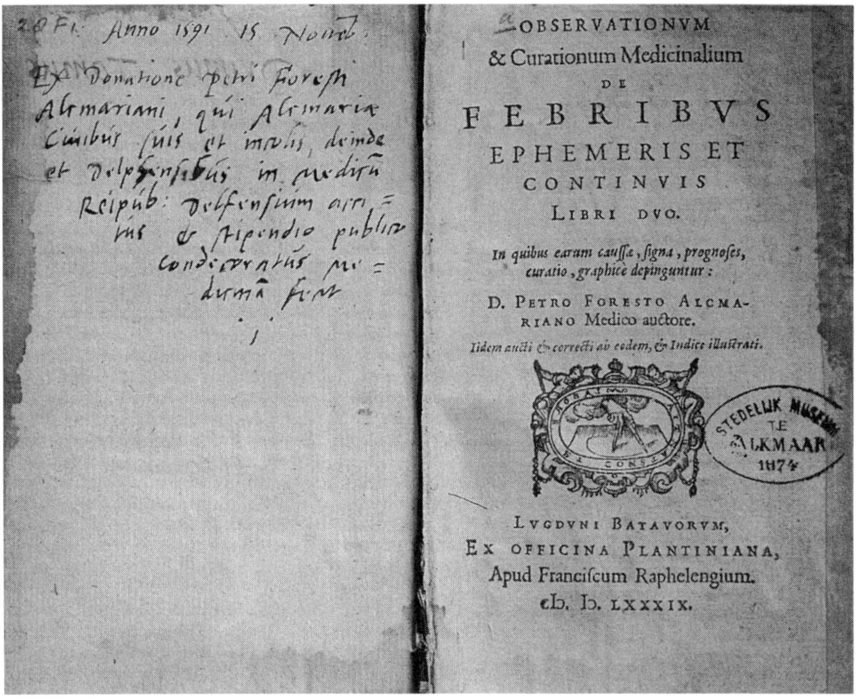

OBSERVATIONVM
& Curationum Medicinalium
DE
FEBRIBVS
EPHEMERIS ET
CONTINVIS
LIBRI DVO.
In quibus earum caussæ, signa, prognoses, curatio, graphicè depinguntur:
D. PETRO FORESTO ALCMARIANO Medico auctore.
Iidem aucti & correcti ab eodem, & Indice illustrati.
LVGDVNI BATAVORVM,
EX OFFICINA PLANTINIANA,
Apud Franciscum Raphelengium.
cIↃ. IↃ. LXXXIX.

Fig. 6.1 The student Pieter van Foreest visits Vesalius in Padua. Watercolour by Alexander Verhuell for Sir C. van Foreest, 1873.

Two other Bolognese medical professors, Luca Ghini (1490–1556) and Benedetto Vettori (1481–1562), seem to have been the teachers who influenced him most. The first taught in Bologna between 1534 and 1544 as the holder of the first chair of simple medicines (*cathedra de simplicibus*), thus teaching the preparation of medicines and their application. Ghini is still known also the inventor of the herbarium of dried plants and the founder of the botanical gardens in Pisa and Florence. Van Foreest mentions that he had followed his lectures on Dioscorides' *Materia Medica*, and had a distinct memory of all the live plants Ghini brought to his lectures to be shown to his students.[25] Throughout his life, Van Foreest maintained a keen interest in pharmacy, and again and again emphasised the appropriate selection of pharmaceutical remedies and their correct methods of preparation and administration. From the start of the University of Leiden he encouraged its authorities to construct a botanical garden presenting up-to-date medical teaching. Particular attention to botanical and pharmaceutical matters is

[25] A.G. Keller, 'Luca Ghini', in Charles E. Gillespie, *Dictionary of scientific biography*, 16 vols (New York, 1970–80), vol 5, pp. 383–4 and Dietrich von Engelhardt, 'Luca Ghini und die Botanik des 16. Jahrhunderts. Leben. Initiativen. Kontakten. Resonanzen', *Medizinhistorisches Journal*, 30 (1995), pp. 3–49. Also *Van der Empiriken*, f. 318.

also reflected in his *Observationes*, where he often describes a remedy, even giving the exact ingredients. In his report on the embalming of William the Silent, which he performed after the Prince's murder at Delft in 1584, for instance, he says that, in addition to plain salt, aloe, terebinth and myrrh had been used, not forgetting, however, to mention that, according to the Evangelist, John Nicodemus had used the same concoction for the preservation of the body of Christ himself.[26] His friend Dirck Kluyt, who was, by the way, married to a niece of his wife and tended his own botanical garden in Delft, supplied the ingredients for this procedure. The two of them together drafted rules and regulations for the local guild of apothecaries to prevent fraud with ingredients. Via the Alkmaar student Wittendellius, both stayed in touch with Hieronymus Mercurialis in Pisa, who sent them seeds from Italy in 1594.[27]

Benedetto Vettori da Faenza, also known as Benedictus Victorius Faventinus (1481–1555), supervised Van Foreest's graduation as *doctor medicinae* on 29 November 1543. Van Foreest's *Observationes* seem to have been profoundly inspired by Vettori's highly successful *Medicinalia consilia ad varia morborum genera* (Venice 1551), later published under the telling title *Empirica*, which makes it obvious that his teacher was famous for his teaching of medical practice. Van Foreest calls him '*Praeceptor meus*' in his *Observationes,* together with a certain Helideus Paduanus Forliviensis, who was the director of the local hospital. Both professors took their students with them into this Nosocomium.[28] In Van Foreest's eyes, Bologna's medical faculty was clearly a centre of medical excellence, as he hailed it later as the place where there 'were precious and learned physicians who cured their patients industriously and conscientiously, thus teaching him the practice of medicine'.[29] It is true that Van Foreest's Italian teachers all were highly professional, innovative and productive doctors. They promoted their works astutely and remained the pre-eminent examples for their northern pupil, although in later life Van Foreest was relieved that Dutch doctors had started to perform equally well. Significantly, in 1594 he praises his friend the Leiden medical professor Johannes Heurnius for 'surpassing in speaking and writing the professors

---

26 *Observationes*, Lib. 29, obs. 29. On this, H.L. Houtzager, 'Pieter van Foreest en de Prins van Oranje', in Bosman-Jelgersma, *Pieter van Foreest*, pp. 119–25, and Lisa Jardine, *The awful end of Prince William the Silent: The first assassination of a head of state with a handgun* (London, 2005).

27 Survey Henriette A. Bosman-Jelgersma, 'Pharmaceutica. Toepassing van geneesmiddelen', in eadem, *Petrus Forestus Medicus*, pp. 293–5, and Heesakkers, 'Gedichten en brieven', pp. 169 and 171.

28 Bosman-Jelgersma, 'Hoe Pieter van Foreest', p. 15 and n. 6. Also *Observationes*, Lib. 1, obs. 17 and ibid., obs. 12. On Vettori see David A. Lines, 'Natural philosophy in Renaissance Italy: The University of Bologna and the beginnings of specialization', *Early science and medicine* 6 (2001), pp. 267–323, esp. biography nr 130, pp. 304–5.

29 *Van der Empiriken*, f. 318.

from Italy'.[30] However, as will be demonstrated hereafter, he maintained contact with some of them throughout his life.

In 1544 he continued his *peregrinatio academica* – in the new sense of acquiring knowledge and gaining extra professional training as well as experience of life. Van Foreest travelled to Rome with a group under the guidance of the German botanist Valerius Cordus (1514–44), whom he had befriended in Padua.[31] The journey was on horseback and the party called at famous places – Venice, Florence, Pisa, Livorno, Lucca, Siena – meanwhile visiting sites that were interesting from either a cultural or a natural philosophical point of view. The travellers examined volcanic stone, minerals and metals, collected botanical specimens and studied various species of birds and fish. The attitude gained on his way south is reflected in Van Foreest's *Van der Emperiken*, in which he scorns physicians whose knowledge of medicinal herbs was completely founded on descriptions and pictures. Although they were not 'empirics' in the sense of unschooled and irregular, as was the case with the abominable quacks, yet their knowledge ought to be based on sense perception in the most literal sense. A true physician had seen the ingredients with his own eyes, and had smelled as well as tasted them. Also he exclaimed that 'it was not enough to sit in schools and bother about lessons, we have to go into the fields, into the woods, into the mountains, hills and valleys to look for medicinal herbs there'.[32]

On their final arrival in Rome, Cordus died in Van Foreest's arms, having caught a fatal fever. Van Foreest was bequeathed the famous collection of dried plants. The rest of his life, he would mourn this dear friend, being convinced that Cordus' knowledge would have changed the medical profession completely if he had made it into old age.[33] In Rome the northern-European network turned out to be indispensable, since Gisbertus Horstius (1491–1556), a physician born in Amsterdam, provided him with a job at the hospital S. Maria della Consolazione, where the latter was in charge.[34] Again, the young doctor exploited his journey and gained as much practical experience as possible. In his *Observationes* Van Foreest discussed the medical problems he went through himself in the Eternal City. Just like Cordus, he suffered there from fevers and caught an inflammation of the throat. In addition to these afflictions, after a week his face also developed problems, as it became thickly studded with solid red swellings. Because he looked a fright, the young doctor was forced to remain inside. At first a laughing Horstius had diagnosed the efflorescences as the unmistakable symptoms of *lues gallica*, the pox. Van Foreest, however, according to Horstius, was not the type to have caught syphilis, and therefore together the two physicians decided on a kind

30 Heesakkers, 'Gedichten en brieven', p. 169.

31 Thomas Archibald Sprague and M.S. Sprague, *The Herbal of Valerius Cordus* (London, 1939).

32 *Van der Empiriken*, f. 317–18.

33 Ibid., f. 320.

34 Bosman-Jelgersma, 'Hoe Pieter van Foreest', pp. 17–18 and *Observationes*, Lib. 2, obs. 13.

of *impetigo*. In the end, the patient healed himself by applying his '*propria salvia*' to the lumps, a cure, he says, already advocated by Avicenna.[35] The fact that his visit to Rome had started under an unlucky star may have induced him to return to the north. In a dedication letter of one his books, his explanation ran that he had become tired of travelling and drifting. Following the advice of his learned Italian friends, he packed his stuff and decided to try his luck in France.[36]

In 1545 the young doctor indeed arrived in Paris, where Guido Guidi (1509–69), alias Vidus Vidius, an acquaintance from Florence, worked as a physician to the French king and taught at the university.[37] Guidi introduced him to the famous Galenist Jacques Dubois, writing under the name of Jacobus Sylvius (1478–1555).[38] This Parisian professor had edited several works by Hippocrates and Galen and wrote a three-volume *materia medica* entitled e *De simplicibus* (Paris 1557). Van Foreest followed his lectures on Galen's book on simple medicines, *De simplicibus*, and became friends with Sylvius. After some insistence, the lofty professor obtained the precious botanical samples that Van Foreest had collected himself in Italy, and those he had inherited in Rome from Valerius Cordus. In return for this costly, probably demanded donation, Sylvius recommended Van Foreest as city physician to the authorities of Pithiviers, a small city near Orléans. It is known from case narratives in the *Observationes* that the young doctor went there, but he seems to have resigned from the position rather soon. In May 1546 he was back home in Alkmaar.[39]

Adolescence was definitely over. At the age of 24 Pieter married and started a medical practice in his home town. Simultaneously, he worked on a semi-official basis as city physician.[40] However, 12 years later a better job came up. The town of Delft required a medical expert because of a serious epidemic of the plague, later to be the subject of the first parts of Van Foreest's *Observationes*.[41] The Delft city council hired him in 1557 and the physician would hold the position for the next 37 years. During this long period he was consulted several times by William

---

35 Bosman-Jelgersma, 'Levensloop', p. 14, and *Observationes*, Lib. 2, obs. 13.

36 Dedication, *Observationes*, Libri 1 and 2, Heesakkers, 'Gedichten en brieven', p. 128.

37 Mirko Grmek, *La période parisienne dans la vie de Guido Guidi anatomiste de Florence et professeur au Collège de France* (Fermo, 1965).

38 Gerhard Baader, 'Jacques Dubois as a practitioner', in Wear, *Medical Renaissance*, pp. 146–55.

39 *Van der Empiriken*, f. 318–19.

40 Vis, 'De Alkmaarse jaren' and idem, 'Alkmaarse stadsdoctoren in de zestiende eeuw', *GEWINA. Tijdschrift voor de geschiedenis der geneeskunde, natuurwetenschappen, wiskunde en techniek*, 21 (1998) pp. 65–80.

41 Burri, *Die Delfter Pest*; Hans L. Houtzager, 'Stadsgeneesheer te Delft', in Bosman-Jelgersma, *Pieter van Foreest*, pp. 99–105, and Vivian Nutton, 'Pieter van Foreest and the plagues of Europe. Some observations on the *Observationes*', in Houtzager, *Pieter van Foreest*, pp. 41–72.

the Silent and his family.[42] His contacts with the family Van Oranje-Nassau may have resulted in the invitation to become professor of medicine at the University of Leiden. During the opening of this newly established university on 8 February 1575, he participated in the formal procession and even delivered a *Laudatio medicinae* (Praise of medicine) (Figure 6.2). A university career was presumably not to his taste, given that he soon returned to nearby Delft and continued his work there. Just like his late sixteenth-century Roman equivalent Angelo Vittori, who also left a huge collection of medical case histories in print, he may have deliberately avoided time-consuming teaching, giving all his energy to his practising and its recording.[43] The position of Delft physician was only given up after the death of his wife in 1595, when Van Foreest returned to Alkmaar. Its town council clearly did not consider him too old to practise, as he became their very well-paid city physician. The assignment, however, did not last long, for within two years, on 10 March 1597, the aged Van Foreest passed away and was buried at the church of St Lawrence in Alkmaar.

Van Foreest and the Renaissance Casebook

In his official portrait, Pieter van Foreest is portrayed jotting down observations on the blank pages of a note book. The details in the portrait are very telling. At first glance we are dealing with a traditional portrait of a scholar. The doctor is clad in a very valuable cloak, trimmed with what looks like panther fur, and sports a heavy gold ring. What are absent, however, are the learned books of his trade, the volumes of Hippocrates, Galen and Vesalius that usually provided the medical sitter with status and authority. Since at the time of his portrayal Van Foreest was at the end of his career, he may have consciously pursued a different style of image building. With the publication of the volumes of his *Observationes* nearing its end, it was time to promote the image of the hardworking medical practitioner who, thanks to an industrious and exact coverage of his treatments, had managed to share his medical knowledge with as many people as possible.

The notebook under his right hand may have been a casebook that did not survive. The casebook was a novel phenomenon in sixteenth-century medicine, although as a professional tool its use goes back to Hippocrates and Galen. There is evidence that the Parisian Guillaume de Baillou (1538–61) and the Italian Girolamo Cardano (1501–76) both used a casebook. Van Foreest was acquainted with both

42 Houtzager, 'Pieter van Foreest en de Prins van Oranje', in Bosman-Jelgersma, *Pieter van Foreest*, pp. 119–24.

43 Henriette Bosman-Jelgersma, 'De Stichting van de Leidse Universiteit', in eadem, *Pieter van Foreest*, pp. 125–9. On Vittori, see Nancy G. Siraisi, '*Historiae*, natural history, Roman antiquity and some Roman physicians', in Gianna Pomata and Nancy S. Siraisi (eds), *Historia. Empiricism and erudition in early modern Europe* (Cambridge Mass., 2005) pp. 343–7.

of these men.[44] Not only his *Observationes*, but also Van Foreest's unpublished manuscripts in the Regional Archive of Alkmaar seem to be primarily reworkings of such notes. It is unimaginable that he would have been able to produce his multi-volume *Observationes* without the backup of detailed and comprehensive patients' records.

Recounting the details of his patient's ailments and working these up, including their theoretical and practical positioning, in the form of *scholia*, must have constituted the centre of his life. In fact, Van Foreest's *Observationes et curationes medicinalium* were published between 1584 and 1606 and they contain as many as 1,350 case histories.[45] The collection reflects more than 50 years of medical practice, the earliest cases dating from his Italian and Parisian student years and his ultra-short time practising in the town of Pithiviers. Vivian Nutton has remarked cunningly that Van Foreest's use of the designation '*observatio*' was a rarity in medical titles of the sixteenth century. The author must have selected it on purpose to call attention to the crucial importance of a doctor's personal experience of disease during the healing process. He examined each medical problem himself and went beyond mere book learning. Each *observatio* was followed by a *scholium*, which involved a detailed scholarly commentary on the case.[46] This format was very common, as university professors concocted such texts by selecting authoritative sentences from classical authors and themselves supplying them with suitable commentaries. Usually these texts had a didactic character and were aimed at (advanced) medical students. Van Foreest's text, by contrast, is much more complete and is clearly addressed to his own kind: academically trained medical doctors of a first-class international level. He considered patient histories the essence of medical science and was self-conscious enough to regard them also as the basis of a proper medical education. 'In search of a medical education' stood in the sixteenth century for eliciting medical data out of patients from all over the world, preferably by yourself, and if that was not possible via descriptions sent to you by colleagues, studying them, providing them with scholarly explanations and ordering them in neat, accessible and publishable surveys.

Nancy Siraisi – and many others, such as Paula Findlen, Anthony Grafton, Brian Ogilvie, Giuseppe Olmi, Gianna Pomata and Jonathan Sawday – have pointed to the 'collectionist' urge of the early modern period and studied the practices of

---

44 Nancy G. Siraisi, *The clock and the mirror. Girolamo Cardano and Renaissance medicine* (Princeton, 1997), and for Baillou see I.M. Lonie, 'The Paris Hippocratics: teaching and research in Paris in the second half of the sixteenth century', in Wear, *Medical Renaissance*, pp. 155–74, 169–74.

45 There are many editions. Therefore here each time the book and the number of the observation will be noted. Also nine books of *Observationes et curationes chirurgicales* (first edition 1610–11) were published. A survey of all editions is published by R. Breugelmans and W.K. Gnirrep, 'Bibliografie van de werken van Petrus Forestus, in Bosman-Jelgersma, *Petrus Forestus Medicus*, pp. 19–116.

46 Nutton, 'Pieter van Foreest', pp. 26–7.

data gathering, which seems to also have been typical of Van Foreest's working methods.[47] Many sixteenth-century scholars presented results of an inquiry, which meant a record of human experience as well as the description of nature. Here, in the case of Van Foreest, are under consideration narratively expressed specific experiences or cases encountered in medical practice that addressed both human experience and natural phenomena in the Aristotelian sense. They were set in order, viz. arranged into thematic groups and provided with commentaries. Traditions and models of medical narrative can of course be found in several contexts, and patients and other people who were not medical practitioners also produced such records, but the present chapter is confined to accounts made by medical practitioners of individual cases or patients.[48] These occur in the very popular *consilia* – some by Van Foreest have also survived – while illustrative cases were also often embedded in general medical or surgical treatises. This is just what Van Foreest tried to do also in his (abortive) handbook that caused him so much trouble and made him lose track in this project.[49] Both genres, the handbook and the *consilia*, developed in the thirteenth century, probably to a large extent independently of ancient antecedents, as the most important ancient examples of medical narrative about individuals were as yet undiscovered.

Medieval accounts of individual cases set out in treatises are relatively rare, even though increasingly common in the fifteenth century. If they were used, the motivation for the insertion of stories from their own practice was claimed to be exemplary or pedagogical. This changed radically in the sixteenth century, when the Hippocratic *Epidemics* with its numerous individual case histories and Galen's

47 Pomata and Siraisi, *Historia*, ch. iii: Gianna Pomata, '*Praxis historialis*. The Uses of *historia* in early modern medicine', pp. 105–46. Also Nancy G. Siraisi, 'Girolamo Cardano and the art of medical narrative', in *Journal of the history of ideas* 52 (1991), pp. 581–602, and eadem, 'Anatomizing the past: Physicians and history in Renaissance culture', in *Renaissance Quarterly* 53 (2000) 1–30. Also Giuseppe Olmi, *L'inventario del mondo. Catalogazione della natura e luoghi del sapere nella prima età moderna* (Bologna, 1992); Paula Findlen, *Possessing nature: Museums, collecting, and scientific culture in early modern Italy* (Berkeley, 1994); Jonathan Sawday, *The body emblazoned: Dissection and the human body in Renaissance culture* (London, 1995); Anthony Grafton and Nancy G. Siraisi (eds), *Natural particulars: Nature and the disciplines in Renaissance Europe* (Cambridge, 1999), and Brian Ogilvie, *The science of describing: Natural history in Renaissance Europe, 1490–1520* (Chicago, 2006).

48 On empiricism and collectionism in other disciplines, see the chapters in Pomata and Siraisi, *Historia*.

49 *Jatrices Petri Foresti Alcmariani medici. Liber Primus introductorius ex Hippocrate Galeno aliisque dogmaticus medicis illustribus descriptus*. Reg. Archief Alkmaar, Library, s.a. (ca. 1590). On this see Catrien Santing, 'Propagating academical medical knowledge and professional practicioning for the sake of the Republic's health', in Annette de Vries (ed.) *Cultural Mediators. Artists and writers at the crossroads of tradition, innovation and reception in the Low Countries and Italy 1450–1650* (Louvain, 2008) pp. 65–86, esp. pp. 70–71.

On Prognosis and *Method of healing* [*Methodus Medendi*], his principle book on therapeutics, were fully edited and commented upon.[50] The reintroduction of the case history after the Greek model not only stimulated changes in therapy but also, and above all, gave evidence of a new interest in observation.[51] In his various books Van Foreest cherished the model of the Hippocratic epidemics, which in fact was combined with the then very popular genre of the *Practica* – handbooks for students and vade mecums for the practising physician, who more and more became literally practical, even prescribing a detailed *curatio* and the ingredients of a prescription – both new elements in the genre. Some years ago Andrew Wear pointed out that in the sixteenth century the *Practica* became 'more and more verbose and concerned to define, divide and discuss their subject matter'.[52]

In sum, in various respects Van Foreest might be called a very typical example of these epistemological changes within the medical profession. He found it extremely difficult to stop collecting information, and wrestled even more to shape his own observations and thoughts into the right form. This is not to deny the claim that his own experiences, i.e. observationally acquired medical knowledge, embodied 'the story of medicine' as such, and this included discussing its theoretical basis.[53]

The 1350 observations that Van Foreest presents comprise, in fact, the histories of his consultations, after the example of Giambattista da Monte and also of Van Foreest's 'praeceptor meus' Benedetto Vettori, who in addition to a handbook of practical medicine had published commentaries on Hippocrates' *Epidemics*. In his introduction to Book 1 the author also acclaimed Symphorien Champier (1471–1538) as an example, who published excerpts of case histories of ancient medical authors, especially from Galen.[54] Apart from these two, he very often quotes and

---

50 A Latin translation of the complete *Epidemics* was included in *Hippocratis Octoginta volumina ... nunc tandem per M. Fabium Calvum Latinitate donata* (Rome, 1525). The Greek text was first printed in the Aldine Hippocrates, *Omnia opera Hippocratis* (Venice, 1526). On this see Gerhard Baader and Rolf Winau (eds), *Die hippokratischen Epidemien: Theorie-Praxis-Tradition, Sudhoffs Archiv*, Beiheft 27 (Stuttgart, 1989), pp. 312–15, and Richard J. Durling, 'A chronological census of Renaissance editions and translations of Galen', *Journal of the Warburg and Courtauld Institutes*, 24 (1961) pp. 230–5. Galen's use of case histories in his *Methodus medendi* is discussed by Vivian Nutton, 'Style and context in the *Method of Healing*'.

51 Lonie, 'The Paris Hippocratics', pp. 169–74, and Vivian Nutton, 'Hippocrates in the Renaissance', in Baader and Winau, *Die hippokratischen Epidemien*, pp. 420–39, esp. 433–9.

52 In general see Andrew Wear, 'Explorations in Renaissance writings on the practice of medicine', in Wear, *Medical Renaissance*, pp. 118–45. Montanus lectured on and edited Rhasis' *Ad Almansorem*, the model for the medieval *practica*.

53 Danielle Jacquart, 'Theory, everyday practice, and three fifteenth-century physicians', *Osiris* 6 (1990), pp. 140–60.

54 Symphorien Champier, *Claudii Galeni Pergameni historiales campi* (Basel, 1532). On him see Pomata, 'The uses of *Historia*', pp. 105–7, 123–4, 130.

even takes over his casuistry and recipes, from a similar collection of 700 cases by the Portuguese Jew Amatus Lusitanus, whom he may have encountered in Ferrara or Rome, where Lusitanus had worked for some time as a papal physician. Lusitanus, whose original name was Joao Rodrigues de Castello Branco (1511–68), however, was also a welcome guest in the Netherlands.[55] The fact that he explicitly mentions and quotes these authors demonstrates that Van Foreest still worked within the Galenic tradition of recording accounts of successful cures. His books are explicitly entitled *Observationes et curationes*, and as a consequence of this and other factors contain a strong component of self-presentation.[56]

The complete Van Foreest series comprises 32 books or *Libri*, which were published either separately or together with two or three other books. Each of them opens with a florid letter of dedication to an important authority, for instance to the Stadholder Prince Maurits, the States of the various Dutch Provinces or the authorities of cities in which the author had professional contacts.[57] In addition, letters to and from friends and colleagues are often inserted. Most of the men mentioned are Leiden scholars – Janus Dousa, Josephus Scaliger, Justus Lipsius, Gerardus Bontius or medical colleagues from the other Holland and Zeeland cities, such as the Middelburg town physician Levinus Lemnius (1505–68) and Bernardus Paludanus (1550–1633), medical doctor and collector of rarities from the port town of Enkhuizen. Some of these men also contributed poetical praises. However, as the dedication letters were meant to promote the author and legitimise his work, his Italian and French student days are frequently mentioned. The names of his Italian professors gave the *Observationes* status as well as authority. Also, they aimed to convince readers that Van Foreest had a thorough command of medical literature. In his introduction he explicitly contrasts himself with the Empiricists, who manoeuvred solely on the basis of observation. As a 'rational physician' he thought out his observations and arranged them in line with his medical erudition.[58] Many books of his colleagues are also mentioned in the salutations. In the letter of dedication to his home town, Alkmaar, of books 26 and 27 on the reproductive organs, the author, for instance, hails the Venetian anatomist Alessandro Benedetti (1452–1512), who had written a book on the subject which he dedicated to the

---

55 Amatus Lusitanus, *Medici physici praestantissimi, Curationum medicinalium centuriae quatuor, quarum duae priores ab auctore sunt recognite, due posteriores nunc primum edite uaria omnes multiplicique rerum cognitione refertae: Quibus praemissa est commentatio de introitu medici ad aegrotantem, deque crisi & diebus decretorijs, medicae rei studiosis utilissima Curationum medicinalium centuriae quatuor, quarum duae priores ab auctore sunt recognite* (Basel, 1556). Biography in Harry Friedenwald, *The Jews and medicine* (Baltimore, 1944) vol. 1, pp. 332–90, see also Pomata, 'The uses of *Historia*', pp. 125–6.

56 Compare Vivian Nutton, 'Style and context', pp. 9–11.

57 On this Heesakkers, 'Gedichten en brieven', and Santing, 'Pieter van Foreest'.

58 Remark by Pomata, 'The uses of *Historia*', p. 137.

Emperor Maximilian. In other words, the reader should not forget that Van Foreest was continuing in a worthy tradition.[59]

The first books discuss fevers such as the plague, the next ones concentrate on the ailments of the organs, starting with the eyes and, via the feet, ending with the human genitalia: in fact this is the traditional Galenic order of *Practica*. Of course, venereal diseases are the lowest of the low and thus should come absolutely last. Basically, the whole series is constituted of short histories of illness followed by *scholia*. In these commentaries, divided into diagnosis, therapy and prognosis, the author makes comparisons with similar cases to support his diagnosis, which might stem from his own practice or from the medical literature. The authors consulted are from a wide range, for in this respect Van Foreest was certainly not prejudiced. In addition to the traditional classical sources, the reader is confronted with lots of Arab writers and many contemporary authors. Quite often remedies are described that he had learned about during his years of travel. For example, the ill Prince William of Orange was prescribed a cinnamon potion for his sore throat, which his doctor had learned in Pithiviers. Weak patients also benefited much from eating *panatella* (a kind of sweetened bread), the recipe for which he had brought with him from Italy.[60] As regards the content, Van Foreest was no innovator, but the *Observationes* certainly show that he kept up with the medical literature, albeit towards the end of his life he seems to lose track somewhat.[61]

The illness report usually starts with a short paragraph on the patient, often identified by name, profession and age – *iuvenis, rusticus, meretrix* – place of residence, sometimes also the date of the illness. Very Hippocratically, the living conditions of the patient are taken into account, as Van Foreest even mentions preferring to visit his patients at home in order to gain an insight into the course of an ailment. Subsequently, the symptoms and complaints are listed, rather concisely by the way. The diagnosis is made, preferably not by uroscopy – Foreest did not want piss brought to his house – and explained. Much attention is paid to the recommended treatment and the prescribed pharmaceuticals. Again in a Hippocratic manner, the individuality or exclusiveness of a treatment is emphasised, ridiculing, for instance, barbers who put their syphilitic patients through massive mercury therapies. In case of recovery from a severe illness, God is thanked, nor does Van Foreest forget to mention that his prognosis had been correct when a patient died. Of course we come across invectives against quacks who had caused much irreparable damage. Again, the emphasis on the prognosis is an example of Hippocratic reasoning.

---

[59] Heesakkers, p. 133. Benedetti became more famous for his *Anatomice* (1502), which by the way was dedicated to the emperor Maximilian, and he also published a collection of consultations. On him see Giovanna Ferrari, *L'esperienza del passato: Alessandro Benedetti filologo en medico umanista* (Florence, 1996).

[60] Luyendijk-Elshout, 'Humanistisch arts', p. 49.

[61] Nutton, 'Pieter van Foreest', esp. 29–30.

Van Foreest's *Observationes* collection mirrors his long medical career, which had included travelling to important centres of medical excellence, such as described above, and attending there the lectures of the most famous medical professors, experiences that found expression in these books. The self-satisfied description (self-advertisement was certainly one of the strongest of the motivations behind Van Foreest's writing, he even records the thank-you presents of patients) of his treatment of illustrious, notorious, as well as perfectly average patients makes up the backbone of the books. This practising brought with it much regional travelling. Next to Prince William the Silent, whom he repeatedly cured of fevers and exhaustion, in the commentaries figure numerous nobles and patricians from over the whole county of Holland and Zeeland. Most names, however, stem from either the neighbourhood of Alkmaar (ca. 300) or Delft (ca. 500), or from cities and villages a day's journey from these, such as The Hague, Leiden and Dordrecht.[62]

Apart from incorporating them in the *Observationes*, Van Foreest also inserted many anecdotes stemming from his professional practice into his other published and unpublished works. These were mainly directed against what Van Foreest considered to be illegal medical practice. Empirics and quacks, in his eyes, chiefly caused chaos and possibly endangered the stability of the wealthy Dutch society. With regard to this, uroscopists, 'urine-monging empirickes' as the 1623 English translation of his *De incerto fallaci urinarum iudicio* calls them [*The arraignment of urines: wherein are set downe the manifold errors and abuses of ignorant urine-monging empirickes, cozening quacksalvers, women-physitians, and the like stuffe*] (Figure 6.4), were his main object of ridicule and denunciation. To this learned, academically trained medical doctor, it was evident that piss, having travelled over long distances in curious containers such as wooden clogs, provided no reliable diagnostic information whatsoever. This is just to mention one the juiciest histories from this treatise, and another example of travelling medical facts.[63]

One might notice that this transformation in the gaining, as well as presentation, of medical knowledge coincides with the (beginning of the) decline of Italian universities and the shift of the intellectual centre to the north-west of Europe. It is noteworthy that Van Foreest's reading of Italian authors was confined to the authors known to him in his student years.[64] The nascent medical faculty at Leiden, established in 1576, is one of the examples of this change. It soon employed active and publishing professors, such as Gerard Bontius, Johannes Heurnius, Pieter Pauw and Rembert Dodoens – all of whom had studied either in Paris, Pavia

---

62 See for a list of patients mentioned and their origin Henry W. van Leeuwen, 'Patiënten en relaties', in Bosman-Jelgersma, *Pieter van Foreest*, pp. 165–78.

63 Pieter van Foreest, *De incerto, fallaci urinarum iudicio* (Leiden, 1589). On this work and on the unpublished *van der Empiriken*, see Vivian Nutton, 'Idle trots', pp. 245–8.

64 Nutton, 'Pieter van Foreest', pp. 28–30.

or Padua.[65] Van Foreest, and probably also Heurnius, who had studied in Padua 1565–71, became acquainted with clinical teaching in Padua through Giambattista da Monte, who is quoted many times in the *Observationes* and who himself had written up his *Consultationes Medicae*, which were later on published by his pupil Crato von Crafftheim.[66] His patients served as both demonstration and touchstone of ancient medical sources and their modern summaries. In Leiden, Jean Fernel's *Universa medicina* (1567) was used, of course in the edition of Van Foreest's friend Heurnius.[67] This handbook presents a synthesis of classical knowledge tested against his own observations, something Van Foreest had envisaged with his own manual, but did not manage to produce.

Publishing collections of case histories became one of Leiden's traditions. Dodoens published a collection, for which the selection criterion seems to have been singularity, as he focused on rare and novel observations.[68] Johannes Heurnius had encouraged his friend Van Foreest to publish the stories of his patients in the service of medical education, to compensate for his refusal to become his fellow professor of medicine, a request the latter fulfilled only hesitatingly. His successors knew no restraints whatsoever in this respect. Between 1659 and 1661, for instance, the clinician François De Boë Sylvius recorded the physical ups and downs of 160 patients in the Leiden St Cecilia hospital that served as the university clinic in extreme (meaning daily) detail.[69]

Travelling Empiric Erudition

Nancy Siraisi has pointed repeatedly to the importance of case histories in early modern medicine or, to be more precise, to the Renaissance medical narrative. In order to demonstrate perceptions about the 'searching out and acquiring the right medical education' held by a sixteenth-century Dutch doctor, it is not necessary here to emphasise the analogy between Renaissance historiography and medicine so rightly advocated by Siraisi, although Van Foreest certainly was historically minded in several respects and clearly thought of his medical

[65] On Leiden, see Willem Otterspeer, *Groepsportret met Dame. Het bolwerk van de vrijheid. De Leidse universiteit 1575–1672* (Leiden, 2000).

[66] Crato von Crafftheim's Basel 1565 edition of the *Consultationes medicae* is illustrated with a portrait of Da Monte on the title page. Da Monte published tables on Galen's *Ars medica* for practical teaching (Venice, 1546); see Stefania Fortuna, 'Galen's *De Constitutione Artis Medicae* in the Renaissance', *The Classical Quarterly*, n.s., 43 (1993), pp. 302–19, esp. pp. 305, 315, and Siraisi, *Avicenna in Italy: The Canon and medical teaching in Italian universities after 1500* (Princeton, 1987), pp. 98–103.

[67] Beukers, 'Theoretische achtergrond'.

[68] Rembert Dodoens, *Medicinalium observationum exempla rara* (Leiden, 1581).

[69] Otterspeer, *Groepsportret*, p. 203.

observations as '*historiae*'.[70] He owned a copy of the works of the third-century Bishop Cyprian, who wrote on heretics and ecclesiastical schismata, which, by the way, he bequeathed to the Public Library of Alkmaar, together with copies of his own *Observationes*, a 1497 *Canon Medicinae* by Avicenna in the translation by Gerardus Cremona printed in Padua, and the 1526 Basel edition of the *Opera Omnia* of Hippocrates.[71] In his works he drew many parallels with circumstances in Antiquity mentioned by Hippocrates and Galen, and used plenty of Arab sources, which he did not despise at all. So, although also in this respect Van Foreest might be typified as a time traveller in the field of medical knowledge, here it has been demonstrated how he collected medical data and established them in extremely loquacious books. Van Foreest seems to have been the type of the collector par excellence – the scholar who accumulates as much data as possible, stores them all, orders them and subsequently nearly succumbs under their load. This must have been the reason why Van Foreest started to publish late in his life – apart from some *Prognosticationes* published in the 1550s, his main works date from the 1580s, when he was well into his fifties. Much of his oeuvre was left unfinished. Even the *Observationes* had to be completed by nephews, who luckily enough had graduated in medicine in Italy, thanks to their uncle's careful coaching. The reason for this incompleteness might also be found in Van Foreest's extremely cautious character, and next to that in his minor ability to retain a text in shape. Besides the loosely constructed *Observationes*, the other treatises are also moulded in the form of dialogues interspersed with many stories from his practice, and are thus likewise case histories, albeit in a less-polished form.

Knowledge of a disease based on personal inspection of the patient, such as is collected and offered by Van Foreest in his *Observationes*, primarily represented expert medical knowledge, which was beginning to constitute the heart of medical education. Medical doctors and students of course had to study medical theory in order to be able to rationalise adequately about ailments, but first and above all they had to set off themselves and follow their path. In the early modern period medical education was therefore an extremely active enterprise. The students went to Italy and France to meet the right people and obtain the right information. Of course, facts and data were to be found also in the books of the ancients and the medievals, but just as much in the object of their profession: the patient. Also in the works of Pieter van Foreest we meet the typically Renaissance interrelation of observational proficiency and philological learning, which led to a direct conciliation of empiricism and book learning. In recent literature this new brand of empiricism therefore has been denominated 'learned empiricism'. As the overall urge to describe the particular began to predominate the medical episteme, the *homo patiens* appeared at the centre of their study and research.[72] It could be the

[70] Siraisi, 'Anatomizing the past', and eadem, '*Historiae*'.

[71] Chris Streefkerk, 'De boekenschenking van Pieter van Foreest aan Alkmaars Librije', in Bosman Jelgersma, *Petrus Forestus Medicus*, pp. 365–8.

[72] Michael Stolberg, *Homo patiens* (Cologne, 2003).

dead body of the anatomists, who explored thousands of corpses from the outside and inside, and mapped their findings in detail. The same was done by practitioners such as Van Foreest, who amassed as well as mastered as many symptoms, conditions and causes as possible and put them in a practical order, as well as in their theoretical context. It therefore seems suitable to end with the words of Pieter van Foreest himself, who in the letter of dedication of his *Observationes*, Books 21–23 on the ailments of the intestines, which he addressed to the town council of Haarlem, started with 'Also in medicine is the phrase of Seneca valid: "Words awaken, but examples draw"'. Clearly, the *homo patiens* constituted that example, but in the sixteenth century he or she could only be treated by calling in additional information from centres of medical excellence all over Europe.

Chapter 7
'Like the bees, who neither suck nor generate their honey from one flower': The Significance of the *peregrinatio academica* for Danish Medical Students in the Late Sixteenth and Early Seventeenth Centuries

Ole Peter Grell

For medical students in post-Reformation Denmark–Norway, study abroad was not only an ambition but a necessity, for the simple reason that the country's only university, the University of Copenhagen (1479), after its post-Reformation refoundation in 1537, remained understaffed and underfunded for decades. Whether students attended a centre of medical excellence or settled for more modest medical faculties closer to home – in Germany – was, of course, dictated by their financial circumstances.

Initially the University of Copenhagen had only one professor of medicine, Christian Torkelsen Morsing (d.1560), who also served as the university's vice-chancellor and therefore had little or no time for teaching. Morsing undoubtedly encouraged prospective medical students to study abroad, if at all possible, having himself undertaken his *peregrinatio academica* in the early 1530s, which had seen him study at the universities of Montpellier and Basle – where he received his MD – and drawn him towards the study of botany and anatomy in particular.[1]

Despite the extensive recruitment drive, by the Reformation King Christian III, of foreign talent to fill the professorships in Copenhagen (of the 41 professors who served the university during the reign of Christian III around half were recruited abroad) in order to add credibility and status to the refounded university, it proved difficult to recruit anyone of quality for the second chair in medicine. It was offered to a number of famous medical men – such as Leonard Fuchs from Tübingen and Johann Guenther von Andernach from Paris, neither of whom was tempted

[1] See O.P. Grell, 'Caspar Bartholin and the education of the pious physician', in Ole P. Grell and Andrew Cunningham (eds), *Medicine and the Reformation*, London, 1993, 78–100.

by what must have appeared to them a cultural and medical backwater. Even more surprising,ly the chair was also offered to Girolamo Cardano, the renowned Catholic physician, then professor of medicine in Pavia, who, while he was far from being an orthodox Catholic, considered the Lutheran faith of Denmark – not to mention its climate – too unappealing to contemplate. Accordingly, Cardano rejected the offer, despite the king's promise of a salary of no less than 800 *thalers* – five times the normal salary for a professor of medicine in Copenhagen.[2] Between 1538 and 1544 the second chair in medicine at Copenhagen was occupied by a certain Thomas Zeger; then the chair remained vacant again until 1547, when the Wittenberg-educated Dutchman Peter Capiteyn, who had been teaching in Rostock, accepted the position while simultaneously becoming royal physician to Christian III; presumably he was able to draw both salaries.[3] Thus, the new university remained a parochial institution during the reign of Christian III (1536–59). It was constantly in need of funds and only managed to attract a few students. Consequently, only a small proportion of the intentions laid down in the Statutes were realised.

However, during the second decade of the reign of Christian's son and successor, Frederik II (1559–88), the university's financial situation improved dramatically. Denmark in particular benefited from the economic boom across north-western Europe during the second half of the sixteenth century, not least because of a growing demand for Danish agricultural produce. This in turn resulted in more money becoming available for the university. Salaries for professors improved rapidly, making these posts more attractive to talented and ambitious individuals. These improvements gathered further pace when the Seven Years' War with Sweden (1563–70) drew to a close, liberating finances which had hitherto been swallowed up by the war effort. Accordingly, in 1569 a Royal Trust was set up, offering stipends for 100 students, modelled – as so much else at the University of Copenhagen – on a similar institution at the University of Wittenberg. That year also witnessed the creation of four Royal Travel Stipends, which were to finance the studies abroad for one student of medicine and three students of theology.

These initiatives corresponded with an explosive growth in the number of Danish–Norwegian students who matriculated abroad. Numbers more than doubled in the period 1571–1600, reaching nearly 1,100, as compared to the 500-plus who had matriculated abroad in the period, 1536–1570.[4] Between 1600 and 1630 numbers fell slightly, to around 1,000, decreasing somewhat further between 1630

---

[2] M. Fink-Jensen, 'Medicine, natural philosophy, and the influence of Melanchthon in Reformation Denmark and Norway', *Bulletin of the History of Medicine*, 2006, **80**, 439–64, especially 440.

[3] M. Fink-Jensen, *Fornuften under troens lydighed. Naturfilosofi, medicin og teologi i Danmark 1536–1636*, Copenhagen, Museum Tusculanums Forlag, 2004, 73–4.

[4] Grell, 'Caspar Bartholin', 86.

and 1660 to around 950,[5] and falling rapidly towards the end of the seventeenth century.[6] This makes a total for the period 1536–1660 of over 3,550 students who matriculated abroad. Of those, the great majority were young noblemen undertaking the Grand Tour, theology students spending one or two years at one of the major Lutheran universities in Germany, especially Wittenberg, and law and arts students securing qualifications for the rapidly expanding bureaucracy of central government.

Medical students constituted only a small minority, a little over 3 per cent of the total. A comparison shows that the pattern and frequency of study abroad presents a totally different pattern from that of other students. Statistically, they constituted a small group, so when compared with the total cohort the results should be taken with a pinch of salt. Still, the numbers of medical students matriculating abroad more than trebled between 1571 and 1600, a total of 20, as compared with the period 1536–70, when only 6 students studied abroad. This trend is similar to, if far more pronounced than, the general trend. However, during the following period, between 1600 and 1630, rather than decline slightly, in accordance with the general trend for students overall, the number of medical students actually doubled, from 20 to 40; and similarly, instead of a registering a further decline between 1630 and 1660, the numbers of medical students abroad peaked, reaching 52. Evidently medical students did not find the Thirty Years' War a hindrance to their travel. Numbers undoubtedly also increased because of much better employment prospects for young medical men in Denmark around this time. Some of the major urban centres had begun to employ town physicians by the beginning of the seventeenth century. This was especially the case in the old cathedral towns, where money previously spent on salaries for canons was now diverted towards the salaries of town physicians. Similarly, doctors were needed by the better-endowed hospitals and orphanages which came into existence during the reign of Christian IV, not to mention the more prestigious positions as regional physicians created by a government increasingly concerned with general health issues and medical regulation, as can be seen from the first national Medical Order issued in 1619.[7] Of the 118 students who studied medicine abroad in the period 1536 to1660, no less than 71 (72 if Johan Rhode's doctorate was an MD) obtained an MD – nearly 65 per cent.

Medical study was a time-consuming business, and accordingly we should not be surprised that the time spent abroad by the majority of medical students was considerable – more often than not a decade or more spent at a number of the best medical faculties available across Europe. Evidently the importance of obtaining

---

[5] V. Helk, *Dansk-Norske Studierejser fra reformationen til enevælden 1536–1660. Med en matrikel over studerende i udlandet*, Odense 1987, 44.

[6] H. Kragh, *Dansk Naturvidenskabs Historie*, vol.1 *Fra Middelalderlærdom til Den Nye Videnskab 1000–1730*, Aarhus, 2005, 187.

[7] Grell, 'Caspar Bartholin', 78–100; for the Medical Order of 1619, see P.R. Kruse, *Lægemiddelpriserne i Danmark indtil 1645*, Copenhagen, 1991, 108–67.

an MD was recognised by these students, but did it pay off in terms of career prospects? If we define success as obtaining either a professorship, preferably in medicine, at the University of Copenhagen, or if not, then a position as royal physician, then the answer is probably yes. Of our 72 MDs, 15 became professors and 6 became royal physicians – a 30 per cent success rate.

The majority of our students obtained their MD from Basle – 20 in total – thereby continuing the trend begun with the first professor of medicine after the Reformation, Christen Torkelsen Morsing. Padua closely followed Basle as the university of choice for MDs – 14 – (15 if Johan Rhode is included). Surprisingly, only four got their MDs from Leiden, to which can be added two in Utrecht, two in Franeker, one in Groningen, one in Harderwijck, giving a total of 10 for the Dutch Republic, while only five students returned home to obtain their MD in Copenhagen. Only one student is known to have received his MD from Montpellier, while a total of at least 13 obtained their MDs in France (two in Caën, one in Angers, one in Valence, eight from unspecified universities) (Table 7.1).

Table 7.1 MDs 1536–1660 for students matriculated abroad[8]

University	Date (number of MDs)	Total
Angers	1660 (1)	1
Basle	1576 (1); 1583 (2); 1591 (2); 1593 (1); 1598 (1); 1602 (1); 1605 (1); 1606 (1); 1609 (1); 1610 (1); 1611 (2); 1615 (1); 1636 (1); 1637 (2); 1645 (2)	20
Bologna	1566 (1); 1617 (1)	2
Caën	1601 (1); 1622 (1)	2
Copenhagen	1603 (1); 1611(1); 1640 (1); 1654 (1); 1667 (1)	5
France (no place)	1560 (1); 1571 (2); 1582/3 (1); 1596 (1); 1614 (1); 1656 (2)	8
Franeker	1648 (1); 1656 (1)	2
Freiburg in Brisgau	1619 (1)	1
Groningen	1646 (1)	1
Harderwijck	1652 (1)	1
Helmstedt	1610 (1); 1617 (1); 1620 (1)	3
Leiden	1624 (2); 1642 (1); 1664 (1)	4

[8] Data collated from Helk, *Dansk-Norske Studierejser.*

University	Date (number of MDs)	Total
Montpellier	1585 (1)	1
Padua	1598 (1); 1623 (1); 1626 (1); 1639 (1); 1645 (1); 1646 (1); 1650 (1); 1654 (2); 1656 (1); 1657 (3); 1659 (1)	14 (15 if Johan Rhode got an MD)
Rostock	1556 (1)	1
Utrecht	1658 (1); 1652 (1)	2
Valence	1653 (1) 1.	
Vienna	1564 (1)	1

Chronologically, it is noteworthy that 75 per cent of the MDs from Basle were awarded between 1576 and 1615 – a total of 15, more or less, corresponding with the golden years of the medical faculty in the University of Basle. Evidently Basle lost some of its lustre for Danish medical students by the second decade of the seventeenth century. The University of Basle had proved unable to replace such prominent medical men as Caspar Bauhin and Theodore and Jacob Zwinger with professors of a similar calibre. The 'Basle connection', however, meant that a number of Danish students of medicine continued to obtain their MDs from Basle for another generation. Irrespective of the decline of medicine in Basle, an MD from there was considered of particular value by Danish students, who clearly believed it would further their career prospects. This is surprising when it is borne in mind that Basle belonged in the Calvinist rather than the Lutheran camp.

Sixty per cent of the MDs from Padua were awarded in the decade between 1650 and 1660. That Padua should have become such an important centre for Danish medical students around the middle of the seventeenth century, despite the confessionalism of the age, is interesting. Despite that confessionalism, these students, nationals of a solidly Lutheran country, do not appear to have been concerned about the possible repercussions of obtaining their MDs from universities situated within the other confessions, such as the Catholic and the Reformed. Obviously, Padua's continued ability to accommodate non-Catholics was important. However the presence in Padua of the learned Dane Johan Rhode from 1622 to 1659 was important. Rhode maintained close contacts with Ole Worm and the Bartholins in Copenhagen and often provided lodging for Danish students studying in Padua. Rhode's contacts among the leading lights at the University of Padua and across Italy were extensive. By 1639, when he obtained his doctorate at the university, until his death in 1659, Rhode remained a highly regarded natural philosopher and physician, much admired by leading Italian colleagues.

Basing oneself on these figures, one would be tempted to conclude that Basle and Padua were the centres of excellence which mattered most to Danish medical students – the first mainly at the start of the period and the latter at the end – whereas the medical faculty in Leiden played only a minor part. That, however, would be a mistake. Bearing in mind that most students matriculated and studied at several universities, a look at the whole cohort reveals that 65 students matriculated at Leiden, 55 in Padua, and only 27 in Basle – only 7 more than were awarded their MDs (Table 7.2). The rationale why some students matriculated where they did is often difficult to understand and was often dictated by non-medical considerations. That Siena features so prominently among the places where medical students matriculated has perhaps more to do with their jobs as tutors to young noblemen than with any personal interest in attending this university – i.e. Siena was a necessary stop on the Grand Tour for young noblemen. Siena also had a reputation of being a 'liberal', open university where foreign students were welcome. If students matriculated on their own, they may well have done so with the same motivation as had Ole Worm, who in 1609 declared his intention to Jacob Zwinger to visit Siena because of its reputation for the finest Italian being spoken there.[9] Likewise Angers in France had a highly esteemed law faculty, while medicine there was not of the same high standard as in Paris, if Worm's student Jacob Svabe can be trusted.[10]

Table 7.2 Universities attended by Danish-Norwegian students of medicine, 1536–1660[11]

University	Number of students
Leiden	65
Padua	55
Basle	27
Wittenberg	24
Franeker	22
Orléans	22
Paris	22
Heidelberg	20
Strasbourg	18
Siena	17
Tübingen	11

9 Schepelern, *Breve fra og til Ole Worm*, vol. 1, no. 8.

10 Ibid., no. 578.

11 Ibid., listed in order of popularity.

University	Number of students
Rostock	10
Marburg	9
Montpellier	9
Geneva	8
Giessen	7
Helmstedt	7
Angers	6
Bourges	5
France	4
Groningen	4
Jena	4
Bologna	3
Utrecht	2

The fact that a good medical training at the best medical faculties was an expensive and time-consuming business may go a long way to explaining the small number who undertook it. When King Frederik II created the four royal travel grants for study abroad in 1569, one of which was reserved for a medical student, he made sure that each successful candidate received 100 *thalers* annually, provided by the three wealthy former monasteries of Sorø, Ringsted and Antvorskov.[12] Of the 12 medical students who received this royal stipend, 5 eventually became professors at the University of Copenhagen and 2 became royal physicians. Being a recipient of the royal stipend and obtaining an MD proved a virtual guarantee of a successful career. The three students who did not obtain an MD received no appointment; and of the nine who did acquire their MD, only two failed to benefit. One was Hans Lauridsen Amerinus, who never sought promotion within the university or at court, but returned to his home town of Ribe to practise as a physician. The other was the gifted mathematician Christopher Dybvad, son of the professor of theology Jørgen Dybvad (d.1612), who repeatedly and unsuccessfully applied for a univrsity position, and who eventually received a life sentence in 1620 for his outspoken criticism of the government, dying in prison a couple of years later.[13]

[12] Helk, *Dansk-Norske Studierejser*, 16.

[13] Fink-Jensen, *Fornuften under troens lydighed*, 305; for Christopher Dybvad, see also *Dansk Biografisk Leksikon*.

Only around 10 per cent of all medical students were able to benefit from the generosity of a royal grant, and the majority were left to find other sources of funding. Cathedral chapters continued to sponsor talented students who had attended their schools during their earlier studies, no longer restricting their funding to students of theology – a post-Reformation change which benefited medical students. Some medical students were supported by salaries from vacant professorships. Thus between 1566 and 1571 the studies abroad of Philip Pratensis and Peter Severinus were financed by the vacant professorship in medicine. In 1578 the salary from the vacant professorship in law was split between the medical students Jacob Hasebard and Eskild Christensen, each receiving 100 *thalers*. From 1579 to 1580 the same salary was split between another two medical students, Eskild Christensen and Anders Christensen, to finance their medical studies in Italy. Others benefited from grants provided by individuals such as professor Thomas Fincke in 1619, and the wealthy nobleman Holger Rosenkrantz the Learned. Otherwise jobs as tutors to young noblemen, or teaching/tutoring at the foreign universities, were the only other avenues for generating money; in fact a considerable proportion of the medical students who studied abroad appear to have financed at least part of their studies by serving as tutors for young noblemen doing the Grand Tour – 39 served as tutors at one time or another, more than 35 per cent of the whole cohort.[14]

Study at centres of excellence under some of the leading medical lights of the age was as essential an ingredient in a successful career for a physician as was an MD from a highly regarded foreign university. However, without good institutional contacts within their home university and government, not to mention an influential family network, all these qualifications mattered little. Thomas Fincke profited from such a family connection. In 1603 he was appointed professor of medicine at the University of Copenhagen, immediately occupying the leading chair in medical theory, due to the sudden deaths of Anders Lemvig and Peter Severinus the Dane. Before accepting the chair in mathematics in 1591, Fincke had spent more than 10 years abroad studying at some of the best German and Swiss universities. He had briefly been back in Denmark in 1582, attending his cousin's marriage to Peter Severinus, who had then served as royal physician for more than a decade and long been an internationally famous physician, not least through his work *Idea Medicinae Philosophicae*, published in Basle in 1571. Fincke evidently recognised the value of this family connection, and it quickly proved useful when Severinus warmly recommended him as an excellent mathematician to his friend and mentor in Basle, Theodor Zwinger. Subsequently Fincke appears to have spent some highly profitable years at the University of Basle, being taught by and befriending some of the leading teachers in natural philosophy and medicine, such as Caspar Bauhin, Felix Platter and Theodore Zwinger, under whose tutelage he obtained his MD in 1587. Before that, however, he had published the only major work he ever wrote, *Geometria Rotundi*, in 1583 in Basle.

---

[14] Data collated from Helk, *Dansk-Norske Studierejser.*

In Copenhagen Fincke proved an extremely talented university 'politician' and administrator and he was able to dominate the medical faculty for more than 50 years. By the second decade of the seventeenth century he also presided over what proved to be a hugely influential dynastic network within the University of Copenhagen. Of his four daughters, one married Caspar Bartholin, who became professor of medicine in 1613, another married Ole Worm, who succeeded Bartholin when he moved on to a professorship in theology in 1624. Both these men became internationally renowned members of the medical faculty. The third daughter of Fincke married the prominent Copenhagen physician Jørgen Fuiren, and the fourth one of the professors of theology. This dynastic dominance over the medical faculty continued for three generations through Thomas and Erasmus Bartholin, and then finally to Caspar Bartholin the younger and Willum Worm.

However, even when all these avenues had been utilised success could not always be guaranteed, as the example of Jens Skjelderup shows. When Peter Capiteyn, who had become second professor of medicine in 1546, died in 1557, his son-in-law Jens Skjelderup, who had been professor in natural philosophy at the university since 1549, clearly had high expectations of succeeding him. Skjelderup had done his best to position himself well for his succession. Thus in 1553 Skjelderup had received his BA in medicine from his father-in-law, and three years later he travelled to Rostock with the king's and the university's blessing to have the MD conferred upon him by the prominent Rostock professor of medicine Jacob Bording. Despite having done his utmost to secure his promotion, Skjelderup clearly no longer had the necessary backing without his father-in-law. Instead, the king recruited Jacob Bording from Rostock.[15]

However, a good career was not the only motivation for studying abroad – the ambition to be able to encounter the best training and be part of the most recent discoveries, experiments and insights would have been just as important to those who spent a decade or more of their lives abroad. Contacts established while on the *peregrinatio academica* proved essential for most of the graduates when they returned home. Peter Severinus the Dane corresponded regularly with his former teacher and mentor in Basle, Theodore Zwinger, and similarly Thomas Fincke remained in contact with his Basle teachers. So, for that matter, did Ole Worm when he returned to Copenhagen in 1613 to take up his first professorship in pedagogy after a decade spent at some of best medical faculties in Europe. Worm's correspondence proved particularly voluminous – more than 1,800 letters written and received by him between 1616 and 1654 have been preserved. He corresponded regularly with some of the leading figures within European medicine and natural philosophy, including some of his former teachers. Between 1617 and 1620 he was in regular correspondence with the botanist and physician Caspar Bauhin in Basle, exchanging information about plants and books, on one occasion

[15] Fink-Jensen, *Fornuften under troens lydighed*, 109.

complaining about the low standard of Danish medicine, which, according to him, was 'practised solely by wise women, barbers, and quacks'.[16]

These ongoing exchanges with prominent medical men across Europe were important to Worm for staying on top of the medical profession and for keeping informed about new developments within the field, but just as important was the constant stream of letters received from students whom Worm had been instrumental in sending on their *peregrinatio academica*.[17] Among the first of Worm's students to go abroad was Hans Andersen Skovgaard, a curate's son from Elsinore who had matriculated at the University of Copenhagen in 1620. Two years later Skovgaard was in Wittenberg, attending the lectures of Daniel Sennert. Writing to Worm in November 1622, Skovgaard took the opportunity to forward a couple of recently published books, while expressing the hope that he might be considered for the royal stipend reserved for a medical student, which had just become vacant due to the death of its holder.[18] Skovgaard succeeded in obtaining the royal stipend that year – Worm evidently proved willing to support him and to intervene with his father-in-law, Thomas Fincke, to secure Skovgaard the grant.[19] Although he supported Skovgaard, Worm was not exactly happy with this student, accusing him of writing infrequently and with considerable delay and, when writing, of not being particularly informative. Worm also pointed out in his letter of May 1623 that some of the professors in Copenhagen had objected to the fact that Skovgaard had not yet obtained his MA, which had now become a prerequisite for those who wanted to receive the royal stipend.[20] Skovgaard was clearly rattled and responded with urgency to Worm's rather sour note, deploring his loss of favour and pointing out that he had posted at least five letters which evidently had got lost on the way. He also claimed to have followed Worm's instructions to the letter. He had reported back to his tutors regularly about his academic progress, as well as his scholarly undertakings in Wittenberg, pointing out that he had written not only to Worm, but also to Caspar Bartholin and Thomas Fincke. As for not having obtained his MA, Skovgaard argued that he would have done so in Copenhagen had he been invited to do so. He would now try to obtain this degree in Wittenberg in the spring, since the winter term would be fully occupied with anatomical studies and Daniel Sennert's 'chemical exercises'. Skovgaard also took the opportunity to inform Worm about the books and catalogues he had sent back to him. With regard to his studies, he pointed out that he expected to be able to take his meals at Dr Sennert's

16 Schepelern, *Breve fra og til Ole Worm*, vol.1, no.42; see also nos. 34, 46, 51, 58, 62, 65, 77.

17 See O.P. Grell, 'In search of true knowledge Ole Worm (1588–1654) and the new philosophy', in P.H. Smith and B. Schmidt (eds), *Making knowledge in early modern Europe. Practices, objects, and texts, 1400–1800*, Chicago, 2007, 214–32 and 330–3.

18 Schepelern, *Breve fra og til Ole Worm*, vol.1, no. 117.

19 Ibid., no. 119.

20 Ibid., no. 130.

table in the near future. Sennert had promised to teach iatrochemistry privately to Skovgaard and a few other students for a fee of 'only 10 *thalers* each', as he put it. Skovgaard had no doubt about Sennert's ability, for only he and Hartmann had a serious reputation in this field, nor for that matter about his honesty, since he had not promised him and his fellow students that they would discover great secrets, but only knowledge and experience of the practical, laboratory processes. Skovgaard declared that he was now ready to focus on iatrochemistry, having examined 'the first four parts of medicine'.[21] Despite finally having received the books Skovgaard had bought for him, Worm first complained about the dilapidated condition in which they had arrived, then he informed Skovgaard that 'a letter, as well as being too short can be too long' – talk about being difficult to please. Even bearing in mind some expressions of support from Worm, such as that 'slaps from your friends are better than kisses from your enemies', Skovgaard could be excused if he felt less than fully convinced of his mentor's support. Worm, however, was full of praise for Skovgaard's iatrochemical undertakings and encouraged him to get directly involved in the experiments and not worry about getting himself dirty, because, as he put it, everything depended on the right artisanal skills. He asked for more information about the experiments and an example of the cure of an illness by 'Sennert's method'.[22]

When Worm wrote to Skovgaard some months later, in November 1623, he was far more positively inclined towards his student, telling him how much he had appreciated his most recent letter, and how impressed he was with the progress Skovgaard had made in his medical studies.[23] Worm also requested Skovgaard to supply him with a copy of Sennert's book on scurvy, which was just about to be published, as well as a couple of recent Paracelsian works he had been unable to obtain in Copenhagen. He also took the opportunity to inform Skovgaard that he had started a collection of natural objects, especially rare animal and minerals, and in particular specimens from the sea. If Skovgaard were to come across such items during his travels, Worm asked him to bear this in mind.[24] In May 1624 Skovgaard forwarded to Worm a medical thesis he had written, and Worm once more praised his progress and promised his support. Realising that the royal stipend he had benefited from since 1622 might soon run out, Skovgaard had taken the opportunity to enquire about the possibility of continuing his studies abroad while acting as a tutor to young noblemen. Worm informed him that this had recently become more difficult, since tutors were now expected to have taught at the newly established Academy for the nobility at Sorø (1623) for a couple of years prior to such appointments. Moreover, Worm was not convinced that such a move would prove suitable in Skovgaard's case. Finally, Skovgaard had complained to Worm about the cost of living in Wittenberg, where prices were increasing rapidly, while

21 Ibid., no. 131.

22 Ibid., no. 133.

23 Ibid., no. 139.

24 Ibid., no. 142.

grain was in short supply. Worm responded by suggesting that Skovgaard travel to either France or Italy to continue his medical education.[25] By January 1625 Skovgaard had finally obtained his MA in Wittenberg, and he immediately posted a number of copies of his thesis to Worm and asked him to distribute them among the professors at the University of Copenhagen. Worm evidently made good his promise of support, and Skovgaard became one of the first recipients of the stipend for medical students studying abroad created by Thomas Fincke in 1619.[26]

In 1625 Hans Andersen Skovgaard returned to Denmark, but his sojourn proved a brief one, and he quickly left for Italy, where he arrived in Padua in January 1626. From here he wrote to thank Worm for all the assistance the latter had given him during his time back home, but he deplored the fact that Worm's many engagements as a physician and professor, combined with his own need to make preparations for his journey to Italy, had conspired to prevent them from discussing matters of mutual interest in any depth.

Despite being delighted with his recent safe arrival in Padua, Skovgaard pointed out that the medical faculty there was no longer as excellent as it used to be, except for three professors, namely the Swiss Nicolaus Prævotius, and Benedictus Sylvaticus and Johan Domenicus Sala, both from Padua. This was due to the fact that all anatomical and surgical dissections had ceased in Padua after the death of Adrian Spigelius the previous year. It had proved impossible to replace Spigelius, who had been a master of both anatomy and surgery. Consequently Skovgaard had been forced to seek out private instruction, particularly in anatomy.[27] The contact between Worm and Skovgaard faded somewhat during the latter's stay in Italy. Despite only writing to his mentor about every six months, Skovgaard still imagined that he was doing enough to stay in touch with his teachers back in Copenhagen, even if his last preserved letter to Ole Worm, in October 1627 indicates that he was feeling distinctly isolated and out of touch with affairs in Copenhagen, especially due to the growing impact on communications of the Thirty Years' War. However, Skovgaard still provided a detailed description of his undertakings in Padua. He reported at length on his extended stay in Pisa, where he had explored the splendid botanical garden of the Grand Duke of Tuscany. He gave details of his journey via Siena and Volterra to Rome, where he had befriended the German physician and natural philosopher Johannes Fabricius, not to mention his trip to Naples, where he had spent considerable time in the company of the botanist Fabio Colonna. Finally, he had returned to Siena in November 1626 to have a rest before returning to Padua. Here he was approached by courtiers of the Grand Duke of Tuscany offering him a salary of 200 *thalers* for conducting public dissections in the anatomical theatre in Pisa during January and February 1627. After some hesitation Skovgaard accepted the offer and given no less than 24 lectures and anatomical dissections for a large audience of 400 people. He

25 Ibid., no. 156.

26 Ibid., nos. 172 and 176.

27 Ibid., no. 193.

was eventually offered a permanent position at the University of Pisa, which he politely declined, pointing out that he was obliged to serve the King of Denmark, having benefited from the royal stipend; furthermore, Skovgaard also maintained that he had religious reservations, fearing for the salvation of his soul if he settled in a Catholic country. Bearing in mind his later actions, Skovgaard's supposed religious qualms about accepting a position in a Catholic country cannot have been that sincere, but were probably intended for his audience back in Copenhagen.

Having returned to Padua, Skovgaard undertook a trip to Verona in the company of, among others, the Danish physician based in Padua, Johan Rhode; here they viewed the museum of Johannes Pona. In Padua Skovgaard befriended the natural philosopher Fortunius Licetus, whose recent publication he recommended to Worm. Skovgaard concluded his letter by emphasising his ambition to return to Denmark as soon as possible, despite the damage the country had suffered in the war. His precise plans for a return, however, were up in the air, owing to the effects of the Thirty Years' War, and he added that he might, against his better judgement, be forced to take his MD in Padua. He was eagerly awaiting Worm's advice on what to do, while being repeatedly offered a professorship in anatomy in Pisa. He asked Worm to promote his case in Copenhagen, especially with his former teachers, Thomas Fincke and Caspar Bartholin.[28]

This may well have been the last letter Worm received from Skovgaard, who appears never to have obtained his MD. When Worm wrote to his friend Johan Rhode in Padua some eight years later, in 1637, asking him when he planned to return to Denmark, he asked for any news about Hans Andersen Skovgaard. Worm added 'that he had heard that he lived in the Greek manner with a Greek woman, which might explain why Skovgaard had forgotten all his friends'.[29] The rumour cannot have been far from the truth, for Skovgaard eventually settled as a physician in Constantinople, where he appears to have served successive sultans as a physician.[30]

Another travelling student with whom Ole Worm kept in touch was his nephew, Henrik Fuiren (1614–59). Henrik's father, Worm's brother-in-law Jørgen Fuiren, a physician who, like Caspar Bartholin and Ole Worm, had married one of Professor Thomas Fincke's daughters, had died in 1628, the year young Henrik matriculated at the University of Copenhagen. As later in the case of Thomas Bartholin, whose father Caspar died in 1629, Worm's role became as much that of a father figure as of a tutor.

---

28 Ibid., no. 223.

29 Ibid., vol. 2, no. 630.

30 Thomas Bartholin refers to Skovgaard's death in 1656 in his *De medicina Danorum domestica dissertationes X. Cum ejusdem vindicis & additamentis*, Copenhagen, 1666, 373 'Skovgaard, who was loved by the sultans, died in Constantinople'. I owe this reference to Mr Niels W. Bruun, The Søren Kierkegaard Research Centre, University of Copenhagen. See also Helk, *Dansk-Norske Studierejser*, 382.

Five years later Henrik Fuiren matriculated in medicine at the University of Leiden.[31] Fuiren was an exceptionally wealthy student who needed no financial support. His grandfather Henrik, who had died in 1628, had been among the wealthiest merchants in Copenhagen. Throughout his *peregrinatio academica* Henrik Fuiren constantly sent gifts back to his uncle and mentor, Worm, in Copenhagen. Among the first things Worm received from Henrik was a recently published work by Adrian Spigelius and seeds for his garden. Worm praised the diligence of his young charge and pointed out that he had heard that Fuiren was neither lazy nor tempted to spend his time amongst 'depraved friends'.[32] Writing to Henrik Fuiren three months later, in May 1634, Worm emphasised that he should pay attention to what his teachers told and demonstrated to him, even if it was in conflict with the teachings of the ancients. In such questions, according to Worm, the present age showed daily progress and Fuiren would eventually benefit.[33] When Henrik Fuiren responded at the end of August that year he apologised for his tardiness. He informed Worm that he had joined a private teaching seminar at Leiden run by Dr Walæus, where Walæus diligently explored the basic rules of medicine and solved disputed points raised by the students. Among those who lectured publicly, Fuiren attended the lectures of Dr Vorstius, Dr Heurnius and Mr Boxhorn. Boxhorn explained Ovid's *Metamorphoses* so excellently, according to Fuiren, that even the professors, who often attended his lectures, never left without having improved their knowledge.[34] Worm lauded Henrik for his undertakings in Leiden, even his attendance at Boxhorn's lectures, pointing out that it was important for students of every subject to be able to express themselves beautifully. However, he did point out to him that the study of chemistry and pharmacy was important and should not be forgotten.[35]

By the beginning of 1638 Henrik Fuiren had moved to Paris. He had evidently hoped to find there the famous French anatomist Jean Riolan, but he had departed in the company of the Queen Mother, Maria de Medici. Despite much activity within the faculty, where every doctor demonstrated his exceptional learning in the weekly disputations and the professors 'illuminated our art through learned lectures', Fuiren found it all somewhat disappointing. He concluded ,'However there is no one here, who through their publications produces evidence about their knowledge, which corresponds with their reputations.'[36]

Six months later Henrik provided his uncle with a detailed report of his undertakings in Paris. Initially he had studied chemistry under the guidance of the 'Scotsman Dr. Davidson', a reference to the Paracelsian iatrochemist and later first professor of chemistry at the Jardin Royal des Plantes in Paris, William Davidson.

31 Helk, *Dansk-Norske Studierejser*, 217.

32 Schepelern, *Breve fra og til Ole Worm*, vol.1, no. 509

33 Ibid., no. 520.

34 Ibid., no. 606.

35 Ibid., no. 616.

36 Ibid., vol.2, no. 695.

Evidently, Worm's advice had borne fruit. Fuiren had then focused on anatomy, because he had decided that this was the best time of the year for that practice and he had realised that the Parisian physicians were excellent anatomists. It would appear that Henrik Fuiren saw dissections of human bodies in Paris for the first time and was able to witness the dissection of no less than seven corpses that winter. He had also found time to get instruction in botany, where he had been taught by Guy de la Brosse, founder of the Jardin Royal des Plantes. Having read De la Brosse's book *De la nature, vertu et utilité des plantes* (1628), Fuiren had expected much from this learned man, but he had been disappointed. He found nothing which could satisfy his thirst for knowledge. De la Brosse had proved unfriendly, not allowing Henrik Fuiren free access to his garden, claiming not to have enough time to show him around, due to his many other engagements.[37] Evidently the experience of reading De la Brosse proved far superior to meeting the man himself. Such experiences cannot have been uncommon among students on the *peregrinatio academica* – famous professors did not always live up to their reputations, and consequently disappointed students who had travelled far to meet them.

Henrik Fuiren did not have a strong constitution and he appears to have suffered from a number of ailments while in Paris. This was enough to be a cause of concern for Worm, who in October 1638 advised his nephew to leave Paris for a healthier place. He suggested Montpellier. Admittedly, Worm had not heard much about the university in Montpellier for a number of years, but if it was anything close to what it used to be, then it was truly a centre of excellence for medical students. It matched the best places in Europe in its teaching of anatomy, botany, practical medicine, not to mention the high standard of its disputations; furthermore, its healthy climate and reasonable living costs had over the years proved attractive to many medical students. In the meantime Worm emphasised to Fuiren the value of taking up lodgings with a well-known practitioner, be it a physician, a surgeon or an apothecary, in order to benefit from his experience.[38]

By January 1639 Henrik Fuiren had resolved to continue his studies in Padua and to visit Montpellier en route. Worm approved of his plan, pointing out that it was easy to get passage by boat from Marseille to Italy if there were no pirates around, otherwise the land route through Savoy was a good alternative. Worm also wrote to Johan Rhode in Padua, requesting him to assist his young nephew when he arrived there.[39] By the beginning of June that year Henrik Fuiren finally arrived in Padua. The journey had passed well and Henrik had avoided any illness en route, the risk of which had caused him far greater concern that the fear of highwaymen and robbers. He provided his mentor with a brief description of his journey:

---

37 Ibid., no. 729.

38 Ibid., no. 753.

39 Ibid., no. 767; for the letter to Johan Rhode, see no. 766.

> After we had left Paris on 15 April we first arrived in Lyon, where we spent four days in the company of the highly refined Dr Henri Gras, the most experienced medical practitioner in the city; we had been recommended to him by Dr Poul Moth [Danish physician and former pupil of Ole Worm]. He showed us all many acts of friendship.
>
> He allowed us into his library which is supplied with the rarest books, he took us with him on his visits to his patients, he lent us his assistant who took us to see the city's adornments, the hospital and the orphanage; over and above that he provided us with letters of introduction to the far-famed Chancellor of the University of Montpellier, Dr Ranchin. Equipped with those, we made for Montpellier, where we arrived on 6 May after having seen the Universities of Valance and Orange. I could list many reasons why the spirit of that place appealed so much to me, but for the sake of brevity I shall refrain. However, among the reasons I am unable to suppress, was the superb breeding of the professors, the capital medical garden, and the frequent disputations performed by both physicians and apothecaries; all these factors might have encouraged me to stay longer, if all things necessary for the study of medicine were not already available in Venezia [Pisa]. To be honest I seriously regret the time I wasted in Paris, because it could have been spent in Montpellier with greater purpose for my studies, and at less expense. After having travelled through Marseilles we arrived in Genoa. Thereupon we visited the University of Pisa and viewed its medical garden; then to Florence and from there via Bologna to Padua, where we reached our destination on 9 June after a difficult journey.[40]

Evidently Fuiren was deeply impressed with the medical faculty in Montpellier in 1639, but a couple of years later his cousin Thomas Bartholin gave a totally different assessment in a letter to Henrik Fuiren:

> After wandering right through France and hurrying towards its boundary, we entered Montpellier, which we had been keen to view for ages because of its ancient reputation for medicine, and which you have seen relatively recently; there we were received into quarters that had once been the royal palace of the Majorcan king. Such are the changes in events. The palace has been transformed into a lodging for commoners, and the School of Medicine, hitherto famous for its large quota of famous men and full of eloquence, has now become well nigh speechless. François Ranchin[41] had departed this life a few days before our arrival. The rest boast few achievements, taken up as they are solely with the disputations of candidates for degrees, which are pleasing and erudite when they

[40] Ibid., no. 796 (my translation).

[41] François Ranchin (1565–1641). Distinguished French physician from Montpellier, who became chancellor of its University in 1612. He wrote on obstetrics and the plague.

> are enlivened by doctors from the school. The King's Garden outside the gates lies neglected owing to the absence of the Superintendant Belleval,[42] who is spending time in Paris with the hope of obtaining the post of chancellor.[43]

Fuiren and Bartholin's descriptions of the medical school in Montpellier could hardly have been more different, despite the fact that they were written little more than two years apart. The rapid deterioration in the fortunes of the medical faculty in Montpellier illustrates the difficulties early modern students of medicine faced in their search for centres of medical excellence. Often, the information they possessed about the places they intended to visit was out of date, in some cases because news of a change in circumstances travelled slowly; in others, as seems to have been the case in Montpellier, the reputation of many of these places rested on the shoulders of just a couple of famous individuals who often had no immediate successors. In other words, when they died or moved away, the rationale for foreign students to go there evaporated overnight, and students such as Thomas Bartholin were disappointed.

Henrik Fuiren had arrived in Padua just when the university broke up for the summer recess, so it was not until he wrote to Worm in late November 1639 that he could report on the activities within the medical faculty. The term had only just begun on 3 November, when all the professors started their lectures. The summer break at the University of Padua apparently lasted for around five months! Since the number of lecture courses came to 15, Fuiren found it impossible to attend them all, not least because he had decided to dedicate his efforts to medicine alone. He also informed Worm that he would limit his description to the statements of those physicians whose lectures he attended regularly.

In the first period in the morning Henrik attended the class of Dr Johannes Vesling, who explained the properties of plants. Then he joined Dr Johannes Domenico Sala's interpretations and explanations of Hippocrates' *Aphorisms*. Subsequently he attended the lectures of Johan Baptista Soncino, dealing with abdominal diseases. After lunch he listened to Dr Benedict Sylvaticus' lectures on fevers, which he considered absolutely essential for anyone who had dedicated their life to medicine. Every day he also turned up for Dr Soncino's private lectures which dealt with female diseases; furthermore Dr Soncino regularly held consultations in the morning, which were open to his students. Henrik Fuiren,

---

42 Martin Richer de Belleval (d.1644). Professor of Anatomy and Botany in the University of Montpellier, where he had succeeded his uncle Pierre Richer de Belleval (c.1564–1632).

43 Letter from Thomas Bartholin to Henrik Fuiren in Padua, 28 September 1641. This letter is part of the forthcoming edition of letters to and from Thomas Bartholin translated into English and edited by Niels W. Bruun. I am grateful to Niels W. Bruun for referring me to this letter and letting me quote from the translation.

however, preferred to escort Dr Marchet during his consultations and had already witnessed this gentleman's surgical interventions on several occasions.[44]

Ole Worm congratulated his diligent nephew on his efforts. However, he encouraged him to do his utmost to join a successful local practitioner, a surgeon or a physician, in order to get the relevant experience with private patients and in hospitals. According to Worm, it was 'possible to acquire knowledge of many things through observation, which cannot be described on paper'.[45]

By June 1640 Henrik Fuiren had taken up lodgings with John Rhode, with whom he now conversed daily about medical matters.[46] The following year Fuiren informed Worm that it was not for his personal pleasure that he remained in Padua, but only to make further progress in his study of medicine. He was determined to make up for the time he had wasted in Paris, and had no intention to return home as someone 'unskilled and ill informed in his field'. He could think of no better place to acquire the necessary medical skills than Padua, where, he argued, it was possible for anyone to accompany the practising physicians, something Henrik was himself totally dedicated to. Likewise, Worm knew better than him the value of the advice gained from former and present patients for 'apprentices'.[47] However, not all Henrik Fuiren's time was spent on improving his medical skills. He still found time for personal pleasure, and during the autumn of 1641 he undertook a journey to Rome. By the end of the year 1642 Henrik Fuiren was finally contemplating his return to Denmark, having been abroad for seven years. He informed Worm that he intended to send his belongings to Amsterdam in the spring of 1643. He himself might be somewhat delayed by visits to patients. Apparently patients came rushing into Padua during the spring, which was considered a particularly fortuitous time to prescribe medicine, and to consult the resident physicians and surgeons.[48]

Towards the end of 1644 Henrik Fuiren had decided to travel via Basle to obtain his MD before he returned home. He informed Worm that he intended to leave Padua when the winter had come to an end. Worm also encouraged him to wait and not expose himself to unnecessary dangers 'in the terribly snow-filled mountain passes'.[49] Fuiren stuck to his plan and must have arrived in Basle in either late June or early July 1645.[50] In Basle he was awarded his MD on 14 October 1645, after three days of giving lectures, which were published that month under the title *Praelectiones Basilienses de ascite* [Basle lectures on dropsy] and included

---

[44] Schepelern, *Breve fra og til Ole Worm*, vol.2, no. 816 (my translation).

[45] Ibid., no. 824 (my translation).

[46] Ibid., no. 847.

[47] Ibid., no. 950.

[48] Ibid., no. 1094.

[49] Ibid., vol. III, nos. 1259 and 1269.

[50] Helk, *Dansk-Norske Studierejser*, 217; he was in Milan en route for Basle on 18 June 1645.

a letter from his cousin, Thomas Bartholin, praising his achievements.[51] Still, it took Henrik Fuiren nearly a year to return to Copenhagen via Paris and Leiden, where he finally arrived in the autumn of 1646. Here he worked as a physician for the next 13 years, until his death in 1659, never showing any interest in a career as either a royal physician or a professor at the university. The fact that he was a wealthy man meant that Henrik Fuiren could pursue his interests in botany, medicine and as a collector of natural objects.[52]

The two case studies of Henrik Fuiren and Hans Andersen Skovgaard show some revealing similarities, despite the different social backgrounds of the two students, one the son of a curate, the other the grandson of one of the wealthiest burghers in Copenhagen. Both studied abroad for a decade, confirming the pattern of lengthy studies abroad for medical students. Both attended and matriculated at a number of universities, confirming the view of the *peregrinatio medica* held by the medical student Jacob Svabe, namely that students had to operate 'Like the bees, who neither suck nor generate their honey from one flower, but from many spread all over the place, so it is with education or the acquisition of skills which have to be obtained from a variety of places.'[53]

Even so, there are some major differences. Skovgaard only attended German and Italian universities, while Fuiren included universities in the Dutch Republic, France and Italy in his tour. Evidently Skovgaard was restricted in his travel by his economic circumstances and depended on grants in order to conduct his *peregrinatio medica*, as opposed to Henrik Fuiren, for whom money was no problem. Skovgaard at one point contemplated becoming a tutor for young noblemen doing the Grand Tour while also taking a temporary, well-paid job as an anatomy lecturer at the University of Pisa. However, Skovgaard still found the necessary money to undertake the highly popular trip to Rome and Naples. Despite having held both the royal stipend and Thomas Fincke's stipend, Skovgaard never obtained his MD, though he did contemplate getting it in Padua. Whether it was personal circumstances, i.e. his Greek mistress, or financial need/temptation, i.e. a lucrative offer to become physician to the sultan of Constantinople, which caused him to settle in Constantinople, is impossible to say. Henrik Fuiren, on the other hand, who was under no particular obligation to obtain an MD, did so successfully, picking it up in Basle, which remained a highly esteemed place among his teachers back in Copenhagen, despite the decline of its medical faculty during the early seventeenth century.

---

51 Ibid.; for the letter see the forthcoming edition of letters to and from Thomas Bartholin translated into English and edited by Niels W. Bruun. I am grateful to Niels W. Bruun for referring me to this letter and letting me quote from the translation.

52 For Henrik Fuiren's life see *Dansk Biografisk Leksikon*.

53 Schepelern, *Breve fra og til Ole Worm*, vol. 1, no. 578 (my translation).

PART III
The Centres of Excellence

Chapter 8
Medical Education in Padua: Students, Faculty and Facilities

Cynthia Klestinec

Padua was the most important centre of study for medical students from 1530 to 1650, approximately. Attracting students from all over Italy, the Continent and England, Padua illuminates the experience of *peregrinatio medica* in the early modern period.

In 1597, Johann Svenzelio, the conciliator or lead counsel of the transalpine nation at the university of Padua, noted the importance of the transalpine students at this famous medical school.[1] His account followed the description of the debates between university professors and the Jesuits: lessons given by the latter were taking students away from the former, and eminent professors such as Cesare Cremonini (1550–1631) were outraged.[2] The debates highlighted the issue of matriculation and the potentially waning presence of a geographically diverse student body. With this in mind, Svenzelio turned to the regular affairs of student life, documenting the outcomes of voting assemblies and the organisation of the annual public anatomy demonstration. For the latter, he claimed that 'certainly' if foreign students (*ultramontanis*), including the members of his nation, had not shown up to the anatomical theatre, where the public anatomy demonstration was held, then it would frequently remain empty.[3] The claim is both suspicious – the anatomical theatre was packed just two years earlier,

[1] On the organisation of geographically designated nations, see Pearl Kibre, *The nations in the mediaeval universities* (Cambridge, Mass., 1948), 3–64 and 116–22. On the role of foreign students at Italian Renaissance universities, see the following and their bibliographies: Richard Kagan, 'Universities in Italy, 1500–1700', in *Les universities européennes du xvi au xvii siècle: Histoire sociale des populations étudiantes*, ed. Dominique Julia, Jacques Revel and Roger Chartier, vol. 1 (Paris, 1986), 153–86; and *Universities in early modern Europe, 1500–1800*, ed. Hilde Ridder-Symoens (Cambridge, 1996). On foreign students in Padua, see Giorgio Fedalto, 'Stranieri a venezia e a padova, 1550–1700', in *Storia della cultura veneta* 4, pt. 2 (1984): 251–79, esp. 271–78.

[2] Cremonini went so far as to compare the rivalry and the factions it produced in the student body to the bloody battles between the Guelphs and the Ghibellines. See Cremonini, *Le orazioni*, ed. Antonino Poppi (Padua, 1948), 59–69; and Lucia Rossetti, 'Cesare Cremonini e la "Natio germanica artistarum"', in *Cesare Cremonini: Aspetti del pensiero e scritti*, ed. Ezio Riondato and Antonino Poppi, 2 vols (Padua, 2000), vol. 1, 131–4. On the original oration, see below, n. 4.

[3] *Atti della nazione germanica artista* [Acta germanicae artistarum], ed. Antonio Favaro (Venice, 1911–12), 2 vols Hereafter, this text will be cited as *Acta*, followed by the

when it opened its doors for the first time – and aggressively self assured. The politics of the student body, however, were as clear to the students as they were to the upper levels of the administration, and even to the Venetian Senate. In a decree on voting privileges (ca. 1591), the Senate called attention to the good behavior of foreign students, the 'great valour' of the foreign student body and the ability of both to enhance the reputation of the university abroad, in *il mondo tutto*.[4] And Svenzelio realised that numbers meant power; the members of his nation were visibly present, registering their interest in anatomical proceedings and instantiating the power they held as a group at the university.

The episode suggests another way of understanding the history of anatomy and medicine, that is, by way of students rather than professors and their published texts. As historians of the university have recognised, students influenced the administration as well as the intellectual and pedagogical culture of the university in both its medieval and Renaissance incarnations.[5] This essay will indicate some of the ways that students shaped the content of their own medical education and impacted on the pedagogical culture of late sixteenth-century Padua. To do so, it will rely heavily on the *acta* of the transalpine students. These notes provide a running commentary on the activities at the university, including the outcomes of voting assemblies, the organisation of the nation's library (and the donation of books for it) and the details of pranks, rituals and festivities as well as the content of medical courses and anatomical exercises. With respect to medical and anatomical lessons, students often described the pedagogical styles of their medical professors, the degree to which such lessons satisfied them and their desire for more frequent lessons on anatomy. These aspects serve as the basis for this essay, illuminating the ways that students engaged with and responded to the materials of their medical education.

In contrast to the early sixteenth century, the later sixteenth century witnessed the growing importance of philosophical anatomy in medical education; and in Padua, where medical students appreciated (and sometimes endured) this training, the emphasis on natural philosophy did not reproduce a stale, scholastic form of medical,

year. *Acta*, 1597, vol. 2, 110: Certo si absque Ultramontanis esset, Theatrum saepe vacuum quin reperiretur, vel Excellentissimo Viro teste affirmare ausim.

4 The decree is accompanied by the inaugural oration that Cesare Cremonini gave on 20 December 1591, in which he lambasted the Jesuits and the divisions they sowed in the student body. See Padova, Studio. Documenti 1467–1625, Cod. Cic. 2525/52, n. 22, Correr Library: Ricerca la dignità è servitio del studio nostro di padoa che li dottori forestieri condotti da queste cons. per erudir li scolari in queste scienze che tal sono necessarie per ben regere ogni Republica, essendo queste persone conspicue di gran valore, è stima appreso il Mondo tutto, sino honorati et ben trattati da ogni anno et spetialmente da gli altri dottori della Citta accioche con tal ragioneval modo aletati si rendino sia pronti ad incontrar le occasione di venir à questo servitio.

5 On the history of the university, see n. 1, n. 8, and n. 10. On pedagogy and science studies, see *Pedagogy and the practice of science: Historical and contemporary perspectives*, ed. David Kaiser (Cambridge, Mass., 2005), especially the introduction, 'Moving pedagogy from the periphery to the center', 1–11.

anatomical knowledge. Quite the contrary, for the new focus on natural philosophical anatomy depended on the practices of contemplation and observation, which together helped to produce a new way of looking at natural (and bodily) phenomena. From student records, we can detect not only the grander historical shifts of the period, but also, more locally, the nature of their experiences at this institution, with its professors, both the eager and the cranky ones, and among their peers, all of which offer insight into what constituted the best medical education at the time.

Foreign students were drawn to the medical faculty and facilities in Padua for a variety of reasons. Svenzelio, for example, embedded his remark about the anatomical theatre in a discussion of the merits of studying medicine at Padua (Figures 8.1 and 8.2). He offered two basic criteria for what constituted the best medical education that European institutions had to offer at the end of the sixteenth century: exact anatomies and practical medicine.[6] In one sense, he merely evoked the two branches of medicine, the theoretical and the practical. The theoretical branch focused on the natural philosophical foundation of knowledge used for the study of medicine; it tended to consider systematic knowledge, such as the structure of causal explanation used to produce *scientia* and especially the purposive or final cause of a condition, phenomenon or anatomical part.[7] Often intersecting with theoretical medicine, the practical branch of the medical curriculum focused on texts related to the diagnosis and treatment of ailments; it included discussions of method and anatomical, pathological and therapeutic knowledge as well as surgery.[8]

In the first half of the sixteenth century, as Jerome Bylebyl has shown, medical students, especially foreign students, came to Padua for its offerings in practical,

---

6 *Acta*, 1597, vol. 2, 109–10: Quam ob causam vero Anatomistam ex nostris quotannis procurare debeamus, pluribus demonstrare possem; hoc solum quaero: Quis nobis est, qui Patavium non tam exactissimarum anatomiarum quam fori tantummodo practici caussa adveniat?

7 Important to medical theory was the study of a range of classical and medieval works by philosophers and medical writers, including Hippocrates, Aristotle, Galen and Avicenna. Paul Grendler provides a sample of the curriculum in Bologna and also the curriculum in natural philosophy in *The universities of the Italian Renaissance* (Baltimore, 2002), 320–21 and 269–79; on the study of medicine in Padua, see Jerome Bylebyl, 'The School of Padua: Humanistic medicine in the sixteenth century', in *Health, medicine and mortality in the sixteenth century*, ed. Charles Webster (Cambridge, 1979), 335–70; on the teaching of Aristotle's texts in Padua, see Andrew Cunningham, *The anatomical renaissance* (Vermont, 1997), 168–70; and for a survey of early medicine and its fairly standard curriculum, see Nancy Siraisi, *Medieval and early Renaissance medicine: An introduction to knowledge and practice* (Chicago and London, 1990), 55–77.

8 Grendler, *The universities of the Italian Renaissance*, 322: 'Using Avicenna's *Canon*, book 3, the professors of practical medicine discussed the head and brain in the first year. They passed on to the lungs, heart, and chest in the second year; moved to the liver, stomach, spleen, and intestines in the third; and finished with the urinary and reproductive systems in the last year.'

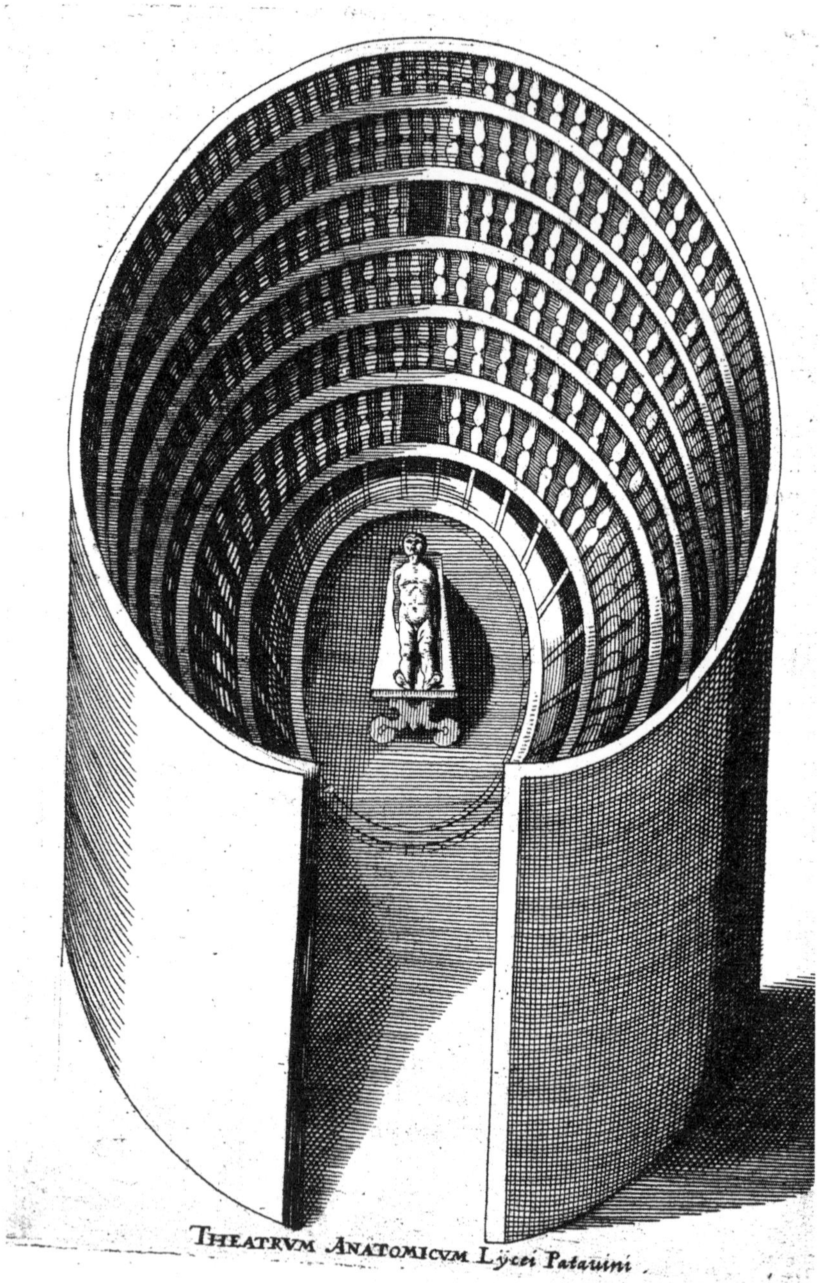

Fig. 8.1 Bird's eye-view of the anatomical theatre at Padua, built in 1595. From J.F. Tomasini, *Gymnasium Patavinum*, Udine, 1654

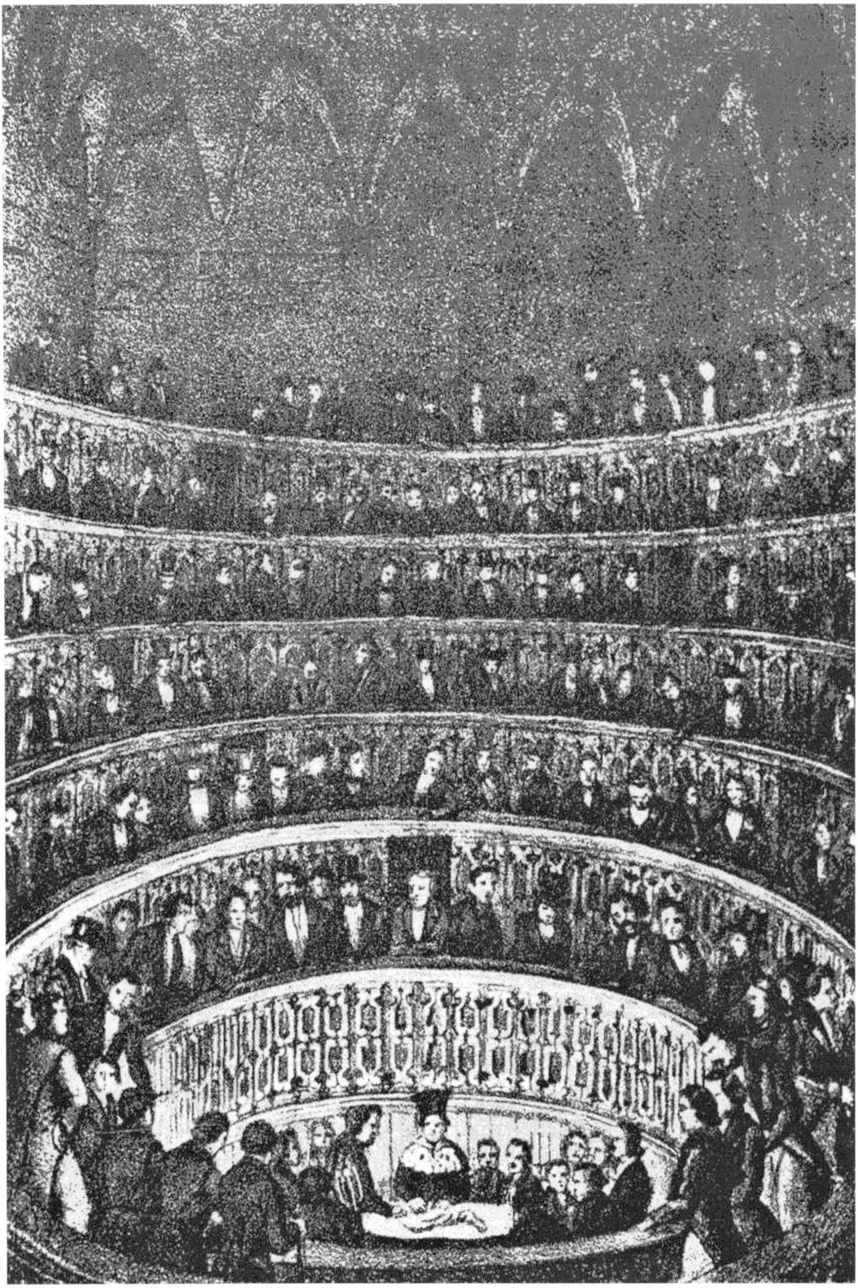

Fig.8.2 The anatomical theatre still in use in the nineteenth century. From P. Tosoni, *Della Anatomia degli antichi e della scuola anatomica padovana Memoria*, Padua, 1842; reprinted 1995

clinical medicine.[9] These flourished alongside and often as a result of medical humanism.[10] After the war of the League of Cambrai (1509–17), an effort was made to hire professors from other institutions and foreign locations. The influx of new professors, which included the Flemish anatomist Andreas Vesalius (1514–64), as well as the expansive printing industry in nearby Venice, allowed intellectual practices associated with medical humanism to prosper. At the same time, professors of medicine such as Giambattista da Monte (1498–1551) emphasised aspects of *materia medica* (herbal remedies) as well as clinical training in their lectures and during their rounds at local hospitals. In the mid-sixteenth century, Bylebyl explains, Venetian and Paduan civic authorities were intensely concerned with hospitals and with their own ability, not that of the clergy, to regulate them.[11] Not surprisingly, then, the domains of *materia medica* and anatomy received a great deal of support in the post-war era, visible especially with the construction of the botanical garden in 1545 (Figures 8.3 and 8.4) and the anatomical theatre in 1594–95.[12] These developments reflected and further encouraged the understanding that a medical education at Padua was second to none.

Many changes, however, took place between the 1540s, when Vesalius taught anatomy, and 1595, when the second anatomical theatre opened, changes which Bylebyl's insightful account is too brief to encompass. In the second half of the sixteenth century and early part of the seventeenth century, students continued to emphasise the importance of clinical medicine, but they also reacted to the intense focus on the natural philosophical aspects of anatomy. Their reactions suggest that the theoretical branch of medicine was the site of a great deal of historical change in the second half of the sixteenth century. Especially prominent was the development of natural philosophical inquiries into anatomy.

The focus on the relationship between natural philosophy and anatomy manifested itself in several areas. Svenzelio used the term *exact* to describe anatomy. In doing so, he referred explicitly to the public demonstrations that the

---

[9] Bylebyl, 'The School of Padua', 335–70.

[10] On medical humanism, *The medical renaissance*, ed. A. Wear, R.K. French, I.M. Lonie (Cambridge, 1985); Bylebyl, 'The School of Padua', and 'Medicine, philosophy, and humanism in Renaissance Italy', in *Science and the arts in the Renaissance*, ed. John Shirley and F. David Hoeniger (Washington, D.C., 1985), 27–49; Vivian Nutton, 'The rise of medical humanism: Ferrara, 1464–1555', in *Renaissance Studies* 11 (1997): 2–19; Cunningham, *The anatomical Renaissance*; and Andrea Carlino, *Books of the body: Anatomical ritual and Renaissance learning* (Chicago, 1999).

[11] Bylebyl, 'The School of Padua', 349.

[12] On the botanical garden, see the following and accompanying bibliography: Vittorio Dal Piaz, 'L'orto botanico e il teatro anatomico di Padova. Indagini e contributi', in *Quaderni per la storia dell'Università di Padova* 31 (1998); and V. Dal Piaz and M. Rippa Bonati, 'The design and form of the Padua 'Horto Medicinale'', in *The Botanical Garden of Padua 1545–1995*, ed. Alessandro Minelli (Venice, 1995). On Padua's anatomical theatres, see below.

professor of anatomy and surgery Girolamo Fabrici (Hieronymus Fabricius of Aquapendente, 1533–1619) gave (Figure 8.5).[13] Beginning his work *On the local motion of animals* (1618), Fabrici explained: 'For this whole time in which we are administering not a popular anatomy, but an exact one, I decided … to deal with the motion by which the whole animal moves with respect to location.'[14] For Fabrici and his students, popular demonstrations covered the general anatomy of the whole body and often served as introductions to the study of anatomy. In contrast, exact anatomies were specific. Organised topically, they focused on the structures and natural philosophical causes related, in this case, to motion (and the sensitive soul).[15] Unlike his predecessors Andreas Vesalius, Realdo Columbo (ca. 1515–59) and Gabriele Falloppio (1523–63), who covered the bones, the muscles, the arteries and the organs in their anatomy demonstrations, Fabrici rarely provided a structural account of the anatomy of the whole cadaver. As Andrew Cunningham has explained, Fabrici's programme of research deepened the relationship between anatomy and natural philosophy; Fabrici had humanist inclinations towards Aristotle, and to a remarkable degree his publications (and research) followed Aristotle's works on the organic soul, the principle responsible for the life functions of the body, that is, the vital operations of digestion, respiration and reproduction (the vegetative soul) as well as sensation (the sensitive soul), motion (the motile soul) and speech (the rational soul).[16]

---

13 Fabrici took the chair of anatomy and surgery in 1565, three years after the death of Gabriele Falloppio (1523–62). Although his responsibilities diminished in the early seventeenth century, he occupied it for nearly six decades, an extraordinarily long tenure and plenty of time to leave his mark on the institution and the field of anatomy.

14 Fabrici, *De motu locali animalium* (Padua, 1618): Toto hoc tempore, quo non popularem, sed exactam anatomen administramus, agere in vestram gratiam, auditores, divino favente auxilio constitui de motu, quo totum animal loco movetur: seu de motu locali totius animalis, seu mavis dicas, de motu, quo totum animal locum, sue positionem mutat.

15 Cunningham, 'Fabricius and the "Aristotle Project", in anatomical teaching and research at Padua', in *The medical renaissance of the sixteenth century*, ed. Andrew Wear, Roger French and I.M. Lonie (Cambridge, 1985), 195–222. This analysis is extended in *The anatomical renaissance*, 167–87.

16 Cunningham, *The anatomical renaissance*, 174. See also Katharine Park, 'The organic soul', in *The Cambridge history of Renaissance philosophy*, ed. Charles B. Schmitt and Quentin Skinner (Cambridge, 1988), 464–84.

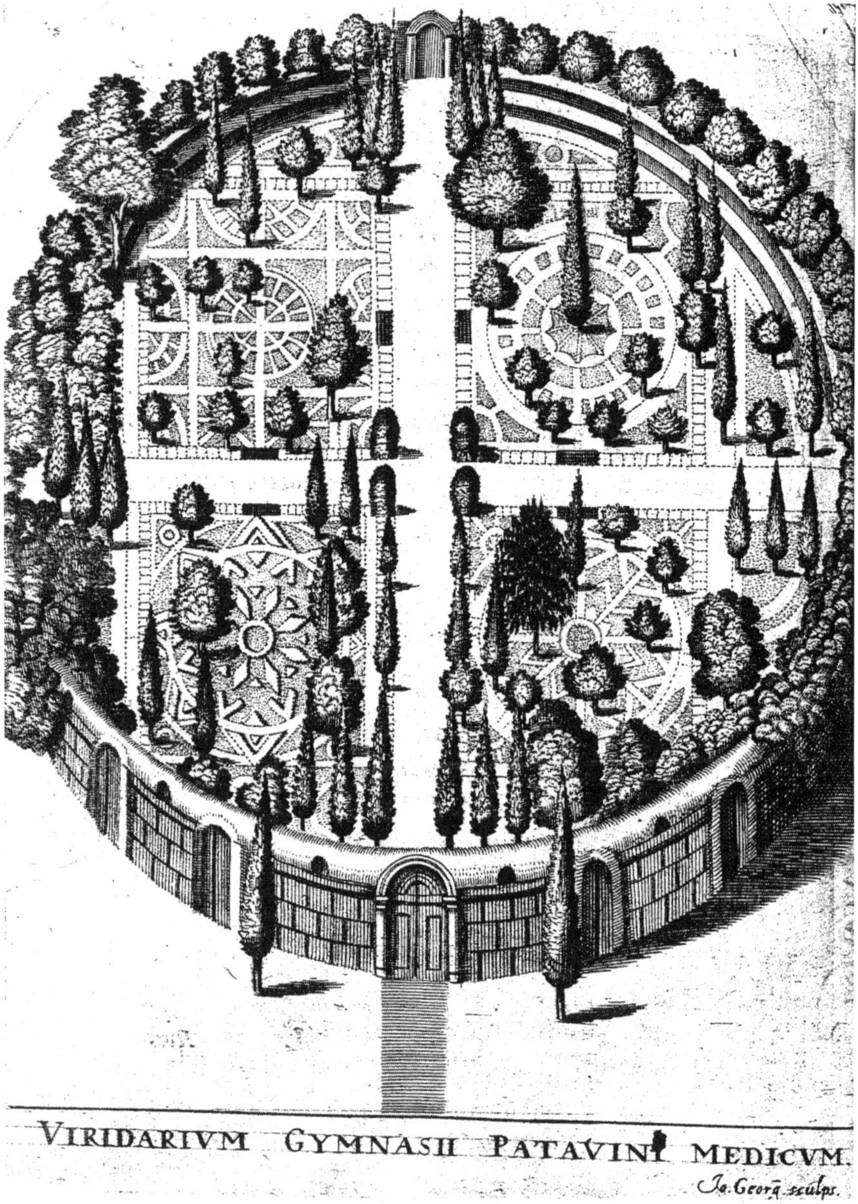

Fig.8.3 Bird's eye-view of 'The medical greenery [***viridarium***] of the Paduan University', or physic and botanical garden, founded 1545. From J. F. Tomasini, *Gymnasium Patavinum*, Udine, 1654

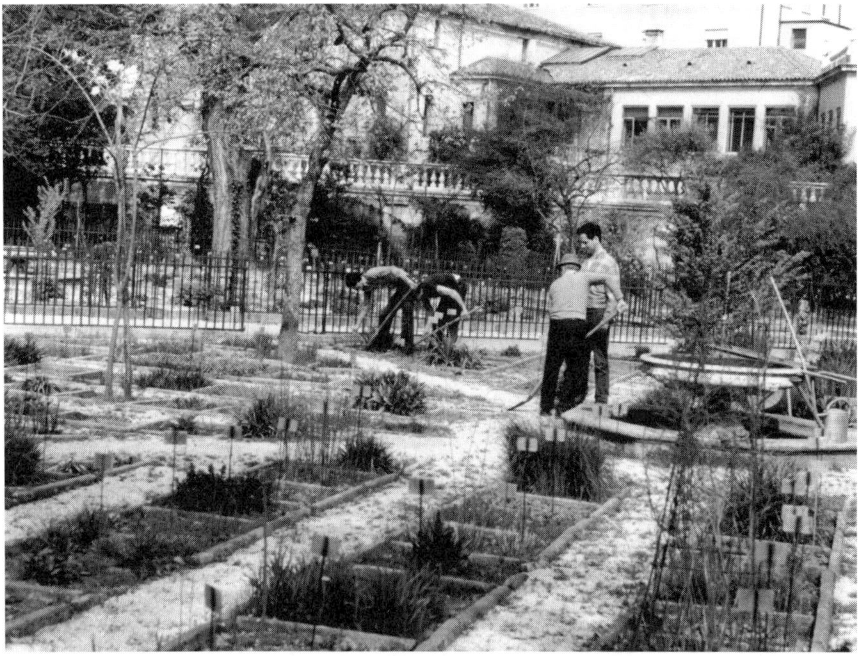

Fig.8.4 The botanical and physic garden at Padua today

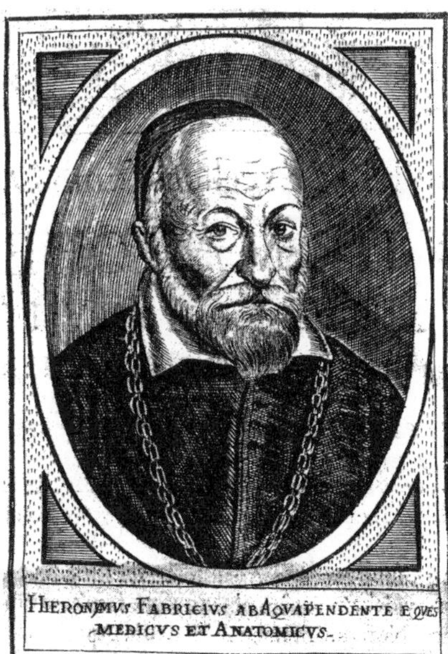

Fig. 8.5 Fabrici (Fabricius ab Aquapendente). From J.F. Tomasini, *Illustrium virorum elogia iconibus exornata*, Padua, 1630

The pursuit of the natural philosophical dimensions of anatomy marked a key difference in anatomical inquiries of the earlier and later sixteenth century. In the late fifteenth and early sixteenth centuries, anatomy lessons, manuals and commentaries might begin with the ways in which anatomy is natural philosophical. Berengario da Carpi (ca. 1460–ca. 1530), for example, begins his commentary on Mundinus's anatomy text by placing it within the context of natural philosophy.[17] In the *Fabrica* (1543), Vesalius describes medicine as a 'sacred art' and assigns anatomy to its foundations and to 'a particular branch of natural philosophy'; it was Vesalius' desire that this branch should be 'recalled from the dead [*ac inferis revocandum*]'.[18] But this was a convention in anatomical writings rather than the beginning of an extensive, rigorously philosophical inquiry into anatomy. Conversely, the early sixteenth-century anatomist Alessandro Benedetti begins his text with the humanist decision to derive his information from Greek sources, especially from directly observed cases documented by classical authors.[19] If Berengario and Vesalius' work used natural philosophy as an appropriate framework for dissection, Benedetti used terminology and the observation of anatomical structures in order to augment the role of discovery in anatomical enquiry (an augmentation visible also in Vesalius's work). In subsequent decades, when Fabrici began to conduct his enquiries, the emphasis on structural discovery waned just as the relationship between natural philosophy and anatomical enquiry became more intimate.

The interest in that relationship came not only from anatomists like Fabrici but also from professors of practical as well as theoretical medicine. In a treatise on anatomical method (1593), Girolamo Capivacci (1523–89), another professor in

[17] Jacopo Berengario da Carpi, *Commentaria cum amplissimus additionibus super Anatomia Mundini* (Bologna, 1521); Roger French, 'Berengario da Carpi and the use of commentary in anatomical teaching', in *The medical renaissance of the sixteenth century*, 42–74, esp. 49; and French, 'A note on the anatomical accessus of the middle ages', *Medical History* 23 (1979): 461–68.

[18] Vesalius, *Fabrica*, dedication: Unde etiam illi potissimum debemus, quod tot conuicris in medicos iaci solitis haec sacratissima ars eluditur, quum tamen ipsius pars, quam liberalibus disciplinis instituti a se turpiter divelli sinunt, praecipua laude illam perpetuo illustret … Caeterum perversissima haec curationis instrumentorum ad varios artifices diductio, adhuc multo execrabilius naufragium, ac longe atrociorem cladem praecipuae naturalis philosophiae parti intulit, 2v … Ac ne, omnibus aliquid communium studiorum gratia tanto successu attentantibus, solus torpescerem, aut etiam a meis progrenitoribus degenerarem, hoc naturalis philosophiae membrum ita ab inferis revocandum putavi, ut si non absolutius apud nos, quam alias unquam apud priscos dissectionum professores versaretur, 3r.

[19] These are two aspects of medical humanism. On the former see French, 'Berengario da Carpi and the uses of commentary in anatomical teaching', 47; and on the latter, see Gianna Pomata, '*Praxis Historialis*: The uses of *Historia* in early modern medicine', in *Historia: Empiricism and erudition in early modern Europe*, ed. Gianna Pomata and Nancy Siraisi (Mass., 2005), 105–46, esp. 115.

Padua, used Aristotle's four causes to distinguish the work of an anatomist from that of a surgeon: the surgeon cuts the body and isolates anatomical particulars, focusing on the material aspects of anatomical structure, while the anatomist, grounded in Aristotelian natural philosophy, moves from material causes to the more abstract efficient, formal and especially, final causes of anatomy.[20] The *demonstratio propter quid*, which gave a knowledge of causes, was seen to develop from the *demonstratio quia*, which was the description of the part; and the anatomist (along with his students) is celebrated for his ability to explain why a thing exists, rather than 'merely' describe it.

Responding to the new intensity of natural philosophical anatomy, students, perhaps more than their professors, struggled with the proclaimed necessity of a natural philosophical foundation for their medical education. Their questions and confusion derived in part from the changing role that anatomy played in their medical education. It was once a minor exercise connected to surgery, and occasionally to therapeutics and the ability to identify the signs and symptoms of disease. Though minor, it served to reinforce the practical training that students received at the university. Increasingly, however, it was aligned with natural philosophy, with the theoretical rather than practical branch of the medical curriculum. The students' experiences of this shift and the quandary it produced were utterly dependent on their physical environment, on the local pharmacies and the hospital of S. Francesco, as well as on the construction of two permanent anatomical theatres (1584–85 and 1594–95). These anatomical theatres were permanent rather than seasonally constructed, and thus established anatomical study as an essential and well-funded component of medical study.

These were the actual venues in which anatomy was studied, the venues where the study of anatomy could illuminate medical as well as philosophical truths. These locations and the interactions between students and professors help to reveal the ways in which the study of anatomy became a major component of medical education, where it reinvigorated pedagogical practices such as observation and vivisection that were used to enquire into the secrets of nature.

Students and Philosophical Anatomies

Medical students were initially frustrated by the philosophical orientation of Fabrici's anatomy lessons. Only two years after his lauded debut (in 1566 his demonstration met with the approval of local and foreign students alike), in 1568 Fabrici gave a demonstration using one male cadaver, one female one and a living animal (a herded animal such as a goat); the Silesian student Lassaro Salio said

[20] Capivacci, *De methodo anatomica* (Venice, 1593). It was published again as *Methodus anatomica, sive, ars consecandi* (Frankfurt, 1594). The *Dictionary of Scientific Biography* indicates that it was formulated between the 1560s and the 1580s. Capivacci explains anatomy in this way: hoc est non modo sensu, sed etiam ratione comparatum (5).

that 'if it was not the most accurate, at least it was tolerable'.[21] Lassaro seemed more impressed by the 'most honourable' burial of the remains, which marked the conclusion of the event, than by Fabrici's demonstration. In 1572, a lack of enthusiasm is again detectable.[22] Fabrici's shortcomings did not revolve around the issue of manual skill. He was not a poor dissector, as the students' descriptions of his inaccuracy might suggest, for only two years later, in 1574, he made the important discovery of the *ostioli* of the veins, a small, delicate ensemble of structures that other anatomists had failed to isolate – which he used to emphasise the importance of causal understanding, not material structure.[23] Rather, Fabrici had failed to meet the expectations of his neophyte audience, to provide his students with a treatment of anatomy that would enhance their medical training. Though students wished to learn how to cut the body, understand the connections between parts, set factures and identify diseases or diseased parts, these features were notably absent from Fabrici's public demonstrations.

Medical students responded by looking to other teachers and alternative lessons for the practical aspects of anatomy and medicine. In 1572, for example, students wanted Niccolò Bucella to offer an anatomy demonstration, because Fabrici's lesson had been so disappointing. Bucella, they said, was a Paduan *medico* and an 'excellent surgeon'; he was 'second to none in all of Italy for learning in surgery and anatomy'.[24] Students emphasised the connection between surgery and anatomy, but they also turned elsewhere for their education in practical matters, even ones related to anatomy.

A range of professors and instructors combined anatomical instruction with a practical focus. These demonstrations, which were considered private, took place in hospitals. During clinical rounds professors taught students how to treat patients, take the pulse, analyse urine and recommend appropriate courses of treatment. During the 1570s and 1580s these private courses were taught by professors of both theoretical and practical medicine: in addition to Capivacci they included Girolamo Mercuriale (1530–1606), Albertino Bottoni (?–1596), Marco degli Oddi (1526–91) and Emilio Campolongo (1550–1604). In 1587–88 Petro Paulo Hochstettero,

---

[21] *Acta*, 1566, vol. 1. 56: Die XVIII Decembris D. Hieronymus Fabricius de Aquapendente, chirurgiae professor, anatomen auspicatus est, quam pro viribus non citra scholasticorum applausu administravit, eamque die 5 Ianuarii anni 1567 absolvit. *Acta*, 1568–1569, vol. 1, 63: Anatome tum administrabatur duorum cadaverum, viri et mulieris, peducisque vivae, si non exquisitissima, saltem tolerabilis, praestita etiam reliquis honorificentissima sepultura. The passage is briefly discussed by Giuseppe Favaro, 'L'insegnamento anatomico di Girolamo Fabrici d'Acquapendente', in *Monografie storiche sullo studio di padova, contributo del R. Instituto Veneto di scienze, lettere ed arti alla celebrazione del VII centenario della università* (Venice, 1922), 125.

[22] On the complaints of Fabrici's students, see Favaro, 107–36.

[23] He explained that other anatomists had missed these membraneous doors because they failed to investigate function (not because they were careless observers).

[24] *Acta*, 1572.

the conciliator of the transalpine nation, described the range of medical courses and their practical emphases. Capivacci taught the 'most exquisite doctrine of the diseases of the head', the diseases of the eye and, 'with his great erudition always showed all these things to us to be connected and not obscure.'[25] Bottoni lectured on the causes, signs, indications and prognosis of diseases, 'setting forth not only the material of the most effective [*accomodatissimas*] remedies but also some things of mystery [*secretis*] that he had added'.[26] Bottoni apparently lectured clearly on all things related to theory, and 'in practice' he was 'accustomed to invite us once more to [attend to] the marvelous [*mira*] felicity and most accurate method of healing'.[27] Degli Oddi lectured for several days at the hospital of S. Francesco on the topic of urine analysis.[28] The list reflects the students' interest in practical courses and texts. During these decades, the transalpine students repeatedly praised these professors for their learning, their pedagogical skill and, with respect to their forays into anatomy, their practical orientation.

The practical orientation of their lessons derived not only from their interest in the medical uses of anatomy (as opposed to the natural philosophical ones) but also from the location of the hospital of S. Francesco. In 1578, when the weather turned cold, both Bottoni and degli Oddi decided, as they were holding lessons in the hospital, to dissect the bodies of two women who had recently died. The decision to open these cadavers was made in order 'to demonstrate to the listeners the affected places and the kindler [or cause] of the diseases'.[29] Subsequently, they dissected the uterus of one cadaver; and Campolongo, professor of theoretical medicine, joined the group and said that in the other cadaver, the body of a woman 'consumed by senility [*marasmo*]', he would 'penetrate the fistula' which resided

25 *Acta*, 1587, vol. 1, 234: Excellentissimus igitur Dominus Hieronymus Capicavius, post absolutam de capitis affectibus exquisitissimam doctrinam, adeo doctum et perfectum de omnibus oculorum malis tratatum nobis praelegit, suasque lectiones ad 11.m. Iulii usque diem produxit, ut maximam ipsius diligentiam cum summa eruditione semper coniunctam esse non obscure nobis omnibus ostenderet.

26 *Acta*, 1587, vol. 1, 235: Quam diligens fuerit Excellentissimus Dominus Albertinus Bottonus in suis quotidianis discursibus, omnibus fere nostris notum est. Nam singulis diebus nos ad novum patientem deduxit, deque illius affectu, causis, signis, indicationibus, ac prognosticis doctissime disseruit, proponendo non solum materias remediorum accomodatissimas, verum etiam semper aliqua quae in secretis habebat adiungendo, ut huius viri singularis benevolentia et humanitas, qua multis nunc annis nostram Nationem prosectus est, hoc quoque et praecendenti anno plurimus perspectissima fuerit.

27 *Acta*, 1587, vol. 1, 235: Etsi enim theoria quam omnes fere ex patria nobiscum adducimus, nos aliquo modo ab illius lectionibus deterrere possit; tamen illius in praxi mira felicitas et accuratissima curandi ratio, nos iterum invitare solet.

28 *Acta*, 1587, vol. 1, 235.

29 *Acta*, 1578, vol. 1, 143–4: Circa finem vero Octobris, cum coeli constitutio frigidior aliquanto esset, decreverunt mulierum quae in nosocomio illo morirentur, cadavera aperire et auditoribus locos affectos et morborum fomites demonstrare. Bylebyl also refers to this episode but does not discuss the specifics ('The School of Padua', 350).

beneath her breast, cutting into it in order to show its parts more clearly.[30] The examination was then interrupted by the complaints of more than one old woman (*anicularum*). Although the authorities threatened Degli Oddi and Campolongo with the loss of their salaries – probably because the dissection was improvised, unregulated and, for the old women, a cause of suspicion and concern – the events treated practical, medical issues. They focused on the nature and cause of diseases and abnormal conditions arising from a fistula; and they also took place in the most practical of locations, the hospital. In contrast, when Fabrici addressed his students in the winter of 1578, the students Samuele Keller and Johann Wolfango Rabus described how he 'filled and elevated their souls with many things'.[31] The contrast reveals the different content of the lessons and the experiences of students. The description also sets Fabrici's anatomy lessons in the context of natural philosophy and its extended discourse on soul.

Competing Faculty and Facilities

The hospital was not the only venue designated for the study of anatomy. In fact, the history of anatomical venues reflects a great deal about the ways in which anatomy and medicine intersected in the second half of the sixteenth century. In 1583, and probably as a result of student complaints, the administration initiated a series of reforms that clarified Fabrici's responsibilities and called for the construction of the first permanent anatomical theatre.[32] Noting the 'utility and great honour' that Fabrici's work brought to the university, the administration

---

30 *Acta*, 1578, vol. 1, 143–4: id consilium feliciter satis ceptum in duobus corporibus subito fuit eversum. Cum enim die sequenti uteros harum mulierum aperire constituissent, et in altera, quae marasmo consumta erat et fistulam sub pectore habebat insignem, incidere et commonstrare quonam penetrasset fistula, Aemylius Campolongus ipsorum aemulus suis eodem die uteri sectionem pollicitus, uteros horum cadaverum abstulerat; unde factum ut re hac, et quaerelis anicularum idem, si morerentur, timentium, ad praefectos nosocomii delatis, interdictum sit et Oddo et Campolongo, sub poena amissionis salarii, ne quod cadaver in posterum aperirent.

31 *Acta*, 1578, vol. 1, 144: De Excellentissimo etiam Anatomico compellando tractatum, quod tantum minus necessarium videbatur, cum ipse non tamen in publicis praelectionibus sed etiam in privatis colloquiis anatomen polliceretur et animos multa spe impleret et erigeret.

32 The series of decrees is recorded in *Acta*, 1583, vol. 1, 192. The administration was also likely motivated to regulate or at least to clarify the nature of anatomical proceedings because private anatomies had begun to occur more frequently, and the issue of obtaining cadavers for them was of greater concern. For the disruption of burial as the origin of this concern, see Carlino, *Books of the body*, pp. 190–94; Katharine Park, *Secrets of women: Gender, generation, and the origins of human dissection* (New York, 2006), chapter 5; and Park, 'The criminal and the saintly body: Autopsy and dissection in Renaissance Italy', in *Renaissance Quarterly* 47 (1994): 1–33.

decided that he would conduct the anatomy as he had done 'year after year' and offer lessons on surgery; and to prevent one lesson from interrupting the other, the two would be held separately.[33] For his anatomy demonstrations, Fabrici received 400 florins, and for his surgical demonstrations another 200 florins, raising his annual income considerably.[34] In practice, however, Fabrici offered surgery demonstrations infrequently because they were included in the private anatomies given by Guilio Casseri (1552–1616), a former student and later rival of Fabrici's, and Paulo Galeotto.[35]

With its decision, the administration distinguished the content of the annual anatomy demonstration from surgery demonstrations. Previously, the same anatomist would move between public and private venues; and in both, he would highlight the admirable form of the body (natural philosophical) and then emphasise the importance of knowing anatomy in order to understand sources of disease (medical) and the ways to set fractures (surgical). The administration's decision helped to distribute these aspects among faculty members: Fabrici gave public anatomy demonstrations that were more philosophical in character; and Casseri and Galeotto administered private anatomies, emphasising the medical and surgical uses of anatomy. In 1585–86 Casseri offered a private anatomy, and the students said that 'by dissecting very carefully all the parts of the body – not only the internal parts but also the external (i.e. the muscles and veins) – and in addition by demonstrating the main surgical operations', he 'acquitted himself excellently and satisfied us all'.[36] Galeotto also gave a private anatomy which students commended for its 'special usefulness'.[37] More consistently than Fabrici, Casseri and Galeotto employed a pedagogical approach that relied heavily on the dissection of the internal and external parts of the body, on the display of surgical

---

33 *Raccolta Minato*. n. 56: 5 February 1583, Et perchè ognuno sa di quantoa utilità, et honorevolezza sia al detto studio il far l'Anatomia ogn'anno … L'andera parte, che'l D. Hieronimo Fabritii sia condotto a legger nello studio nostro di Padoa l'Anatomia ordinamente di anno in anno, et la Chirurgia insieme in questo modo però, che tutti li mesi dell'Inverno sia tenuto leggere, tagliare, et mostrare l'Anatomia come lettura ordinaria, passati veramente i mesi d'Inverno non possendosi per li tempi caldi maneggiare si corpi morti, che si puovefanno sia tenuto legger per ordinaria la Chirurgia non intermettendo però quando si possa tagliare, mostrare, e trattare anco le cose di essa Anatomia.

34 Ibid.

35 Giuseppe Sterzi, 'Guilio Casserio, anatomico e chirurgo (c. 1552–1616)', in *Nuovo archivio veneto*, ser. 3, 18 (1909): 207–78; 19 (1910): 25–111. Though Galeotto was immensely popular with the transalpine students, I have been unable to find him in the academic roster.

36 *Acta*, 1585–1586, vol. 1, 210: In qua sane diligentissime omnes non modo internas corporis partes, sed et externas, id est musculos atque vasa dissecando, insuperque praecipuas operationes chirurgicas monstrando optime sese gessit, nobisque omnibus satisfecit.

37 *Acta*, 1585–1586, vol. 1, 211: Rogamus itaque universos et singulos, ut benevolentiam et labores huius clarissimi viri, propriamque utilitatem considerando, frequentes huic interesse velint.

operations and often on the participation of students (a feature made possible by the more intimate setting of the private lesson). Thus, while private lessons focused on manual techniques such as surgical manoeuvres, the public anatomy demonstration could focus on the natural philosophical dimensions of anatomy, demanding from the students a new, conceptual sophistication.

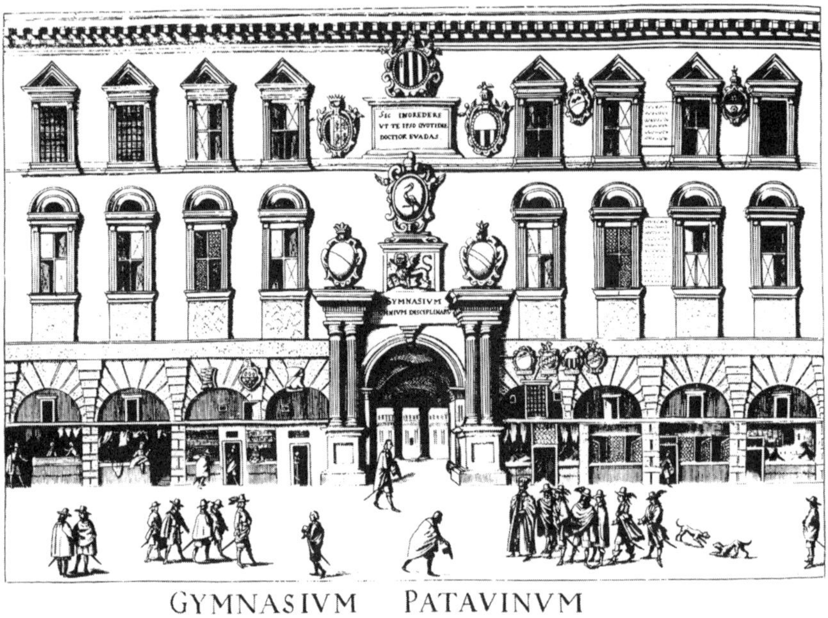

Fig.8.6 The Bo, façade. The anatomical theatre is behind the blind windows of the top two floors on the left. From J.F. Tomasini, *Gymnasium Patavinum*, Udine, 1654

Conceived as a part of these reforms, the first permanent anatomical theatre in Padua was completed by 9 January 1584.[38] A small wooden structure, much like scaffolding, that was built in a corner of Palazzo del Bò, the theatre was described as a *theatrum publicum et perpetuum*, literally a place for seeing that was public and permanent (Figure 8.6).[39] It was called public because it was intended to hold

[38] Antonio Gamba, 'Il primo teatro anatomico stabile di Padova non fu quello di Fabrici d'Acquapendente', in *Atti e Memorie dell'Accademia Patavina di Scienze, Lettere ed Arti* XCIX (1986–87): 157–61.

[39] *Acta*, 1584: Theatrum et cubiculi ad usum anatomiae agendae ex serenissimi Dominii benignitate de publico aerario eiusdem Dominii costructi sunt, ut in perpetuum preseverent ad ipsum usum destinati. See also Jacopo Tomasini, *Gymnasium Patavinum* (Udine, 1654), p. 77; and Gamba, 'Il primo teatro anatomico', 158.

the public anatomy demonstration, while temporary theatres would continue to host private anatomical exercises.[40] It provided not only a material space that was permanent but also a formal arrangement, a permanent seating order and the hierarchical display of academic posts: 'in the new theatre, the frontmost seats had been assigned to the Venetian grandees along with the Rector and the professors, and the next nearest seats to the conciliators'.[41]

In addition to emphasising formal codes of conduct (rather than the students' ability to observe anatomical minutiae), the theatre encouraged rather than quelled competition between professors. In 1586–87, in late January, Galeotto gave a demonstration, amidst 'a throng of spectators', in the church of St Catherine, which was appreciated because he had shown a special concern for his students. So great was his concern that he could elicit and receive funding from both the Italian and the transalpine students to pay for the construction of the temporary theatre.[42] Whereas Fabrici oriented his demonstrations around his own, topical interests, Galeotto seems to have treated anatomy more comprehensively, covering what was 'useful' for students before turning to a specific topic. In 1587 he explained 'the external lineaments of the body' before focusing on the eye, when he 'lectured so clearly and so learnedly on its action and structure that he conducted himself as a man most experienced in anatomical matters and in optics'.[43] In 1588–89

---

[40] While this theatre was visited by Venetian authorities, it does not seem to have been of interest to the local community, except in one instance, which I discuss below.

[41] *Acta*, January 23, 1584, vol. 1, 193: initium anatomicae publicae coepit h. 16 matutina, praesentibus aliquot doctoribus medicis, philosopho item Mercenario et metaphysico, ubi in novo illo theatro magnificis Venetis, una cum Rectore et professoribus primae sessiones, Consiliariis vero proximae fuerunt assignatae. See also Gamba, 'Il primo teatro anatomico', 159. While *theatrum* means a place for seeing and would seem to imply a more concentrated focus on the dissected corpse, the description of the seating arrangement suggests that the spectators who could see the most were the dignitaries rather than the students. The practices of intense, visual scrutiny were not immediately present in the new theatre.

[42] *Acta*, 1586–1587, vol. 1, 225: Absolvit interim anatomiam suam Galeotus, quam multis diebus diligenter satis et in excitante eum auditorum frequentia hactenus administraverat. Cumque paulo post sponte Italos nonnullos gratitudinis ergo in theatri anatomici exstructionem contulisse symbola praedicaret, a nostris idem sese sperare haud obscure significabat; potissimum cum sciret nostram prae reliquis Nationem anatomicis ut plurimum delectari studiis, haecque res omnis non in suam sed auditorum suorum utilitatem esset redundatura.

[43] *Acta*, 1586–1587, vol. 1, 225–6: Excellentissimi Anatomici tam lauta fuisse promissa dixi, ut nihil praeter anatomica exercitia totam hyemem expectaverimus… potissimum cum sciret nostram prae reliquis Nationem anatomicis ut plurimum delectari studiis, haecque res omnis non in suam sed auditorum suorum utilitatem esset redundatura… Facto autem principio, post declarata externa corporis lineamenta cadaveris ratione protinus ad oculum aggressus Anatomicus, de eius actione et fabrica ita plane ita erudite multis disseruit lectionibus, ut virum sese gesserit anatomicarum rerum et opticae peritissimum.

Galeotto gave a private lesson *in officina al Corallo*, which was a pharmacy, a setting of considerable, practical importance to the study of medicine[44]:

> [Galeotto] conducted in the workshop *al Corallo* for three whole weeks a thorough and complete anatomy, in which not only did he demonstrate most clearly and with amazing facility and beautiful method the way to dissect bodies, the structure of all the parts and their actions and functions, but he also showed us the ways … through the whole body of the veins, arteries and nerves, to the great delight of us all.[45]

Students appreciated Galeotto's attention to the techniques of dissection and the isolation of anatomical parts. In 1588, and again in 1591, they recorded their desire to commend in any way possible in all subsequent years the 'generous industry' of Galeotto.[46]

While the competition between Galeotto and Fabrici increased, the students' remarks suggest that Galeotto spent considerable time on the processes of dissection and on the comprehensive study of anatomy. Fabrici, however, seems to have radically shortened the time spent discussing anatomical structures (the stage of the demonstration called *historia* or *observationes*). This pedagogical tendency is reflected again in Fabrici's final demonstration in the first anatomical theatre. In 1588–89 the demonstration relied on two male corpses, the bodies of criminals executed for their 'evil deeds'.[47] Fabrici spent only the first two days of

---

44 *Acta*, 1589, 271.

45 *Acta*, 1588–1589, vol. 1, 248: His itaque peractis, et publica anatome tandem ad finem perducta, Eccellentissimus vir Dominus Paulus Galeoti ne quid a pristina sua de scholaribus bene merendi voluntate recessisse videretur (quam vis iniuriis publici Anatomici theatrum ipsius esset destructum, ipse variis modis ab eodem fuerit lacessitus et in minus commoda carnisprivii tempora reiectus), in officina *al Corallo* per integras tres septimanas luculentissimam et absolutissimam habuit anatomiam, qua non solum mira facilitate ac pulchra methodo, modum secandi corpora, partium omnium structuram ac earundem actiones et usus evidentissime monstravit, sed etiam venarum, arteriarum et nervorum in universo corpore ductus et propagines, non sine maxima omnium nostrorum iucunditate, sine ullis nostris impensis (quamvis ad eas ut aequum erat a spectatoribus exigendas a nobis hortaretur) nobis ostendit.

46 *Acta*, 1591: Conveniens certe fuisset et gratis auditoribus dignum, Galeoto pro immensa et liberali sua industria si nobis nullus modus reprehensione et invidia carens occurrebat alius, is constituebatur, uti verbis saltem Nationis nostrae nomine ipsi gratiae agerentur, merita ista ipsius perpetuae nostrorum memoriae commendarentur, sique alia de nostra Natione in ipsum proficisci possent gratitudinis munia, ea prompta parataque offerrentur omnia.

47 *Acta*, 1588–1589, vol. 1, 267: Ad ultimum Massarii etiam admoniti fuerunt, ut diligenter observarent, me loca illa, quae Consiliariis in anatomia destinata sunt, ab aliis occuparentur, atque illi vel abire vel de alio sibi loco prospicere cogerentur. XIIII die eiusdem mensis a magnifico huius urbis magistratu duo hominum propter furta et

the demonstration on the dissection; by the seventh day, 23 January 1588, he was lecturing on the topic of generation and fetal development (a subject that seems unrelated to his male specimens). The students noted that Fabrici could have been more diligent about the administering of this anatomy, but 'he hardly kept his promises'.[48] In other words, though Fabrici could have focused more attention on the dissection of the body and its particular structures, he did not.

In addition to pedagogical variations, the atmosphere inside Galeotto's temporary theatre was one of considerable discipline and learning. But the same could not always be said of the atmosphere inside Fabrici's theatre. As Fabrici began his afternoon lecture in 1588, the theatre was 'besieged by many people, friends of the student-assistants [*massariorum amicis*] and members of the local community [*popularibus*]'.[49] Although the Syndic tried to lead the Doctors and Professors into the theatre, many people arrived late, and the noise and confusion interrupted Fabrici's lecture.[50] Suddenly, two murderous thugs (*sicarius*) broke into the theatre and threatened the spectators; a fight and a fire broke out; while both were extinguished, the damage from the fire helps to explain why this theatre was never used again and why it was destroyed sometime between 1589 and 1592.[51]

maleficia perpetrata ad furcam damnati sunt; et quo minus anatomia publica impediretur aut differeretur, istorum corpora eadem statim die Universitati concessa fuere.

48 Ibid.: Ad XVI diem huius, Aquapendens hora XVI dissectionem structurae humani corporis aggressus est. Quamvis autem Aquapendens in huius anatomes administratione XIIX dies integros consumpserit, atque paulo diligentionem atque superioribus annis se gesserit, aureis tamen suis pollicitationibus minime satisfecisse videbatur.

49 *Acta*, 1588–1589, vol. 1, 267: Anatomicus audita iam hora lectionis initium fecisset, loca illa, quae tantum pro Consiliariis retinenda essent, a pluribus aliis vel Massariorum amicis vel popularibus obsiderentur, ut ita advenienti Domino Syndico apud Consiliarios nullus relinqueretur locus. On class categories, see Brian Pullan, *Rich and poor in Renaissance Venice: the social institutions of a Catholic state, to 1620* (Cambridge, Mass., 1971).

50 *Acta*, 1588–1589, vol. 1, 267–8: Syndicus autem Universitatis atque amplissimi sui offitii ratione statim ab initio anatomiae apud Doctores et Professores in theatro locum obtinere potuerat; ne se ipsum tamen ingerere videretur, Dominis Consiliariis se adiungere maluit. Cum igitur se aliquantulum tardius accessisse, atque loca, facto lectionis initio, replete videret, potius sibi abeundum quam strepitum aliquem excitandum aut legentem Anatomicum interturbandum esse, cogitavit.

51 *Acta*, 1588–1589, vol. 1, 268: Sed bidellus Universitatis, qui ad theatrum expectare atque advenientes Professores ad assignatas sessiones deducere soelabt, videns in theatro quaedam Professorum loca vacua superesse, Domino Syndico locum dari Massarios iubet…Etenim Domino Syndico vix theatri limina transgresso, duo Siculorum, seu ut rectius dicam siccariorium, ex quatuor illis Massariis obviam fiunt, qui non solum posthabita omni Universitatis et praesentium Excellentissimorum virorum authoritate, sibilis et ignominiosis verbis ipsum ut hoc loco indignum explodere tentabant, sed etiam alter ipsorum exuto omnis humanitatis offitio, stricto pugione impetere nequaquam subverebatur. Contra tamen Dominus Sapiens, ut vere sapientem atque fortem virum decet, sufficienter refutatis atque convitiis in adversaries retorsis, strenue se opposuit, neque latum quidem unguem ab eo

As Fabrici began to develop his philosophical inquiries and to use the permanent anatomical theatre to explore the relationship between natural philosophy and anatomy, the study of anatomy achieved considerable visibility. It became a point of interest for the wider community and, as this episode indicates, questions of discipline began to plague the anatomical theatre. The sensational episode foreshadows what would become a repeated theme in descriptions of anatomical theatres, namely, their regulatory function – to control not only students but also members of the local community, including adversarial interlopers.[52]

Completed and in use by 1595, the second permanent anatomical theatre was larger than the first and more capable of providing crowd control. It was an elliptical arena, a wooden stadium with surprisingly sheer verticality; stairs encircled the shell and served the elliptical structure with various means of access; and there were eight windows, which provided ventilation and illumination.[53] Described as 'exquisite', 'most honourable' and 'dignifying', this theatre celebrated the academic tradition of anatomy and witnessed the emergence of a dramatic tradition of public anatomy demonstrations.[54] For medical students, however, the second theatre more fully separated the processes of dissection from the demonstration. It did not immediately provide a visual experience of dissection; rather, like much

---

quem occuparat loco dimoveri passus fuit. : Ubi Anatomicus intelligeret, rem hanc ad arma devenire, atque hunc ignem in immensum incendium quod postmodum quam difficillime consopiretur, excrescere et hinc propter vicinum malum ad se quoque aliquid mali pervenire posse, confestim Siculis serio interdixit, ne quid ulterius contra Syndicum, cui maxime hic locus competeret, susciperent. On the destruction of the theatre, *Acta*, 1592, vol. 11, 32; and Gamba, 'Il primo teatro anatomico', 159, n. 12.

[52] Following this episode, however, administrators wondered if students shouldn't carry more weapons into the theatre so that, in the future, potential crimes could be averted.

[53] The second theatre was completed in 1594, according to F. Abriano, *Annali di padova* (a manuscript collection of chronicles of Padua, the library of the Civic Museum, Padua, BP 149), 135v. The architect of the theatre remains unknown. Critics have suggested Fabrici as well as Dario Varotari, a friend of Fabrici, who in addition to being a painter was also the architect of Fabrici's villa. They have also underscored the theatrical elements of the space and the demonstration. See V. Dal Piaz, 'L'orto botanico e il teatro anatomico di Padova, indagini e contributi,' *Quaderni per la storia dell'Università di Padova* 31 (1998): 63–73, 69; M. Rippa Bonati, 'L'anatomia 'teatrale' nelle descrizioni e nell'iconografia', in *Il teatro anatomico: storia e restauri*, ed. Camillo Semenzato (Padua, 1994), 74–6, and 'Le tradizioni relative al teatro anatomico dell'Universita di Padova con particolare riguardo al progetto attribuito a fra' Paolo Sarpi,' *Acta Medicae Historiae Patavina* 35–6 (1988–90): 145–68; and G. Cagnoni, 'I Teatri anatomici dell'Università di Padova', tesi di laurea, IUAV, Venice (unpublished).

[54] *Acta*, 1594, vol. 2, 32: iam splendide satis extructum; and *Senato Terra Registro 66* (ASV): il theatro per farla in esso stabile, et honoratissimo, resta nondimenso à farsi provisione, esse non sia disturbata, come per l'aversoro si è fatto ogn'anno con maleficio de'scolari, et con non poca indegnità nosora pero.

Renaissance drama, the performance relied on the verbal skills of the anatomist and the listening skills of the audience.[55]

Spectators came to watch and listen to Fabrici as he expounded upon the (initially anatomical) causes of human nature. The architecture of the theatre reinforced this point. In 1606, Cesare Malfatti described the theatre as beautifully constructed in walnut and containing two rooms, one for the anatomists and the demonstrations, and one for the cadavers and their dissection.[56] In his history of the university, *Gymnasium Patavinum* (1654), Jacopo Tomasini (1595–1655) extended this description: the second anatomical theatre contained two chambers, an inner one where 'the cadavers and the dissected parts were worked upon', which also contained 'skeletons, instruments and other things likely to be used by the anatomist', and an arena where the cadavers were 'demonstrated publicly before the presence of various student nations', university officials and statesmen[57] The separation of the two chambers meant that the demonstration privileged the display of a previously dissected cadaver rather than the process of its dissection. While such display depended on seeing the cadaver, it did not lend itself to scrutinising the structures and shapes of anatomical particulars. By 1599, moreover, it was standard for the student-assistants (*massari*) to dissect the specimens in the inner chamber before the demonstration began. As Giuseppe Sterzi has noted, in that year they were renamed *anatomistae*, anatomists, indicating that the process of dissection was not only prior to and separate from the demonstration but also largely removed from Fabrici's responsibilities.[58]

While it is somewhat startling to learn that Fabrici let his students undertake the dissection, we should remember that his programme of research did not depend on the discovery of new anatomical structures. Instead, it depended on normative structures, the features of anatomy that were typically present in the specimens. Fabrici was here following Aristotle, whose study of nature began

---

[55] Richard Andrews, *Scripts and scenarios: The performance of comedy in Renaissance Italy* (Cambridge, 1993), 31–63, and for Padua and Venice, 121–68.

[56] Cesare Malfatti, *Descrizione particolare della città di padova et del territorio padoano*, [1606], 54.

[57] Jacopo Tomasini, *Gymnasium patavinum*, xxxi, De anatomia et anatomicus, 78: Adversa altera conclave aperit, in quo praesentibus variarum nationum studiosis, quae publicae demonstranda sunt, apertis cadaveribus exscindi ac praeparari consueverunt. Huius fores et parietas Anatomicorum insignia exornant, grata Universitate, tum ingenio docentium, tum laboribus naturae arcana scrutantium, honorem hunc exhibente. Ex eo in spatium aliud porta ducit, in cuius secretiore angulo cadavera, eorumque partes dissectae asservantur. In eodem arrae sunt et conditoria, vestimentis, sceletis, instrumentisque Anatomicorum custodiendis aptata.

[58] Sterzi, 'Guilio Casseri', 213, 232–5. In the previous year, the transalpine students had thought it necessary to elect a *consigliere anatomico*, a kind of preparer, to help Fabrici with the labours of dissection.

with common, not rare, experiences and sense perceptions.[59] While the study of common phenomena would eventually give way to the study of particular, highly circumstantial phenomena, the Paduan tradition of anatomy, as it was embodied in Fabrici and practised in the late sixteenth century, was dedicated to normative anatomy. The extraordinary and the monstrous lay beyond the bounds of Fabrici's programme and the Aristotelian coordinates of explanation. As Fabrici himself explained: 'even if certain extraordinary animals form exceptions, they do not invalidate the truth of my statements'.[60] Thus, even if students, in the course of their preparations, failed to isolate the entire set of structures under discussion, Fabrici could verbally describe them and get on with the business of their functions and natural philosophical uses. The structures were normative; they were, for the most part, already known.

At the end of the sixteenth century, the public anatomy demonstration was not a spectacle of corporeal dismemberment, but rather a natural philosophical presentation, suitably popularised and dramatic. It occasionally included music;[61]

---

59 Lorraine Daston, 'Baconian facts, academic civility, and the prehistory of objectivity', in *Rethinking objectivity*, ed. Allan Megill (Durham, N.C., 1994), 37–63. With respect to Aristotle and anatomical methods, Andrea Carlino notes that Aristotle's works made observations more significant, and analogies between animal and human physiology legitimate. See *Books of the body*, 133.

60 Fabrici, 'De formatione ovi et pulli', in *The Embryological treatises of Hieronymus Fabricius of Aquapendente*, ed. trans. Adelmann (Ithaca, 1942), 142.

61 On music, *Acta,* 1597, vol. 2, 111: A.d. 12 Xbris ad exhilarandos anatomiae spectatores recreandosque ex tristi aspectu animos, ex vetusta consuetudine (quae tamen superioribus aliquot annis proximis interrupta) fidicines ab Anatomistis conducti et in Theatrum reducti fuere, procurante hanc rem sedulo D. Placotomo; aderantque musici isti etiam sequentibus diebus quamplurimis, sumtus certe qui illis irrogantur minime poenitendi, si quidem dum ipsis attendunt et auscultant spectatores, ab omni tumultu et calcitratione supersedere solent, cuius tranquillitatis gratia Theatrum anatomicum aliquot annos diutius inconcussum durare poterit. See also Gamba, 'Il primo teatro anatomico,' 160. See also *Acta*, 1600, vol. 2, 171: [8 January] Ingruentibus iam magnis frigoribus, coeloque iam nives, pruinas, glacies que demittente, Excellentissimus Aquapends absoluta prius absolutissima in publico auditorio tam humanorum quam ceterorum animalium, ut et volucrium seu pennatorium ossium ostensione, postea quam tria extarent corpora seu subiecta, duo virilia, muliebre unum, ad sectionem solemni pompa cum fidicinibus ab Anatomisticis conductis accessit, eamque aliquot dierum spacio, frequenti sempre auditorum corona admodum evidenter administravit, et tandem post luculentam oculi dissectionem sectioni finem imposuit. Tomasini also explains that students took part in musical exercises as well as dancing lessons, military exercises and phyiscal ones. See *Gymnasium patavinum*, xxxvii, De aliis exercitiis gymnasticis, p. 133. For Francesco Portenari, a music educator and performer in Padua, see Bruno Brunelli, 'Francesco Portenari e le Cantate delgi Accademici padovani', in *Atti del Reale Istituto Veneto di Scienze, Lettere ed Arti*, 79, pt. 2 (1919–20): 595–607; and Brunelli, 'Due accademie padovane del cinquecento', in *Atti e Memorie della R. Accademia di scienza, lettere ed arti in Padova*, nuova serie, v. 36, disp. I. (1920): 43–57.

and Tomasini refers to the decoration of the 'elegantly crafted' arena and to the ways that the anatomist laboured, scrutinising 'the secrets of nature [*naturae arcana*]'.[62] Tomasini did not elaborate on the details of corpses or the processes that were used to display their interiors. Rather, (like Fabrici), he stressed the philosophical dimensions of anatomy, which were intelligible against the longer tradition of the secrets of nature.[63] In addition, travel writers highlighted the dramatic connotations of the theatre. In his guide to Padua (1623), Angelo Portenari describes the anatomical theatre in the section on Palazzo del Bò but mentions it later in his list of the modern theatres (in addition to the ancient arena) that existed in Padua.[64] In his guide, Francesco Schott (1548–1622) called the anatomical theatre one of the marvels (*maravigliosa*) of Padua: it was a celebrated space used by professors of medicine and an ingredient that enabled the university to be 'a market of the sciences', one that rivalled the ancient Athenian academy.[65]

Students seemed aware of the potential for the theatre to celebrate their medical school as well as the role they played in it. The theatre opened its doors in 1595 to 'Jews [perhaps Jewish scholars], teachers, tailors, shoemakers, sandal-makers, butchers, fishmongers, and, lower than these, porters [perhaps funereal] and basket-bearers'.[66] The transalpine student who furnished this description

---

[62] Tomasini, *Gymnasium patavinum*, 78: Patentibus valvis, geminae sese offerunt portae, quarum quae a latere dextro est, aream ostendit, e qua affurgentes ex oppositis locis ligneae scalae, in cuneos amphitheatri turba spectatorum perducunt. Adversa altera conclave aperit, in quo praesentibus variarum nationum studiosis, quae publice demonstranda sunt, apertis cadaveribus exscindi ac praepari consueverunt. Huius fores & parietes Anatomicorum insigna exornant, grata Universitate, tum ingenio docentium, tum laboribus naturae arcana scrutantium, honorem hunc exhibente. Ex eo in spatium aliud porta ducit, in cuius secretiore angulo cadavera, eorumque partes dissectae asservantur. In eodem arrae sunt & conditoria, vestimentis, sceletis, instrumentisque Anatomicorum custodiendis aptata.

[63] On the secrets of nature, see Katharine Park, *Secrets of women*, 77–120; and Monica Green, 'From "Diseases of women" to "Secret of women": The transformation of gynecological literature in the later Middle Ages', in *Journal of Medieval and Early Modern Studies* 30 (2000): 5–39.

[64] Angelo Portenari, *Della felicità di padova* (Padua: Pietro Paolo Tozzi, 1623), 96–7.

[65] Francesco Schott, *Itinerario, overo nova descrittione de'viaggi principali d'Italia* (Padua, 1659), 42: Et è cosa celebre l'Anfiteatro Anatomico drizzato in esse Scole ad uso de'Professori di Medicina: è lo Studio di Padova un famosissimo mercato delle Scientie, non altrimente, che si fosse anticamente l'Academia d'Athene. This passage is reprinted in *Padova: Diari e viaggi*, ed. Giuseppe Toffanin (Milan, 1990), 32.

[66] *Acta*, 1595, vol. 2, 58: Confluxerat eo tota quasi civitas, et extremae etiam farinae homines tanquam ad forum cupedinis: subsellia occuparunt hebraei, sedentarii magistri, sartores, calceolarii, solearii, carnarii, salsamentarii et his inferiores baiuti et corbuli illi, adeo ut in dubium relinqueres plus ne collegii scholares anatomici sectioni ac dexteritati attenderent, an haintia huiusmodo homuncionum ora aspicerent.

noted the presence of almost the 'whole citizenry' and the specific professions of the members in the audience. This was a special moment in the history of this university. The number of foreign students in Padua reached a record high at the end of the sixteenth century, a level that would not be maintained, due to Counter-Reformation politics and the opening of new universities in the alpine lands in the late sixteenth and early seventeenth centuries.[67] In the sixteenth century, foreign students graduating with distinction could still hope to obtain one of the academic posts that the university reserved for foreigners; but in the seventeenth century, the number of such opportunities decreased.[68] Inside the theatre, students assumed their places with their respective nation. The theatre, that is, allowed the hierarchy between student nations to assume material existence – the transalpine students had a large, visible presence inside the theatre that would have reinforced the importance of their nation within the academic community.[69] And this was no small thing, for the transalpine students were increasingly wary of the dangers of counter-reform initiatives.[70] They sought direct protection from professors as well as the Venetian authorities, a protection more readily given when the reputation of foreign students was a good one.

Conclusion

> We cure with herbs not with words [*Non enim verbis sed herbis aeger curatur*].
> Where the philosopher ends, there begins the physician [*Ubi desinit physicus, ibi medicus incipit*].[71]

---

[67] See n. 1.

[68] Richard Kagan, 'Universities in Italy, 1500–1700'; M. Saibante, C. Vivarini and S. Voghera, 'Gli studenti dell'Università di Padova dalla fine del '500 ai nostri giorni (studio statistico)', in *Metron* 4 (1924–25): 163–223; and more generally, Maria Rosa di Simone, 'Admission', in *Universities in Early Modern Europe*, 302–10. On the cultural conservatism of seventeenth-century Venice, see Peter Burke, 'Early modern Venice as a center of information and communication', in *Venice reconsidered: The history and civilization of an Italian city-state, 1297–1797*, ed. John Martin and Dennis Romano (Baltimore, 2000), pp. 389–419.

[69] M. Saibante, C. Vivarni and G. Voghera, 'Gli studenti dell'università di padova dalla fine del 500 ai nostri giorni (Studio Statistico)', in *Metron* 5 (1924): 163–223, especially the matriculation graphs.

[70] Biagio Brugi, *Gli scolari dello Studio di Padova nel Cinquecento* (seconda edizione riveduta, con un'appendice su gli Studenti tedeschi e la S. Inquisizione a Padova nella seconda metà del secolo XVI) (Padua, 1905).

[71] The first is cited from Bartholin, *Enchiridion metaphysicum*, though it appears much earlier in Baldassar Heseler's notes, see below nn. 69 and 70; probably Galenic in origin, the dictum can also be found in Celsus, *De medicina*, book 7, which deals entirely with surgery. The second comes from numerous sources. On both, see Charles Schmitt, 'Aristotle among the physicians', in *The medical renaissance of the sixteenth century*, 1–15.

Attached to the permanent venue of the anatomical theatre, the study of anatomy became more significant to medical education in the late sixteenth century. Dominated by Fabrici himself, the theatre repeatedly cast the innovative aspects of anatomy as natural philosophical. This reflects a change from the earlier part of the century, when anatomy was a minor component of medical education and more frequently considered to be a part of practical medicine and important to understanding surgery, diseases and treatments. This change was important for students, who earlier seemed especially eager to pursue the practical dimensions of anatomy and medicine and the lessons in clinical medicine that professors such as Da Monte regularly offered. The mindset is captured by Baldassar Heseler, a Silesian student who observed in Bologna in 1540 the anatomical lectures and demonstrations of the eminent professor Matteo Corti (Mattheus Curtius, 1475–1542), and the dissector Andreas Vesalius.[72] Lavishing praise on Vesalius, Heseler criticised Corti for the complicated and highly rhetorical nature of his lecture. Such rhetorical flourish was unnecessary in discussions of anatomy and medicine, according to Heseler, because 'we cure with herbs not with words'.[73] The contrast (or conflict) between practical medicine and rhetoric recalls Mundinus' introduction to anatomy, where he offered knowledge of the human body and its parts: in providing this knowledge 'I shall not look to style but shall merely seek to convey such knowledge as the chirurgical usage of the subject demands'.[74]

By the end of the sixteenth century, however, students were less inclined to associate (the content and rhetoric of) public anatomy demonstrations with surgery. Instead, they reflected on the prominence of natural philosophy in discussions of anatomy and in general, in the medical curriculum; for them, 'where the philosopher ends, there begins the physician' seemed more provocative. Drawn from Aristotle's *De Sensu et Sensato* and parts of *Parva naturalia*, the dictim was quoted by numerous Paduan philosophers and professors of medicine: Jacopo Zabarella (1533–89), Cremonini, Da Monte, Degli Oddi, Fabrici, Casseri and others.[75] As Charles Schmitt has explained, the university curriculum intended a student to pass from logic to natural philosophy, on his way to medical studies.[76]

---

72 Baldassar Heseler, *Andreas Vesalius' first public anatomy at Bologna, 1540: An eyewitness report by Baldassar Heseler*, ed. trans. Ruben Eriksson (Uppsala, 1959).

73 Heseler, 52–5.

74 Charles Singer, *The Fasciculo di medicina, Venice 1493*, 2 vols (Florence, 1925), I, 59. The original of the *Fasciculo* states: e perche la cognitione delle parti del subiecto nela medicina e el corpo humano el qual si chiama li luoghi dele dispositioni e una delle parti della scientia dela medicina. e de qua nasce che fra tucte laltre cose dovemo haver cognitione del corpo humano e delle parti de esso: la qual cognitione in surge e procede dalla anathomia. la quale ho preposto de dimostrare: non observando stile alto: ma secondo la manuale operatione vene daro notitia (vol. II, 65).

75 Charles Schmitt, 'Aristotle among the physicians', 12.

76 Ibid. As early as the thirteenth century, via the works of Taddeo Alderotti (c. 1215–95) in Bologna and Pietro d'Abano (1257–c.1315) in Padua, philosophy was

Schmitt suggests that philosophers considered their inquiries independent of the field of medicine: 'the place of natural philosophy and medicine in the overall schema of arts and the relation between the two had already been given serious attention in many discussions from the early middle ages onward. By the time we get to the philosophers of the sixteenth century it was a commonplace known to all.'[77] Though a commonplace for professors, the relationship between natural philosophy and medicine was a more ambiguous (and thus productive) one for students.

Students recognised both aspects of medicine, the theoretical and the practical, and although they continued to appreciate the practical components of their education perhaps more than the philosophical ones, the latter were increasingly influential. In 1598, Johann Svenzelio described the way Fabrici spoke of 'universal rather than particular' aspects of anatomy, especially the understanding of the organs of respiration; by contrast, Casseri treated particularities in 'an ape and a living dog' and in the dissection of nine cadavers, which was 'most illuminating' and for which he received great applause.[78] With so many specimens, Casseri must have spent considerably more time than Fabrici did on dissection, vivisection and the study of anatomical particulars.[79]

Observation, however, did not override natural philosophical speculation. The transition from Fabrici to Casseri, which took place during the first decade of the

---

conjoined to medicine.

[77] Ibid, 3–7.

[78] *Acta*, 1597–1598, vol. 2, 114: Circa initium Februarii, postquam Eccellentissimus Aquapendens anatomiam maxima ex parte absolverat (de universalis enim uti vocat ipse iam loquor, non de particulari et exactiori, quam nostro hoc anno de apprehensionis scilicet progressionis respirationisque organis … [Casseri] Id quod revera praestitit, non tantum seorsim in simia a nobis oblata, qua plurimum excitatus fuit, sed et in vivorum canum aliquot apertione, tum vero in novem humanorum cadaverum consectione, quam quidem luculentissime maximo cum appl[a]usu et ingenti aliorum quoque Nationum concursu ultra 5 septimanas adminnistrasse ipsum nemini obscurum esse debet, praesertim quomodo integram totius animalis fabricam in tribus distinctis subiectis totidem horis…maximo cum honore monstraverit. The fact that Casseri covered the 'fabric of the whole animal' is especially interesting because Fabrici used the phrase for his research and collected publications. Perhaps Casseri sought to integrate his work with Fabrici's; or perhaps the phrase was an Aristotelian flag, meant to encompass a wider approach to anatomy at the end of the sixteenth century. A crucial difference, though, is Casseri's attention to dissection, vivisection and anatomical particulars and Fabrici's lack of attention to those features and emphasis on the 'apprehension' of universals.

[79] The whole ordeal lasted five weeks, which was typical for demonstrations involving one or two cadavers and a number of animal specimens, but perhaps less typical for a demonstration done with nine cadavers. Casseri's attention to dissection was also visible in 1595–96, when he gave a private anatomy that included the dissection of an umbilical vessel, an explanation of foetal development, and various surgical operations (which students loved). See *Acta*, 1594–95, vol. 2, 60.

seventeenth century, was not one from natural philosophy to a new, observation-oriented empiricism. Instead, we must consider the ways in which universal ideas about anatomy, what anatomists called the final or purposive causes of anatomy (those that clarified the relationship between anatomical parts and the soul), were intended objects of contemplation. How does contemplation, a process of conceptual rigour that was grounded in sense perception, relate historically to observation? As the lessons of humanist pedagogues such as Stefano Guazzo, Bartolomeo Meduna and Orazio Lombardelli indicate, this kind of contemplation helped to train students to listen and to behave quietly.[80] Students maintained their contemplative habits even in Casseri's ocular demonstrations. When Casseri substituted for Fabrici in 1604, one student described his demonstration as useful because 'he read to the students and demonstrated this anatomy ocularly ... everyone was able to see particularly all the parts ... [and] the ways of treatments'; and for this, Casseri earned 'the greatest attention every morning' from his audience.[81] For Casseri, students were both silent and attentive (rather than disruptive), a posture that encouraged visual scrutiny.

Contemplation, we may consider, was a necessary precursor to the development of sensitive observers. In his *Syntagma anatomicum* (1649), Johann Veslingus (1598–1649), who joined the faculty in Padua in 1632, described the anatomical theatre as a place to 'behold' rather than 'dispute' the causes of anatomy.[82] In doing so, he indicated the lasting influence of Fabrici's style of demonstrating anatomy: Fabrici taught students to contemplate the philosophical truths of anatomy, and Veslingus coupled this with a lack of dispute or, in other words, with quieter, more reserved forms of participation. Veslingus wished to elongate the divide between disputation, the rehearsal of old knowledge, and the discovery or formulation of new knowledge. Disputation, though, was not the only culprit. These men, Veslingus explained, spent too much time looking at anatomical illustrations as if they were 'contemplating the siege of Troy'.[83] Though change was afoot – we

80 I have discussed the relationship between humanist pedagogy and anatomy in 'Civility, comportment, and the anatomy theatre: Girolamo Fabrici and his medical students in Renaissance Padua', in *Renaissance Quarterly* 60 (2007): 434–63.

81 The testimony is transcribed by Giuseppe Sterzi. 86–7: April 23, 1604: Hora essendo da questi inteso quanta utilità habbia apportato l'havere letta ed ocularmente mostrata questa Anatomia, così per la sua diligenza et cura usata, come per la comodità che dava ad ogn'uno in farli vedere particularmente tutte quelle parti che in così breve spatio di giorni si potessero mostrare, e vedere, non curandosi di tralasciare le proprie cure, che di qualche notabile utile li erano, per dare questa sodisfattione, e per comunicare parte della sua profonda dottrina, a quelli che con grandissima attenzione ogni mattina procuravano ascoltarlo.

82 Johann Veslingus, *Syntagma anatomicum* (Padua, 1647), To the Reader.

83 Ibid.: Est cuius memoriam operosa librorum moles fatigat: est qui laqueis controversiarum misere implicitus, pedem expedire sentibus tricisque vix potest. Detinetur alius in figuris, tanquam halosin Troiae contempletur, *rerumque ignarus imagine gaudet*.

hear in Veslingus's remarks something of the standard critique of Aristotelian learning that came from men of the New Science – the habits associated with natural philosophical anatomy persisted. Students contemplated philosophical truths; they gave Casseri their rapt attention; they contemplated anatomical illustrations. These instances of visual focus reflect the habits of contemplation associated most strongly with natural philosophical inquiry. They derive from the interaction between practical and theoretical medicine, from the movement and exchange between the clinic and the anatomical theatre. They also attest to the ways in which anatomical inquiry, as it became a more deeply philosophical pursuit, continued to orient the field of medicine. As students contemplated the philosophical truths of anatomy, they helped to promote change in the tradition of natural philosophy and in the practices and habits of thought that were pivotal to early modern medical education (Figure 8.7).[84]

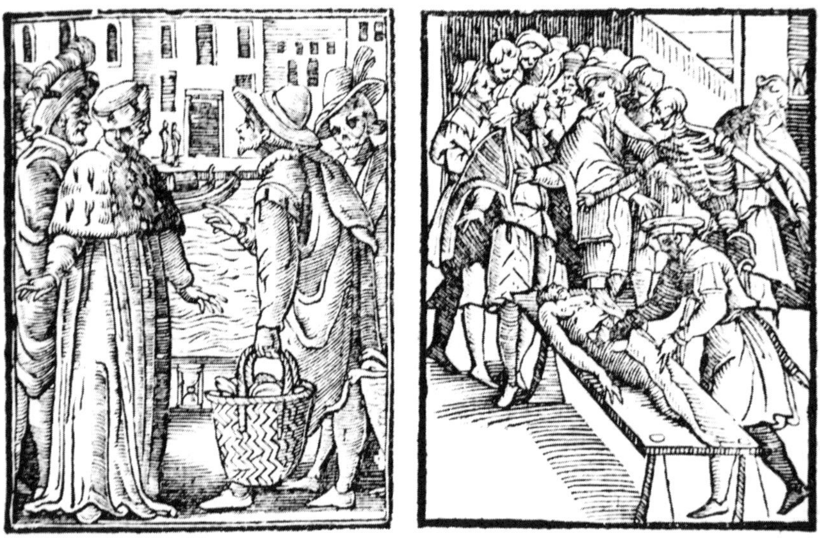

Fig.8.7 Dissection scene from F. Glissenti, *Discorsi morali contra il dispiacer del morire*, Venice, 159

[84] [84] This apparent street dissection scene is from a work in the *ars moriendi* tradition, but includes dialogue between a philosopher and a courtier who go around Venice interviewing artisans and professionals.

Chapter 9
Paris: 'certainly the best Place for learning the practical part of Anatomy and Surgery'

Toby Gelfand

Was Paris a 'centre of excellence' for the study of medicine in early modern Europe? If so, what specifically was 'excellent' about the French capital? For whom? Were there changes over the course of the eighteenth century? Such questions resist unqualified generalisations. They are inevitably difficult to measure objectively. Judgements about excellence varied according to the perspectives of diverse historical actors who did not necessarily agree on the definition, criteria and goals of the ideal medical education, much less where, if indeed anywhere, such could be had. Rather, the evidence suggests that no single institution nor city fully satisfied the aspirations of medical students in the eighteenth century.

The uncertainties voiced by the Philadelphia surgeon Thomas Bond illustrate how elusive excellence could be. In 1771, Bond asked his friend and fellow citizen Benjamin Franklin, then resident in London, to recommend a European centre for furthering his son's medical studies. The son, Richard, had shown much promise in the study of 'Physic and surgery' and would soon be graduating from the medical school in Philadelphia: '… where to send him [in Europe] is with me a doubt'. Bond senior had fond memories of his own studies in Paris. But that had been more than 30 years ago; all his mentors there were now dead. He knew nothing of the current state of teaching in Paris and had misgivings about the schools in Leiden and Vienna. Bond praised the Paris Academy of Surgery for 'uniting science to their profession'. While he acknowledged that most young American medical men opted for Edinburgh and London, Bond judged London surgery 'a mere *mechanic art*'; and he faulted the Scottish capital for 'extraordinary novelties' 'better calculated to please the fancy than to form the judgment'.[1]

Franklin replied that, in his candid opinion, there was 'more valuable to be learnt from the honest candid observations of an old practitioner … than from all the formal lectures of all the universities on earth'.[2] In a circuitous way, elite

---

[1] Bond to Franklin, 6 July 1771, *The papers of Benjamin Franklin*, 37 vols (New Haven, CT, 1959–), 18, 164–6 (emphasis in original).

[2] Franklin to Bond, 5 February 1772. Ibid., 19, 61. Franklin did note that he had heard excellent things about London's anatomical lectures and hospitals, where students had opportunities of 'conversing with the most eminent Practitioners and Reading under their Advice and Direction: And yet the general Run is at present to Edinburgh'. He added

eighteenth-century medical education would come round to a version of Franklin's bluff reply. Middle-class educated young men, often in possession of university medical degrees, like Richard Bond, came to the European medical centres, in Bond senior's word, to 'finish' their training. They paid fees to accompany recognised teachers for relatively short periods, perhaps just a few months. Above all, they sought practical experience in hospitals and in private courses.[3] This was a far cry from the traditional apprenticeship of the guilds in which callow youths in their early teens began the multi-year labours of learning a craft as little more than domestic servants under the direction (and orders) of a 'master'. But it was nonetheless an apprenticeship, if under higher social and less formal economic conditions.

Paris offered a multiplicity of institutional settings to students of the healing arts. In addition to separate and distinct schools of medicine and surgery, free public lectures and fee-paying private lessons in anatomy, surgical operations, accouchements or midwifery, chemistry, physiology, pharmacy etc. were available. Quality varied. The Paris medical Faculty remained staunchly committed to ancient Galenic medicine and resistant to innovations in medical theory, chemistry and therapeutics long after its rivals at Montpellier and other European medical centres had broken with traditional classical medicine.[4] By conforming until late in the eighteenth century to the medieval custom of rotating professors every two years, the Paris Faculty's statutes effectively prevented the best teachers from establishing ongoing public courses. Those who came to study medicine in Paris, as we shall see, were attracted to other venues.

---

that he had seen at the opening of the school at Edinburgh the previous November: 'a much greater number of medical students than had ever been known before'.

[3] I have discussed private dissection courses in 'The “”aris manner' of dissection: student anatomical dissection in early eighteenth-century Paris,' *Bulletin of the History of Medicine* 46 (1972): 99–130. Of course, mature medical men and natural philosophers visited Paris, among other cities, on the 'grand tour'. Normally their time in the French capital was briefer than that of fee-paying younger men, and they were considered guests rather than clients. Nonetheless these 'tourist' accounts of contacts with colleagues and impressions of Paris teaching remain useful sources for the historian.

[4] See Guy Patin, *Lettres*, 3 vols ed. J.-H. Réveille-Parise (Paris, 1846) for ample illustration of this leading representative of the Paris medical Faculty's commitment to ancient tradition. On the eighteenth century, see Paul Delaunay, *Le monde médical parisien au XVIIIe siècle* (Paris, 1906). The Faculty's statutes are reproduced in Auguste Corlieu, *L'ancienne Faculté de médecine de Paris* (Paris, 1877). I have discussed the inadequacy of the structure and content of the Paris Faculty's public teaching in *Professionalizing modern medicine. Paris surgeons and medical science and institutions in the 18th century* (Westport, CT, 1980), esp. 94–106, 131–5, 174–6. L.W.B. Brockliss, 'Before the clinic: French medical teaching in the eighteenth century', in *Constructing Paris medicine*, ed. Caroline Hannaway and Ann La Berge (Atlanta, GA, 1999), 71–115, has challenged this interpretation. See my reply in *Canadian Bulletin of Medical History. Bulletin Canadian d'histoire de la médecine* 17 (2000): 273–4.

The 25-year-old Théophile de Bordeu, a graduate of Montpellier with a degree in medicine and surgery, arrived in 1747 intent on furthering his career prospects in surgery. For a fee, Bordeu took lodgings with and became 'assistant' to the most famous surgeon in Paris, if not all Europe, Jean-Louis Petit (1674–1750). Bordeu's correspondence makes abundantly clear that he valued the prestige of his affiliation with the elderly Petit as much as, if not more than, the acquisition of surgical experience. Paris, he wrote, in anticipation of his voyage, was no place for beginners: 'there, one improves, acquires polish, and that look of competence, even impertinence, which we need'.[5] Bordeu was pleased that his father, a physician, was spreading the news back home that he was 'chez Petit'. The rabble [*canaille*] of surgeons from his home region, he reported, were wide-eyed when they saw him with the great man in his carriage on the way to visit patients.[6]

'No city in the whole world equalizes it'

Then as now, Paris held out a certain inherent, if not easily definable, attraction to visitors. The Englishman John Evelyn noted in his Paris diary in 1644: 'I think no city in the whole world equalizes it.'[7] Evelyn's praise, echoed by numerous others during the ensuing centuries, went particularly to the Parisian urban landscape and architecture – the 'streets, suburbs, common buildings, public edifices, some of the hospitals are fair foundations and handsome piles'.[8] Experience of the sights and pleasures of the French capital elicited admiration and conferred prestige: 'To have seen the cities of Italy, Germany, and other kingdoms, that's nothing', wrote an enthusiastic German tourist, 'what grabs attention is when a man announces that he has been to Paris.'[9]

Studying medicine, or at least certain aspects of medicine, in Paris conferred its own prestige. In 1750 an envious English medical writer deplored the notion, outmoded in his opinion, but still generally entertained, 'that a man cannot

5 Théophile de Bordeu, *Correspondance*, 4 vols, ed. Martha Fletcher (Montpellier), 1: 113.

6 Ibid., 152. See Elizabeth Williams, *A cultural history of medical vitalism in enlightenment Montpellier* (Burlington, VT, 2003), 115–20.

7 John Evelyn, *Diary*, 6 vols, ed. E.S. de Beer (Oxford, 1955), 3, 637.

8 Ibid.

9 Quoted in Albert Babeau, *Les voyageurs en France depuis la renaissance jusqu'à la révolution*, (Paris, 1885), 27 (no source named for quote from mid-seventeenth century). Neglecting the obvious attractions of Paris in favour of exclusive attention to serious studies risked being considered a 'kind of misanthrope', wrote an eighteenth-century surgeon about one such foreign medical student. See Antoine Louis, 'Éloge de Molinelli' (1766), in *Éloges lus dans les séances publiques de l'Académie royale de chirurgie de 1750 à 1792* (Paris, 1859), 77 (hereafter cited as *Éloges*).

be a good surgeon and accoucheur without a tour to Paris'.[10] According to the anonymous author of *A short comparative view of the practice of surgery in the French hospitals*, some of his countrymen absented themselves for about three months (the approximate duration of a course of instruction abroad) while circulating the spurious rumour that they had gone to study in the French capital: 'they have return'd at the appointed Time, accoutered *à la mode de Paris*, talk of the *Practices, Customs*, and large *etc*'s; which they never see; and thus pass in the Neighborhood as accomplish'd *Surgeons* and *Accoucheurs*, or what not?'[11]

Hospitals: 'A measure of a nation's civilisation'[12]

Its population of around 700,000 inhabitants at the end of the eighteenth century (an increase of about 40 per cent during the course of the century) placed Paris second only to London among European cities. But the population density of the French capital exceeded that of its geographically more capacious English counterpart, leading an eighteenth-century English medical visitor to observe: 'whereas London lies long, Paris lies round'.[13] Numerous hospitals sustained by the Church and the central government stood within a relatively compact perimeter. If, in the words of the leading European authority on the subject, the Paris surgeon Jacques Tenon, hospitals were a 'measure of a nation's civilisation', then Paris potentially could claim first rank.[14] At the centre of the city, adjacent to Notre Dame Cathedral, stood the most populous hospital in Europe, the Hôtel-Dieu, housing an average of 2,500 sick poor, a figure that could swell to nearly 4,000 during epidemics (Figure 9.1). Twenty-one other hospitals brought the total to more than 6,000 patients. The most important as far as learning opportunities were concerned were the Charité, a 200-bed hospital for men run by the monks of Saint Jean-de-Dieu and renowned for cleanliness and providing each patient with his own bed (unlike the Hôtel-Dieu in both respects), and the Invalides hospital for incapacitated veterans, with more than 400 beds set aside for the sick. Another nearly 30,000 indigent homeless

---

[10] [John Harrison], A short comparative view on the practice of surgery in the French Hospitals: with some remarks on the study of anatomy and midwifery. The whole endeavoring to prove that the advantages to students, in these professions, are greater at London than at Paris, (London, 1750), 4–5.

[11] Ibid., 5–6 (emphasis in original).

[12] Jacques Tenon, *Mémoires sur les hôpitaux de Paris* (Paris, 1788), 1.

[13] Thomas Baker, 'A Tour in France, 1732,' MS. 5780, fol. 14r, Wellcome Library, London. I thank Amanda Engineer, archivist and manuscripts librarian, for making available to me a copy of this item. See also Martin Lister, *A journey to Paris in the year 1698*, ed. by Raymond P. Stearns (Chicago, 1967), 7.

[14] Statistics on the numbers and capacities of the Paris hospitals are from Tenon, *Mémoires*, 1–25; see also Marcel Fosseyeux, *L'Hôtel-Dieu de Paris au XVIIe et au XVIIIe siècle* (Paris, 1912).

persons, many of whom were elderly and/or suffering from chronic illness or other disabilities designated as 'incurable', found refuge in hospices; of these, the Hôpital Général's two huge divisions, the Salpêtrière hospice for women and the Bicêtre for men, housed a total of 10,000 persons, 7,000 at the former alone.[15]

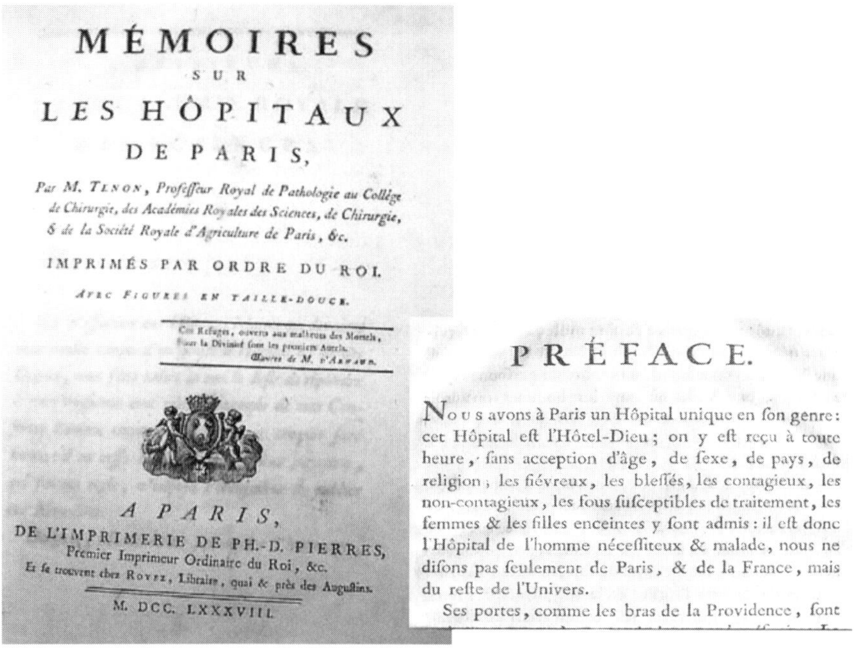

MÉMOIRES
SUR
LES HÔPITAUX
DE PARIS,

Par M. Tenon, Profeſſeur Royal de Pathologie au Collège de Chirurgie, des Académies Royales des Sciences, de Chirurgie, & de la Société Royale d'Agriculture de Paris, &c.

IMPRIMÉS PAR ORDRE DU ROI.

Avec figures en taille-douce.

Ces Refuges, ouverts aux malheurs des Mortels,
Pour la Divinité sont les premiers Autels.
Œuvres de M. d'Arnaud.

A PARIS,
DE L'IMPRIMERIE DE PH.-D. PIERRES,
Premier Imprimeur Ordinaire du Roi, &c.
Et ſe trouvent chez Royez, Libraire, quai & près des Augustins.
M. DCC. LXXXVIII.

PRÉFACE.

Nous avons à Paris un Hôpital unique en ſon genre: cet Hôpital eſt l'Hôtel-Dieu; on y eſt reçu à toute heure, ſans acception d'âge, de ſexe, de pays, de religion; les fiévreux, les bleſſés, les contagieux, les non-contagieux, les fous ſuſceptibles de traitement, les femmes & les filles enceintes y ſont admis: il eſt donc l'Hôpital de l'homme néceſſiteux & malade, nous ne diſons pas ſeulement de Paris, & de la France, mais du reſte de l'Univers.

Ses portes, comme les bras de la Providence, ſont

Fig.9.1 Title page and preface to Jacques Tenon, *Mémoires sur les hôpitaux de Paris*, Paris, 1788. The opening line of the preface declares: 'We, in Paris, possess a hospital of a unique kind: this hospital is the Hôtel-Dieu; admissions take place at any hour of the day, with no discrimination as to age, sex, national origin or religion.'

In addition to practical learning in hospitals, students in Paris could avail themselves of an array of free public courses. During the eighteenth century, public lectures in various medical subjects took place in four principal venues: the schools of medicine and surgery, both of them medieval foundations, and the Collège Royal and the Jardin Royal (Jardin du Roi), founded in the sixteenth and seventeenth centuries respectively. Although these were separate and distinct institutions, nothing prevented a student from frequenting several sites, along with paying for privatc instruction, visiting the hospitals and perhaps witnessing

[15] Tenon, *Mémoires*, 15, gave the numbers of sick at the Salpêtrière and Bicêtre as 450 and 788 respectively. He counted another 300 patients at the Pitié, a third division of the Hôpital Général.

sessions of the Academy of Sciences, whose sections of anatomy and botany admitted physicians and surgeons to the classes of distinguished anatomists. One student found, for example, that he was able to take advantage of the different times of day at which lectures took place to attend the Jardin du Roi, the surgical school and the Hôtel-Dieu and Charité hospitals, all located within easy proximity of one another.[16] Few, if any, European centres could match this concentration of resources for studying medicine.

In what follows, I consider four 'cross-sections' or samplings spanning the eighteenth century. By means of examples of foreign medical visitors, I seek to illustrate what attracted them to Paris, where they went, what they saw and whether and how this changed over the course of the century. I then take a closer look at the reputation and reality of the French capital as the European centre in which learning by human dissection could best be pursued.

The Jardin du Roi at the Turn of the Eighteenth Century

At the turn of the eighteenth century the Jardin Royal or Jardin du Roi was the most important site in Paris for a variety of medical studies.[17] Created by royal edict in 1626 as a result of the efforts of the king's physician, Guy Labrosse, the primary purpose of the Jardin's extensive botanical collection was its medicinal uses, as indicated by the full designation 'Jardin des herbes médicinales'. When John Evelyn visited in 1644, just four years after the long-delayed opening, he praised the 'famous Jardine royale [*sic*]' for 'all varieties of ground for planting and culture of medical simples'.[18] English visitors spoke of the royal 'physic Garden'.[19] Until 1718, the Jardin remained under the direction of the king's physician (Figure 9.2).

In 1673, the Jardin inaugurated practical anatomical and surgical instruction with the appointment of Pierre Dionis, a surgeon, as 'royal demonstrator'. Louis XIV intervened to grant the Jardin's anatomist first claim to the cadaver of an executed criminal, a privilege that had formerly belonged exclusively to the Paris medical Faculty. Dionis taught for the remainder of the decade of the 1670s to large audiences, some 400 to 500 onlookers by his own estimate.[20] Texts of his courses of anatomy, surgery and midwifery went through numerous editions and

---

16 Louis, 'Éloge de Roederer' (1765), *Éloges*, 61

17 See Yves Laissus, 'Le Jardin du Roi', in *Enseignement et diffusion des sciences en France au XVIIIe siècle*, ed. Rene Taton (Paris, 1964), 318–41.

18 Evelyn, *Diary*, vol. 2, 102 (8 February 1644); Laissus, 'Jardin du Roi', 288–92.

19 Lister, *A journey to Paris*, 65.

20 Pierre Dionis, 'Préface', *L'Anatomie de l'homme*, 2nd edn (Paris, 1694), 8 (non-paginated).

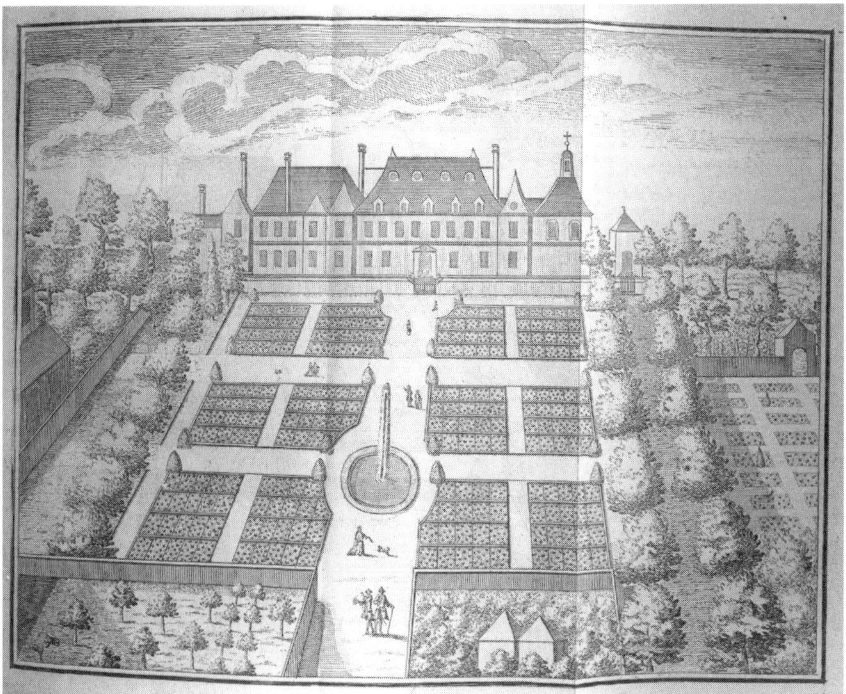

Fig.9.2 The Jardin du roi or Jardin royal [King's Garden]; engraving from Pierre Dionis, *Cours d'opérations de chirurgie, démontrées au Jardin du Roi* [*Course of surgical operations demonstrated at the Jardin du roi*] (Paris, 1708)

translations into Latin, various European languages and even, for the anatomy text, into the 'tartar language' (Figure 9.3).[21]

In 1682 Joseph-Guichard Duverney, a physician and member of the Academy of Sciences, took over anatomical teaching at the Jardin. His courses over the following decades enjoyed a wide popular following among society, in part owing to his dramatic style of lecturing. He reportedly attracted as many as 140 foreign visitors in a year.[22] Martin Lister, an English physician, gave a detailed account of his visit to the Jardin in 1698. Lister, who had studied in Montpellier some 30 years earlier, intended to meet Duverney. But when the anatomist did not appear, he climbed up to the Jardin's 'dissecting room' where he saw a Mr Bennis, 'working

[21] Antoine Louis, 'Histoire de l'Académie royale de chirurgie,' *Mémoires de l'Académie royale de chirurgie*, 4 (1768) 29–30.

[22] [Fontenelle], 'Éloge de M. Duverney', *Histoire de l'Académie royale des sciences*, 1730 (Paris, 1732). Duverney did not yield his post to his son until 1718.

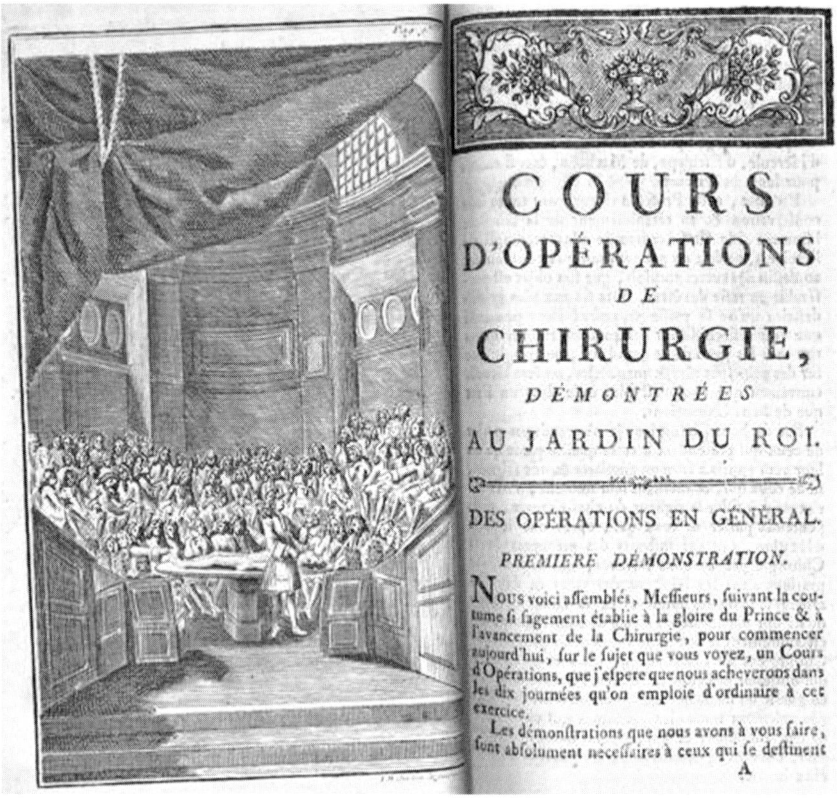

COURS
D'OPÉRATIONS
DE
CHIRURGIE,
DÉMONTRÉES
AU JARDIN DU ROI.

DES OPÉRATIONS EN GÉNÉRAL.

PREMIERE DÉMONSTRATION.

Nous voici aſſemblés, Meſſieurs, ſuivant la coutume ſi ſagement établie à la gloire du Prince & à l'avancement de la Chirurgie, pour commencer aujourd'hui, ſur le ſujet que vous voyez, un Cours d'Opérations, que j'eſpere que nous acheverons dans les dix journées qu'on emploie d'ordinaire à cet exercice.

Les démonſtrations que nous avons à vous faire, ſont abſolument néceſſaires à ceux qui ſe deſtinent

A

Fig.9.3 First page of Pierre Dionis, *Cours d'opérations de chirurgie, démontrées au Jardin du Roi* [*Course of surgical operations demonstrated at the Jardin du roi*] (Paris, 1708). With engraving depicting amphitheatre lesson on the cadaver

by himself upon a dead body, with its breast open and belly gutted'.[23] Bennis and another 'English gentleman', a Mr Probie, had followed Duverney's winter course of three months which 'showed all the parts of the body'. 'He [Duverney] had for this purpose, at least twenty human bodies from the Gallows, the Chatelet (where those are exposed who are found murthered in the Streets, which is a very common business at *Paris*) and from the hospitals.'[24] 'Mr' suggests that Bennis and Probie were surgeons and that the dissection material for these English students greatly exceeded the two cadavers officially allotted for the Jardin's public lessons.

---

23 Lister, *A journey to Paris*, 65.

24 Ibid., 69.

Martin Lister also visited the home of Jean Méry (1645–1722), one of the first surgeons to gain membership in the Academy of Sciences. He was much impressed with the surgeon's private anatomical 'cabinet', consisting of two rooms:

> in the outward were [a] great variety of Skeletons; also entire Preparations of the Nerves; in two of which he shewed me the mistake of *Willis*, and from thence gathered, that he was not much used to dissect with his own Hand … But that which much delighted my Curiosity, was the Demonstration of a blown and dried Heart of a *Fetus*; also the dried Heart of a *Tortoise*.[25]

At the time of Lister's visit, Méry was surgeon at the Invalides hospital. In 1700 he became chief surgeon at the Hôtel-Dieu, where he established regular dissection courses in anatomy and surgical operations. Although hospital regulations forbade the attendance of outsiders, Méry and his successor chief surgeons of the Hôtel-Dieu were known to admit fee-paying students.[26]

The Hôtel-Dieu and the Charité Hospitals in the 1720s

Opportunities for foreigners to see operations in hospitals went back well before the eighteenth century. Most daring and well-attended were the lithotomies, or procedures for the extraction of urinary stones, which took place on specified days: 'I saw the whole operation of lithotomie namely 5 cut of the stone', wrote John Evelyn on 3 May 1650, of his visit to the Charité hospital.[27] Edward Browne, a physician, described another 'lithotomy day' at the Hôtel-Dieu, 'where in a short space I saw six cut'.[28] Both Englishmen had good enough views to describe in much the same terms the instruments employed. In 1698 Martin Lister observed operations (and their fatal sequellae) at both the Hôtel-Dieu and the Charité performed by the travelling empiric Frère Jacques, who demonstrated his new method, the lateral approach, of cutting for the stone.[29] The Scottish-born surgeon James Houstoun gained access to the Hôtel-Dieu around 1714 after studying in Edinburgh for two years and Leiden (where he received a medical degree) for three. Many years later, Houstoun recalled:

---

25 Ibid., 66. Méry's preoccupation with anatomy led one commentator to describe him as 'more accessible to the dead than the living'. De Ratte, 'Éloge de Lamorier' in R.-N. Desgenettes, *Éloges des academicians de Montpellier* (Paris, 1811), 223–4.

26 See Gelfand, *Professionalizing modern medicine*, 53, 229 n. 33.

27 Evelyn, *Diary*, vol. 3, 3–4.

28 Edward Browne, *Journal of a visit to Paris in the Year 1664*, edited by Geoffrey Keynes, repr. from St Bartholomew's Hospital Reports, vol. 56 (London, 1923), 24–5.

29 Lister, *A journey to Paris*, 236–40.

> Paris is certainly the best Place for learning the practical part of Anatomy and Surgery, from the frequent Opportunities of seeing Chirurgical Operations of all Sorts perform'd in the Hospitals.[30]

The Charité established a formal arrangement for clinical teaching of surgery in the 1720s. In 1724 a royal edict authorised the Paris surgical corporation, rather than the religious brothers who otherwise administered the hospital, to name the chief surgeon. The edict called for this individual to set up an *école pratique* of anatomy and surgery within the Charité. The following year, Henri-François Ledran (1685–1770) inaugurated this practical school.

One of Ledran's private students was the 19-year-old Swiss physician Albrecht Haller. In 1727 Haller completed his MD at Leiden and, after studying in London, at the end of the year came to Paris, where he became a live-in student or *pensionnaire* with Ledran. He witnessed the surgeon's operations at the Charité and in private practice, along with the autopsies routinely performed after all deaths of hospital patients.[31] These served as the basis for Ledran's books (later praised by Haller) on methods of lithotomy (1730) and his two-volume general surgery (1731) comprising 115 operative procedures. While in Paris, Haller was able to purchase cadavers for his own study. As well, he visited the Jardin du Roi to follow J.-B. Winslow's anatomy course and Antoine de Jussieu's botany course. Haller also attended Jean-Louis Petit's inaugural lecture at the surgical school.

The Hôtel-Dieu enjoyed an unrivalled reputation as a place for gaining practical experience in midwifery or accouchements. In the early eighteenth century surgeons and physicians took advantage of the opening-up of this field to male practitioners. James Houstoun considered the Hôtel-Dieu maternity wards 'the only place, for thorough instruction in this business'. Houstoun recalled working alongside the hospital's four female midwives to deliver about 10 children in a typical 24-hour period: 'I continued in this hospital four months without setting my foot out of it four times … I brought nearly three hundred women to-bed in the

---

30 James Houstoun, *Memoirs of his own lifetime* (London, 1747), 74. Houstoun went on to declare the French 'to be more dextrous and expert operators in surgery and cutters in anatomical dissection (I speak in general) than any I have seen'. 'But', he added, 'as for their theory, that I did not want,' ibid., 75. In 1718, 20-year-old Alexander Monro of Edinburgh journeyed to Paris, where he studied surgical operations under the chief surgeon of the Hôtel-Dieu and attended the Charité as well as private courses.

31 Albrecht Haller, *Tagebuch der Studienreise nach London, Paris, Strasburg, und Basel 1727 bis 1728*, ed. E. Hintzsche (Bern, 1942), 25–34; Louis, 'Éloge de Haller' (1778), *Éloges*, 267–78, esp. 266–7. See also Louis, 'Éloge de Ledran' (1771), *Éloges*, 160–74, esp. 165–6. Haller's friend, compatriot and fellow Leiden MD Johannes Gessner entered into a similar arrangement with Ledran. On one occasion, the two young men went to the Charité at 5 a.m. to attend Ledran's course of surgical operations on the cadaver. *Johannes Gessners Pariser Tagebuch. 1727*, trans. and ed. Urs Boschug (Bern, 1985), 201. See also 189–92. I thank Hubert Steinke for sending me this reference.

time.' A 'mistress midwife' ran the service, but 'in very extraordinary cases, we called in the master-surgeon of the hospital's assistance'.[32]

During the French regency period (1715–23) at least five more medical men from Great Britain gained admission to the hospital's vast maternity wards.[33] Despite the hospital board's insistence in December 1720 that it was 'indecent' for men to deliver babies, less than a year later a 'docteur Campbel' from Scotland was admitted to the labour room for three months to observe and 'even to work if the surgeons so agreed'. A letter from the king of England to the regent of France was needed in Campbel's case to overturn the administrator's objections. Similar kinds of patronage opened doors for other foreigners, while those lacking influential support and funds met with refusal.[34]

In 1730 the chief surgeon's post at the Charité hospital, a five-year appointment, passed to Sauveur-François Morand (1697–1773), who had been Ledran's assistant during the latter's tenure.[35] Like his predecessor, Morand was a university-educated son of an unlettered surgeon. Born at the Invalides hospital, where his father served as chief surgeon, Morand received his surgical mastership at the precocious age of 19 and, even more remarkably, gained entry to the Academy of Sciences just six years later. His various other posts – chief surgeon at the Invalides, demonstrator at the surgeon's school and secretary of the Academy of Surgery, made Morand a

---

32 Houstoun, *Memoirs*, 73–4. After months of recruiting influential backing to gain entry to the Hôtel-Dieu maternity wards, Houstoun finally succeeded, probably around 1714. See Adrian Wilson, 'William Hunter and the varieties of man-midwifery', in *William Hunter and the eighteenth-century medical world*, ed. W.F. Bynum and Roy Porter (Cambridge), 358.

33 *Délibérations de l'ancien bureau de l'Hôtel-Dieu*, ed. Leon Brièle, 2 vols (Paris, 1881–83), 1: 274, 284–5, 287, 288, 289. In 1786 Tenon counted 175 women either pregnant or delivered at the Hôtel-Dieu, *Mémoires*, 236. R. Campbell, *The London tradesman* (London, 1747), advised the young surgeon after completing apprenticeship to study midwifery in Paris. See Joan Lane, 'The role of apprenticeship in eighteenth-century medical education in England', in *William Hunter and the eighteenth-century medical world*, 65.

34 See Fosseyeux, *L'Hôtel-Dieu*, 286–95. Private obstetrical courses given by Grégoire père et fils attracted foreigners, such as Alexander Monro of Edinburgh in 1718, during this and subsequent periods. As Adrian Wilson has noted, private courses presented many more opportunities to gain experience in difficult deliveries than did ordinary hospital practice. Wilson, 'William Hunter', 358. See also Kees van Strien, 'A medical student at Leiden and Paris: William Sinclair (1736–38): Part III,' *Proceedings of the Royal College of Physicians, Edinburgh* 25 (1995): 639–51.

35 Ledran continued to attract foreign students. When he visited Montpellier in 1746 he told Théophile de Bordeu that foreign physicians and surgeons overwhelmed him with their requests for instruction, Bordeu, *Correspondance*, 1: 117. William Hunter evidently took his course in the early 1740s. The English surgeon William Cheselden said of Ledran's *Traité des opérations de chirurgie* (1742): 'I have never read any book of surgery from which I learnt so much as from his' in *The operations in surgery of Mons. Le Dran*, trans. Thomas Gataker (London, 1749), 445.

highly sought-after teacher (Figure 9.4). His son, a physician, estimated that he took in more than 70 foreign students *en pension* over a 20-year period, beginning in 1726. Among the 'many from England and Scotland' were the future royal surgeon Caesar Hawkins, and the military physician John Pringle.[36] According to a contemporary surgeon, most of Morand's foreign students received stipends from their governments to study in Paris during the protracted period of peace in Europe.[37]

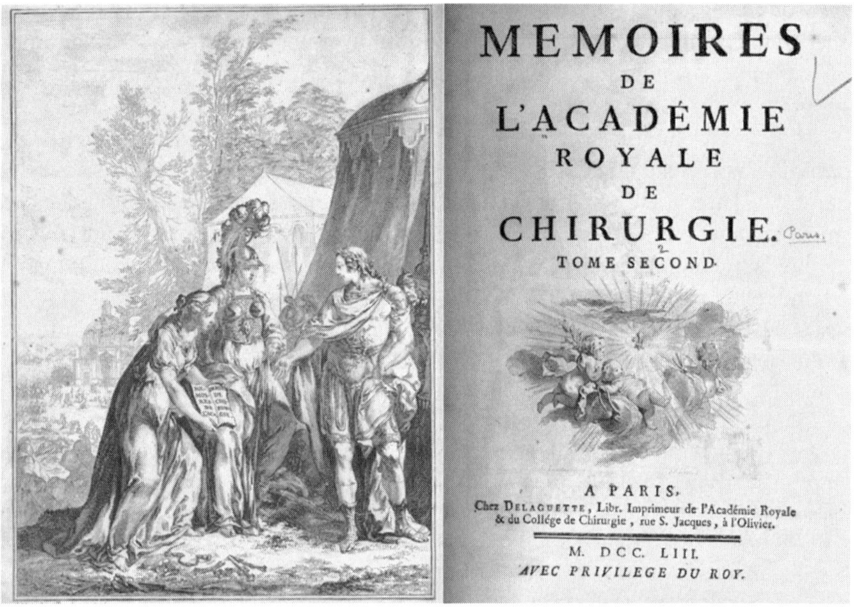

MEMOIRES
DE
L'ACADÉMIE
ROYALE
DE
CHIRURGIE.
TOME SECOND.

A PARIS,
Chez Delaguette, Libr. Imprimeur de l'Académie Royale & du Collége de Chirurgie, rue S. Jacques, à l'Olivier.

M. DCC. LIII.
AVEC PRIVILEGE DU ROY.

Fig. 9.4 Title page of *Mémoires de l'Académie royale de Chirurgie. Tome second* [*Memoirs of the Royal Academy of Surgery*, vol. 2] (Paris, 1753), with allegorical figures presenting volume to warrior-king Louis XV. Five quarto volumes were published between 1743 and 1774

Pietro Paulo Molinelli, a Bologna graduate in medicine and surgery, came to France at the age of 28. Following six months in Montpellier, where he concentrated on the study of venereal diseases, he spent two more years in Paris. Living *en*

---

[36] *Lettre traduite du latin sur feu M. Morand* (Paris,) 12, notes (a). Others who had studied with Morand were Gaubius of Leiden, the chief surgeon of the empress of Russia and the chief surgeon of the king of Spain. In his roll call of places from which his father's students came, Morand fils named Piedmont, Savoy, Malta, Spain, Portugal, Germany, Russia, England, Scotland and Italy. See P. Huard, 'Les échanges médicaux franco-anglais au XVIII siècle, *Clio medica* 3 (1968) 45.

[37] Louis, 'Éloge de Morand' (1774), *Éloges*, 209.

pension with Morand, the Italian had access to the surgeon's public and private courses and to the Charité and Invalides hospitals. Molinelli returned to Bologna to become professor and chief hospital surgeon. He persuaded Pope Benedict XIV to establish public courses modelled after those he had seen in Paris. As well, on Molinelli's urging, the pope requested and received on behalf of the surgeons of Bologna a fine set of surgical instruments from La Peyronie, the French king's chief surgeon.[38]

An Englishman, Thomas Baker, in all likelihood a medical practitioner, recalled Morand's warm welcome and training of another countryman during his brief visit to Paris in 1732:

> I went one morning to this hospital [the Charité] to see the patients [wounds] dressed when I was introduced to Mons. Morand at that time chief surgeon of the hospital by Mr. Freeman, an English gentleman bred up under Mons. Morand in that hospital and since gone surgeon to the Earl of Essex ... Mons. Morand used me with the utmost civility and respect.[39]

Baker accepted the Paris surgeon's invitation to return to the Charité that same afternoon 'to see him lay open two or three fistulas in ano'. He described Morand's handling of the instruments in this procedure as well as operations for cases of facial abscess and fractured skull. Morand then took his guest to a session of the Academy of Sciences, where, from the gallery, he admired the anatomist Winslow and the surgeon 'M. [Jean-Louis] Petit himself'.[40] After more medical touring, Morand invited Baker to his house, where, on the following day, Baker complimented the 'neat' library and 'curious collection of diseased bones ... shells, several other curiosities'.[41]

Mid-century

By 1750 lecture courses at the surgical school, newly designated as a 'Collège', had overtaken the Jardin du Roi as the preferred site for public instruction in anatomy, surgery and related subjects. Medical visitors continued to visit the Jardin (and the Collège Royal) to hear distinguished physicians such as Antoine Petit and, later, Félix Vicq d'Azyr. But, after 1718, when the royal physician Fagon died, and especially with the arrival of Buffon as director

---

[38] Louis, 'Éloge de Molinelli' *Éloges*, 84–5.

[39] Baker, 'A tour in France', fol. 13r. Baker noted parenthetically that in the Paris hospitals the chief surgeons did the wound dressings, perhaps unlike their English counterparts. He visited the Hôtel-Dieu also.

[40] Ibid. fol. 13v.

[41] Ibid., fol. 14r.

of the Jardin in 1739, natural history rather than medicine became the main focus of research and teaching there.[42]

During the first half of the century, the Paris surgical profession underwent a dynamic evolution. By 1750 the former guild of barber-surgeons had become a liberal profession generously endowed by the royal government, which established an autonomous school of surgery, an Academy, and a prerequisite of university studies for the surgical degree. The occupants of five surgical teaching chairs established in 1724 had obvious advantages over the medical Faculty's randomly named professors, who fulfilled in turn briefly, reluctantly and with poor remuneration, their teaching obligations. Instructors at the surgical school came from the elite of the profession; they held permanent or tenured positions endowed by the government. The number of professorial chairs at the College of Surgery steadily grew, eventually to 10, with a total of 18 instructors who taught the following courses: physiology and hygiene, pathology, therapy, anatomy, operations, accouchements, eye diseases, chemistry, botany and bone diseases. Hundreds of students from all over France as well as from abroad registered for courses at the College of Surgery.[43] While the vast majority would return to the provinces for careers as village and small-town barber-surgeons, future physicians and city surgeons also attended.[44] For a select few students, a dissection school, founded in 1757, and a small research hospital set up within the impressive new buildings constructed in 1774, completed the surgical school's resources (Figure 9.5).[45]

[42] Laissus, 'Le Jardin du Roi,' 288–99. See also Louis, 'Éloge de Benomont' (1773), *Éloges*, 191.

[43] Lists of registrants by name and place of origin are in Bibliotheque de la Faculté de Medecine, Paris, Mss 50–69. See Toby Gelfand, 'Deux cultures, une profession, les chirurgiens français au XVIIIe siècle', *Revue d'histoire moderne et contemporaine* 2 (1980) 468–84. For listing of courses and professors at the College of Surgery, see Pierre Huard, 'L'enseignement médico-chirurgical', in *Enseignement et diffusion*, 224–6.

[44] Haller, Gessner and Bordeu, among other physicians, mentioned going to the Paris surgical school.

[45] See Gelfand, *Professionalizing modern medicine*, 85–92. Of 1,566 inscriptions for Sabatier's course of surgical operations at the College in 1785, nearly 100 (just over 6 per cent) were foreigners. R.-B.Sabatier (1732–1811) taught at the surgical school for 30 years before receiving a surgical professorship at the new École de santé in 1794. He gave private courses as well and was said to lecture to English and Italian students in their own language, while he employed Latin for German students. Ibid. 78.

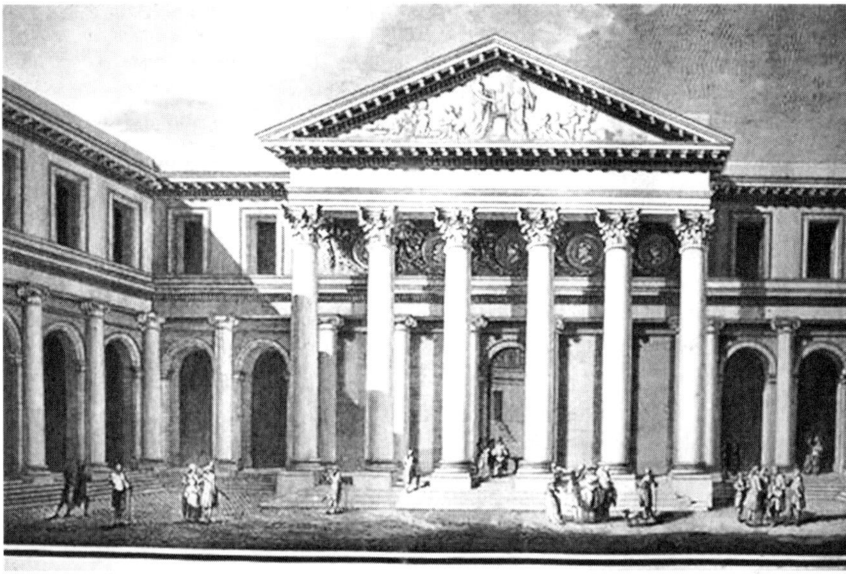

Fig.9.5 Façade and courtyard of Royal College and Academy of Surgery, Paris. Jacques Gondoin, architect's plan (1774)

Foreign students, as noted earlier, typically came to Paris after completing medical degrees elsewhere, often in Leiden. They sought instruction from leading practitioners, whom they paid for private lessons and access to their hospitals. That pattern continued at and after mid-century. The place of the French capital as an important destination on a European tour of medical studies remained secure but perhaps less essential than it had been earlier in the century.

The 27-year-old Peter Camper arrived in June 1749 for three months, following completion of a medical degree from Leiden three years before and extensive studies in London.[46] In Paris, Camper became acquainted with the surgeon Antoine Louis, who at the time was completing six years' service as chief resident at the Salpêtrière hospice. Although no older than his guest and not yet formally qualified to practise, Louis, as he later recalled, possessed a crucial asset: 'as chief of the Salpêtrière … where there were then more than eight thousand persons, I always had cadavers at my disposal'.[47] Despite the warmth of the season, the two men

---

[46] Louis, 'Éloge de Camper' (1790), *Éloges*, 378–88. Camper spent two further years in Leiden after taking his medical degree. His studies in London took in a broad range of sciences, from electricity to natural history and two courses of accouchements taught by William Smellie.

[47] Ibid., 352. Louis slightly exaggerated the extent of his authority and perhaps also the size of the population. As *gagnant-maîtrise*, he served six years as a means to receive his surgical degree. He was the resident surgeon in the hospice whose population Tenon

spent several hours together nearly every day while Louis instructed his Dutch colleague on different surgical procedures, before demonstrating rapidly in just a few minutes how to perform an actual operation on the cadaver. He also escorted Camper to see Buffon at the Jardin du Roi and Réaumur, Winslow and Jean-Louis Petit at the Academy of Sciences. As well, Camper had 'long conversations' with the accoucheur André Levret.[48]

Twenty-one-year-old Jean-Georges Roederer spent the year 1747–48 in Paris. A native of Strasbourg, Roederer had trained for three years in the military and civil hospitals in his home territory. In Paris he divided his time between 'public lectures and practical work' at four sites: the Jardin du Roi, the surgical schools, the Hôtel-Dieu and the Charité. He devoted special attention to a course on accouchements with Grégoire. Roederer then went on to London to study with the man-midwives William Hunter and William Smellie. After visiting Oxford, Leiden and Göttingen he returned to Strasbourg to take his medical degree in 1750.[49]

Desault's School at the Hôtel-Dieu: The End of the Old Regime.

In 1780 Benjamin Franklin, America's venerable ambassador to France, came to the aid of a young medical graduate of the University of Pennsylvania, then visiting Paris. Twenty-three-year-old John Foulke carried letters of introduction stating his wish to 'improve himself in Surgery and Physic'. A 'perfect stranger in Paris', the Philadelphian sought 'recommendations to the most eminent in the Medical branches' and 'favorable introductions into the Hospitals'.[50] Franklin called upon the services of a Paris physician of his acquaintance to secure Foulke an advantageous place *en pension* with Pierre-Joseph Desault (1738–95), a surgeon well embarked on a very promising career.[51]

---

estimated at about 7,000 persons. No doubt there were 'at all times' many deaths among the elderly female population suffering from chronic ailments.

[48] Ibid. Louis stated that Camper, having already engaged in a wide variety of other studies in London, wanted to concentrate on surgery in Paris.

[49] Louis, 'Éloge de Roederer', *Éloges*, 59–72. Jacques Gélis has described an 'obstetrical grand tour' of Europe beginning around 1750 in which prospective accoucheurs sought out in sequence individual masters of the art rather than schools or locations. In this connection he mentions Fried at Strasbourg, Smellie and Hunter in London, Levret, then Baudelocque in Paris, etc. Gélis, *La sage-femme ou le médecin* (Paris, 1988), 293–7.

[50] *Franklin papers*, 32: 317–18.

[51] Ibid. 33: 67–8. Desault had earlier taken *en pension* another young Philadelphia medical man. Franklin also put in a good word on Foulke's behalf with the influential physician Félix Vicq d'Azyr, ibid: 282. Foulke studied in England and Holland while abroad. Writing from Leipzig, he deemed that school 'much inferior to that of Paris and in no way superior to that young seminary which owes its birth to you', a reference to Franklin's role in establishing the future University of Pennsylvania, ibid., 586.

During the early 1780s Desault (Figure 9.6) moved up the ranks of the Paris surgical profession, from taking in students like Foulke for private instruction and serving at the College of Surgery's small hospital, to chief surgeon of the Charité hospital and, finally, in 1785, at age 47, to chief surgeon of the Hôtel-Dieu.[52] Within two years, he had, over the protests of the hospital's religious nursing sisters, won the support of the hospital administrators for important innovations in teaching. Desault made surgical operations on patients, in a new amphitheatre constructed for that purpose, the focal point for elaborate clinical lessons. Four hours every day throughout the year were given over to teaching during ward rounds, outpatient consultations and the amphitheatre lesson.

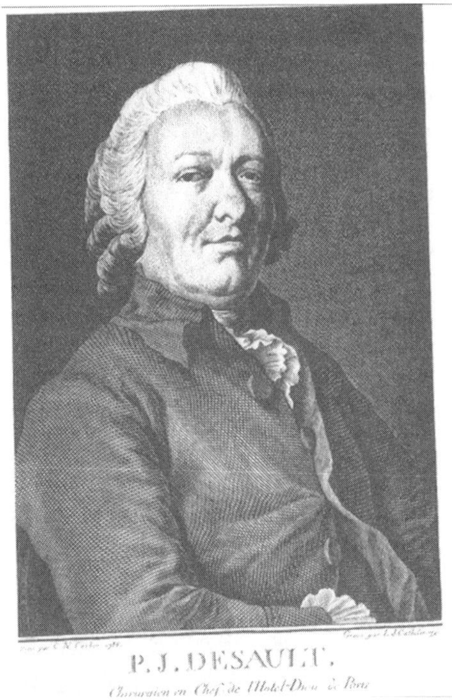

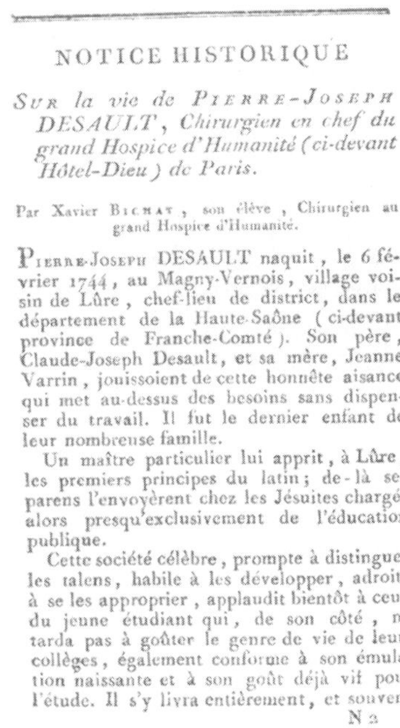

NOTICE HISTORIQUE

Sur la vie de Pierre-Joseph DESAULT, Chirurgien en chef du grand Hospice d'Humanité (ci-devant Hôtel-Dieu) de Paris.

Par Xavier Bichat, son élève, Chirurgien au grand Hospice d'Humanité.

Pierre-Joseph DESAULT naquit, le 6 février 1744, au Magny-Vernois, village voisin de Lûre, chef-lieu de district, dans le département de la Haute-Saône (ci-devant province de Franche-Comté). Son père, Claude-Joseph Desault, et sa mère, Jeanne Varrin, jouissoient de cette honnête aisance qui met au-dessus des besoins sans dispenser du travail. Il fut le dernier enfant de leur nombreuse famille.

Un maître particulier lui apprit, à Lûre, les premiers principes du latin; de-là ses parens l'envoyèrent chez les Jésuites chargés alors presqu'exclusivement de l'éducation publique.

Cette société célèbre, prompte à distinguer les talens, habile à les développer, adroite à se les approprier, applaudit bientôt à ceux du jeune étudiant qui, de son côté, ne tarda pas à goûter le genre de vie de leurs collèges, également conforme à son émulation naissante et à son goût déjà vif pour l'étude. Il s'y livra entièrement, et souvent

N 2

Fig.9.6 First page of Xavier Bichat's obituary of his teacher: 'On the life of Pierre-Joseph Desault, chief surgeon of the great Hospice of Humanity (formerly the Hôtel-Dieu) of Paris', with portrait engraving of Desault on facing page. From *Journal de chirurgie*, 4 (Paris, 1796)

[52] On Desault's career see, Gelfand, *Professionalizing modern medicine*, 116–27.

By 1791 Desault could plausibly boast to have trained more 'genuine surgeons' than his predecessors had produced over the course of the preceding century.[53] Three hundred students attended his lessons – two hundred fee-paying outsiders in addition to the corps of young surgeons working at the hospital. How many of the outsiders came from abroad can only be surmised. According to Xavier Bichat, Desault's former student assistant and collaborator, foreign governments had awarded stipends for surgeons to attend the Hôtel-Dieu clinic. In 1801 Bichat affirmed that his mentor's former students occupied prestigious posts in many European centres.[54] As the Revolution turned increasingly violent, menacing Desault himself, foreigners would have had difficult access at best.[55] But at least 50 students from Montpellier testified that Desault's course, which they attended in 1791–92, far excelled any other available in Paris or Montpellier.[56]

Desault's hospital clinical teaching represented a significant turning point in European medical education. At the same time, the surgeon perceived his innovation as a continuation on a vastly expanded scale of eighteenth-century private medical instruction. Although he gave up private practice and teaching after becoming chief surgeon at the Hôtel-Dieu, Desault vigorously defended the principle of charging fees to outside students who attended his hospital lessons. 'Experience has shown', he asserted in concluding a letter in November 1791 in defence of his hospital instruction, 'that free education is the worst of all ... it destroys the professor's zeal and it destroys the student's initiative; and, if more proof is needed, it could be found at the Hôtel-Dieu of Paris, where those having the right to attend the lessons gratis, are the least diligent.'[57]

---

53 Toby Gelfand, 'A confrontation over clinical instruction at the Hôtel-Dieu of Paris during the French Revolution', *Journal of the History of Medicine and Allied Sciences* 28 (1973): 268–82, esp. 276.

54 'Éloge de P.-J. Desault', in *Oeuvres chirurgicales de P.-J. Desault*, 1 (1798) 26, 48. Bichat's eulogy was dated 1801.

55 The British surgeon Astley Cooper managed to attend in the summer of 1792. Cooper left a mixed assessment of Desault, describing him as 'a good anatomist and an excellent manipulating surgeon, but as far as I could judge, not possessing the higher scientific principles, which are necessary to constitute a surgeon of the first order'. Bransby Blake Cooper, *The life of Sir Astley Cooper, Bart.*, vol. 1, 1843, 219–20.

56 'Lettre de M.J.-B. Mayet, médecin au mairie de Paris', in Alexandre Tuetey, *L'Assistance publique à Paris pendant la révolution* (Paris, 1895–97), 4 vols, 3: 137–9.

57 'Réclamation de M. Desault ... contre une pétition présentée à l'Assemble Nationale', Archives nationales de France, MS 538: 3, 47. Quoted in Gelfand, 'A confrontation over clinical instruction at the Hôtel-Dieu', 280. Desault's letter to the Committee of Public Instruction of the Revolutionary National Assembly responded to a challenge from a deputation of 'citizen-students in surgery' claiming to represent 2,000 petitioners demanding free admission to his hospital lessons. A few years earlier Jacques Tenon used similar reasoning in arguing for the superiority of private teaching. Tenon considered fees for service from the perspective of the instructor rather than the student. The best private instructors of anatomy, he wrote, were 'so much the better as their fortune

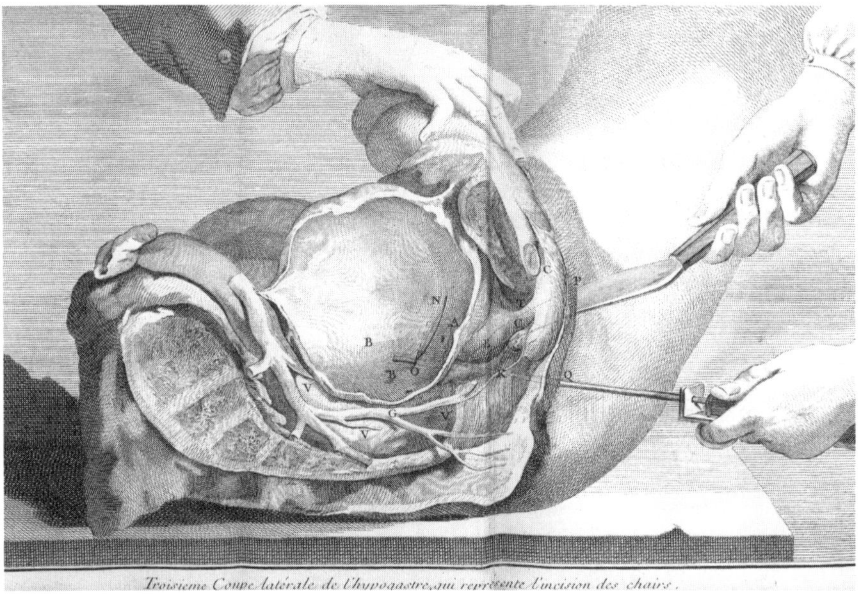

Fig.9.7 Practising surgery on the cadaver: the lithotomy operation. From *Mémoires de l'Academie royale de chirurgie*, vol. 1 (Paris, 1743)

Cadavers for Dissection: An Enlightenment Mission

The attraction of Paris for medical students throughout the eighteenth century was closely connected to the ready availability of specimens for human dissection, particularly in the setting of private courses. As Diderot remarked in contrasting public lectures with private medical instruction, 'private schools [are] more instructive, where the student works by himself and practises operations' (Figure 9.7).[58] When William Hunter introduced individual dissection into London private medical education, he advertised that he would be offering students 'the same manner as at Paris', thus referring to an evidently generally understood linkage between Paris and student anatomical dissection as well as to his recent personal experience with such lessons in the French capital.[59] Even the mid-century British pamphleteer who denied the superior teaching reputation of Paris hospitals over

depends on the good quality of their teaching and the well-deserved reputation earned by it'. Tenon, *Observations sur les obstacles qui s'opposent aux progrès de l'anatomie* (Paris, 1785), 30.

58 Quoted in Jean Mayer, *Diderot, homme de science* (Rennes, 1959), 39.

59 Gelfand, 'The "Paris manner"', esp. 121–3. Hunter's advertisement appeared in the *London Evening Post* on 16 September 1746, ibid., 99.

their London counterparts conceded: 'they [the Paris hospitals] have a greater plenty of subjects for dissection'.[60]

Enlightenment ideology had much to do with promoting the reputation of Paris as the preferred place for learning anatomy and surgery, a reputation not yet firmly established prior to the eighteenth century. Exmellin, a French Protestant surgeon, accused Catholic authorities of restricting the supply of available cadavers to the Paris medical Faculty. On registering to study in Amsterdam and Leiden in January 1677, he remarked: 'the surgical teaching I receive here is very different from that given in Paris where dissection is very hard to come by'.[61] If the Protestant's testimony may have been biased, François-Joseph Hunauld (1701–42), a prominent Paris physician and anatomist, expressed similar concerns in the late 1720s. After a year in Vienna, where he had been unable to do any dissection, Hunauld longed to return to his anatomical work in Paris. But, he added, 'My only wish would be to get them [cadavers] a little easier than in the past.'[62]

Enlightenment spokesmen, by mid-century, had taken up the cause of human dissection as an essential prerequisite for medical progress. Nowhere was this more evident than in the great *Encyclopédie* of Diderot and D'Alembert. In the article 'cadaver', D'Alembert approved the illegal practice of obtaining specimens by robbing graves and he pleaded that 'magistrates shut their eyes to this abuse [graverobbing] which results in considerable benefit'.[63] Diderot characteristically called for more radical reform. In a well-ordered society, he wrote, autopsies would be performed after all deaths; the priest would receive remains for burial only after the anatomist had finished with his studies.[64] In his contribution to the article 'anatomy' in the first volume of the *Encyclopédie* (1750) Diderot went even further. Here the philosopher pleaded for surgical experimentation on condemned criminals while they were still alive. In return, the subject, if he happened to survive, would be granted freedom. Diderot praised the historical precedent of this sort of human vivisection, said to have been performed by the ancient Alexandrian physicians.[65] The pre-Revolutionary popular writer Restif de la Bretonne echoed

[60] *Short comparative view*, 8–9. The author noted, however, that he had to pay exorbitant sums for 'bodies' in Paris. See Marcel Fosseyeux, 'Le prix des cadavres a Paris aux XVIIe et XVIIIe siècles', *Aesculape* 3 (1913), 52–6. Martin Lister, *Journey to Paris*, 69, thought the frequency of murders in Paris provided the anatomists with more bodies than elsewhere.

[61] Pierre Vallery Radot, 'Exmelin (1646?–1707) Navigateur, historien et chirurgien des flibustiers', *Histoire de la médecine* 11 (1961): 24–45, quote on 41. Exmelin studied in Paris in the early 1660s.

[62] Quoted in Fosseyeux, ' Prix des cadavres', 56.

[63] 'Cadavre', *Encyclopédie ou dictionnaire raisonné des sciences, des arts et des métiers*, 20 vols (Paris, 1753), 3: 511.

[64] Ibid. Diderot added his comment to d'Alembert's article.

[65] 'Anatomie', *Encyclopédie*, 1: 409–10. Diderot suggested several experimental surgical interventions: extirpation of the spleen, removal of some portion of the brain,

Diderot's thoughts on the subject, noting that in this manner the death of criminals would be made 'doubly useful'.[66] That such ideas could be entertained – there is no evidence that they went further – made the advocacy of distributing dead bodies for dissection seem by comparison a modest Enlightenment proposal.

Did magistrates in fact 'turn a blind eye' to grave robbing, as d'Alembert recommended? Although such actions remained formally illegal, contemporary discussion of the flourishing market in cadavers suggests a degree of official tolerance. Purchasing or receiving contraband anatomical specimens was not, in itself, a violation of the law, a distinction that Albrecht Haller apparently failed to appreciate. (In 1727, Haller departed Paris hastily, but mistakenly, 'an error understandable in a foreigner', according to his well-informed eulogist, fearing to be arrested for purchasing disinterred cadavers from surgeons.)[67] Duverney managed, at least for a time, to keep his anatomy course at the Jardin du Roi supplied far beyond the official limits on cadavers.[68] The physician-anatomist Winslow gratefully acknowledged the court physician Adrien Helvétius' 'special permission' in according specimens for his private dissection courses.[69] During most of the second half of the century, the surgeon Jean-Joseph Suë (1710–92), in addition to teaching public courses at the College of Surgery, conducted a private dissection school, known to attract foreigners. The American John Morgan for example, after receiving his MD from Edinburgh, studied under Suë and lived in his house during the winter of 1763–64.[70]

Alongside these relatively few well-established private schools directed by prominent teachers on a long-term basis, were many other private courses which advertised annual offerings of a range of subjects. At the bottom of the hierarchy, and doubtless most numerous, young surgeons improvised lessons in garrets pompously designed 'amphitheatres'. These marginal enterprises, centred around the Place Maubert (since medieval times a place of execution), depended upon a steady flow of anatomical specimens either purchased from grave robbers or disinterred by the surgeons themselves. Desault's private teaching began in this modest way. Diderot, among many others, recognised that grave robbing sustained

and blood transfusion. Given the practice of interrogation and capital punishment, which routinely involved torture of a 'patient' (the word had currency in this judicial sense), Diderot's proposal that the condemned criminal serve society as a medical patient may be taken as more than a rhetorical ploy.

66 Restif de la Bretonne, 'Les débris de cadavres', in *Les nuits de Paris* (Paris, 1960), 54–5 (originally published, London, 1788–89).

67 Condorcet, 'Éloge de Haller', *Histoire de l'Académie des sciences*, 1777 (Paris, 1778), 130.

68 See above.

69 J.-B. Winslow, *Exposition anatomique de la structure du corps humain* (Paris, 1732), xv.

70 See Gelfand, 'Paris manner', 118–19, n. 52.

such private dissection courses: 'the private schools ... where the student works by himself and practises operations have recourse to the cemeteries'.[71]

Given their rates of mortality, the Paris hospitals potentially could have easily satisfied the needs of medical instruction.[72] However, hospital authorities were reluctant to supply cadavers to outsiders. In 1749 Hôtel-Dieu administrators reaffirmed their long-standing policy of refusing requests of this kind, citing their fear of 'arousing reproach and public outcry ... disgust and revulsion', among the common folk [*le peuple*] whom the hospital served.[73]

The attitude and, indeed, the policy of the huge Salpêtrière hospice appeared less sensitive to public sentiment and more open to the surgeon's needs. In 1731 the administrators of the Hôpital Général (of which the Salpêtrière was the main division) reminded inmates that they owed their sustenance to charity. In return, the poor were expected to 'overcome their revulsion' against their bodies being used for instruction, specifically for post-mortem dissection.[74] James Houstoun attributed this policy to direct government intervention: 'the King has ordered, that every Body of those that dies in the *Sale Petrier* [*sic*] (a very large Hospital for the Reception of the *Poor*) should be subjected to *Anatomical Dissection*, for the Improvement of *Physick and Surgery*'.[75] On the eve of the Revolution, Nicolas Chambon de Montaux, physician at the Salpêtrière, accoucheur and future mayor

---

[71] See above, n. 63. See also Louis-Sébastien Mercier, articles 'Anatomie', 'Clamart', 'Jeunes chirurgiens', 'Tableau de Paris', in *Paris le jour, Paris la nuit*, ed. Daniel Baruch (Paris: Robert Laffont, 1990), 71–2, 139–40, 278–9; Restif de la Bretonne, 'Les débris des cadavres', 'Les violateurs des sépultures', 'L'assassin', 'La morte vivante', *Les nuits de Paris*, 54, 55, 63, 136–8.

[72] The mortality rate at the Hôtel-Dieu exceeded 20 per cent, worse by far than that at hospitals in other European cities. See Tenon, *Mémoires*, 278. Fosseyeux, *Hôtel-Dieu*, 339, calculated an average rate of 14 deaths per day during the 1780s. Death rates at the Salpêtrière were probably considerably higher.

[73] *Délibérations... de l'Hôtel-Dieu*, 1: 352. For a detailed discussion of the Hôtel-Dieu's policy on distribution of cadavers, see Gelfand, 'Paris manner', 106–7, 111–15. Significantly, the Hôtel-Dieu administrators left out the phrase 'wounding Christian charity' that appeared in their mid-17th-century prohibition of furnishing cadavers for outside study, ibid., 111.

[74] 'Délibération du bureau de l'Hôpital Général ... 12 mars 1731', Archives Préfecture de Police de Paris, Collection Lamoignon, t.30, fol. 281. The surgeon S.-F. Morand described the availability of bodies for dissection as 'the best thing that the dead can do for the living'. 'Éloge de Cheselden', *Mémoires de l'Académie royale de chirurgie* 3 (1757) 107–8. As early as 1684, the anatomist Alexis Littre, a physician, thanks to his 'connection with a surgeon of the Salpêtrière', was said to have dissected, together with his colleague, more than 200 cadavers during an exceptionally cold winter.

[75] Houstoun, *Memoirs*, 74–5 (emphasis in original). Houstoun, it should be recalled, worked at the Hôtel-Dieu around 1714. Houstoun's sweeping generalisation does not rule out the possibility that the Salpêtrière, like the Hôtel-Dieu, opposed providing cadavers for dissection courses *outside* the hospice.

of Paris, wrote: 'the government, convinced of the need for these studies, has *for a long time* facilitated the transport of cadavers'.[76]

Conclusion

Paris appears to have been the European centre of excellence for the study of surgery and related clinical subjects, such as accouchements, during the first half of the eighteenth century. The unrivalled reputation of the French capital derived from the relative ease with which anatomical studies could be pursued. Anatomy, of course, had obvious relevance for surgical training. But, from the time of the Renaissance, knowledge of the structure of the human body took on increasing importance for physicians as well.[77] Anatomy was the fundamental subject upon which physiology (Haller's 'animated anatomy') and much of pathology came to be based. 'He told me that I should learn anatomy *par coeur*', Théophile de Bordeu wrote to his father of the surgeon Ledran's first words of advice on how to succeed in medicine.[78]

Enlightenment medical men and philosophers alike privileged learning anatomy by personal dissection of the cadaver. There were, of course, alternative methods. In the early eighteenth century eloquent public lecturers, like Duverney (1648–1730) and Winslow (1669–1760) at the Jardin du Roi, Bernhard Albinus (1653–1721) and Johann Jacob Rau (1658–1719) in Leiden and Alexander Monro *primus* (1698–1767) in Edinburgh, earned fame (and monetary rewards) with students of the healing art as well as a wider public audience. They made do with relatively few cadavers. Dramatic lectures supplemented by displays of injected preparations of the vessels and nerves, wax models, engravings and other artistic representations of the anatomical parts served instead of hands-on dissection by students. Philosophical and moral reflections suggested by the anatomical revelations added to the appeal of the presentation.[79]

Anatomists at the Jardin du Roi and the Collège Royal continued to offer public demonstrations of this kind. But by the second half of the century medical

---

[76] Nicolas Chambon de Montaux, *Moyens de rendre les hôpitaux plus utiles* (Paris, 1787) 211–12 (emphasis added). Hospital patients were by definition poor and not working, Chambon noted. But 'the suffering man does not cease to be a citizen; if there is a way in which he can contribute to the public welfare, his infirmities do not exempt him from a duty which gratitude and humanitarianism likewise impose upon him'. See Gelfand, 'A clinical ideal: Paris 1789', *Bulletin of the History of Medicine* 51 (1977): 397–411, esp. 406–9.

[77] See Andrew Cunningham, *The anatomical renaissance: the resurrection of the anatomical projects of the ancients* (Aldershot, 1997).

[78] Bordeu, *Correspondance*, 1: 117.

[79] See Christopher Lawrence, 'Alexander Monro *Primus* and the Edinburgh manner of anatomy', *Bulletin of the History of Medicine*, 62 (1988): 193–215.

students wanted hands-on training in surgical anatomy.[80] Private dissection courses combining the two disciplines (and sometimes accouchements as well) flourished in Paris and elsewhere.[81] After mid-century, London emerged as a serious rival to the French capital, in part due to the rise of private teaching in newly established voluntary hospitals.[82] As well, the results of a transfer of knowledge, techniques and methods of instruction from Paris to London became evident. William Smellie and William Hunter were but two of the most successful British 'man-midwives' who, having profited from studies in Paris, then established private courses, rendering it unnecessary for the younger generation to make the same trip.[83] French-authored texts in anatomy and surgery no longer were the undisputed standards of reference they once had been. Translation, which had been predominately from French to English, became a two-way exchange after mid-century.[84]

Paris nonetheless remained an important centre for clinical instruction in the late eighteenth century, notably at Desault's Hôtel-Dieu school. Private dissection courses consistently attracted students. Public lectures at the Jardin du Roi and the College of Surgery added to the prestige of the city as an indispensable stop on the medical 'grand tour', or a longer stay *en pension*. Thanks to government backing for their professional project, the Paris surgeons had a seminal role in the promotion of the capital as a place for foreign physicians as well as surgeons to advance their studies.

For a variety of reasons, the reputation of the Paris medical Faculty continued to decline over the course of the century.[85] However, individual physicians attracted students. Physician anatomists at the Jardin du Roi – Duverney, Hunauld and Winslow during the first half of the century and Antoine Ferrein, Antoine Petit, Vicq d'Azyr and Antoine Portal thereafter – earned European-wide reputations for

---

80 For William Hunter's dismissal of Ferrein's anatomical lecture course at the Collège royal, see Gelfand, 'Paris manner', 103. See also Lawrence, 'Alexander Monro', 212–14.

81 Delaunay, *Le monde médical parisien*, 18–19 itemises private courses offered in 1776.

82 See Susan Lawrence, 'Entrepreneurs and private enterprise: the development of medical lecturing in London, 1775–1820', *Bulletin of the History of Medicine* 62 (1988): 171–92.

83 John Hunter, for example, boasted that his brother William 'was the only one that stem'd the course of our young Gentlemen going to Holland and France for their medical education, he even inverted the stream'. In Samuel Foart Simmons and John Hunter, *William Hunter 1718–1783, A Memoir*, ed. C.H. Brock (Glasgow, 1983), 6.

84 See Toby Gelfand, '"Invite the philosopher as well as the charitable": hospital teaching as private enterprise in Hunterian London', in *William Hunter and the eighteenth-century medical world*, 129–51, esp, 138–41.

85 The Royal Society of Medicine, rather than the Paris Faculty, represented progressive reform in medicine and public health, but this academic body came into being only in 1776 and had no jurisdiction over medical education. See Caroline M. Hannaway, 'The Société royale de médecine and epidemics in the "ancien régime"', *Bulletin of the History of Medicine* 46 (1972): 257–73.

public teaching and, more importantly, for their more instructive private courses.[86] The English translator of Winslow's *Exposition anatomique* (1732), for example, claimed that the author's courses had long afforded students of anatomy the 'best opportunities' in Europe. He added, however, that 'those who have been his scholars at Paris' might be sorry not to find in the *Exposition* what they had heard in Winslow's private courses about the implications of anatomy for understanding physiology.[87]

Thomas Bond of Philadelphia was one of those who took courses with Winslow and his colleagues. I began this essay with Bond's uncertainty in 1771 about where in Europe he should send his son to complete his medical education. It seems fitting to conclude with the same witness's unambiguous satisfaction in 1739 with his own choice of medical studies abroad. In an enthusiastic letter, Bond aptly summarised the opportunities he had found in Paris:

> I have now spent three months in Paris, the most diligently I ever did any [in] my life and I fear at the Prejudice of my tender Constitution, but if I was almost sure 'twould kill me I could not avoid tending the Curious Courses of Anatomy, Surgery, Midwifery, Physiology etc and in short 'tis impossible there can be better if so good schools in the world.[88]

---

86 Ferrein and Portal also lectured at the Collège Royal. See Jean Torlais, 'Le Collège royal', in *Enseignement et diffusion*, 261–86. On the popularity of Antoine Petit's private teaching in the 1760s compared with arid lectures at the medical Faculty, see Gilbert Chinard, 'The life of a Parisian medical student in the eighteenth century', *Bulletin of the History of Medicine* 7 (1939): 374–80. See also Alfred Rouxeau, *Un étudiant en médecine quimpérois (Guillaume-François Laennec) aux derniers jours de l'ancien régime* (Nantes, 1926), 35–70, for a range of private courses in Paris, including Petit's, followed by a medical student between 1769 and 1771.

87 G. Douglas, 'Translator's preface', to Winslow, *An anatomical exposition of the structure of the human body* (London, 1749), xvii.

88 Letter of Bond to John Bartram, 20 February 1738/39. Quoted in Elizabeth H. Thomson, 'Thomas Bond, 1713–84. First professor of clinical medicine in the American colonies', *Journal of Medical Education* 33 (1958): 614–24. Quote on 616–17.

Chapter 10
Medical Education in Eighteenth-century Montpellier

Elizabeth A. Williams

In October 1739 a 17-year-old Théophile de Bordeu left his home in Izeste in the Pyrenees on the journey that would take him to Montpellier for four years of medical study. During his time in Montpellier Bordeu studied with distinguished professors; learned the fundamentals of both medicine and surgery; taught private courses; and formed lasting associations with other students. Six years later, in September 1745, another to-be-famous physician, Samuel-Auguste-André Tissot, like Bordeu aged 17, left his home in the village of Grancy in Switzerland and wended his way to Montpellier. Tissot stayed four years and his experience resembled that of Bordeu in many ways: he too studied with celebrated physicians, gained knowledge through hands-on experience and established ties that would continue throughout his career. Of both these famed doctors we can say, without hesitation, that they received in Montpellier a good medical education, perhaps an 'excellent' one, depending on the criteria by which one judges. Yet in accounts that Bordeu and Tissot left of their student years in Montpellier both expressed complaints about the dull and unimaginative teaching, the paucity of training opportunities and the exploitation of students by greedy professors and locals.[1]

The contrast between what some historians have said about the high quality of medical education in eighteenth-century Montpellier and what these testimonials of Bordeu and Tissot indicate helps to highlight problems that historians face when they try not only to describe medical education in former times but to make judgements about quality.[2] Assessments of quality often ineluctably merge with

---

1 *Théophile de Bordeu: Correspondance*, ed. Martha W. Fletcher, 4 vols (Montpellier: Université Paul Valéry, n.d.), 1: 26–145, especially 1: 36, 38, 106–7, 113, 122, 126, 128; on Bordeu's overall attitude toward Montpellier, see Elizabeth A. Williams, *A cultural history of medical vitalism in Enlightenment Montpellier* (Aldershot: Ashgate, 2003), 114–15, 208–9; on Tissot, see Antoinette Emch-Dériaz, *Tissot, physician of the Enlightenment* (New York: Peter Lang, 1992), 13–19.

2 For praise of Montpellier in contrast to Paris, see, for example, Charles Coury, 'The teaching of medicine in France from the beginning of the seventeenth century', in *The history of medical education*, ed. C.D. O'Malley (Berkeley: University of California Press, 1970), 121–72, esp. 124, 128–9, 137; Charles C. Gillispie, *Science and polity in France at the end of the Old Regime* (Princeton: Princeton University Press, 1980), 217–18. In arguing

discussions of the appeal exerted over students by given institutions, yet much evidence indicates that the search for excellence was not always foremost in students' minds. Students selected universities for all kinds of reasons and, as I will show in respect of Montpellier, their motives were often unrelated to academic 'excellence'. In any event, using the term 'excellence' raises a number of questions: given the competing imperatives of practitioners, patients and society at large, not everyone agreed on what medicine or medical training ideally should be. Much of the literature on medical education has focused on what has been judged a slow and uncertain shift in the early modern period from 'theoretical' or purely didactic training to a more 'practical' style of education, and my discussion here will attend in good part to this problematic.[3] I will look at Montpellier's mixed record in this regard while also suggesting that historians need to develop a more nuanced set of categories than the stark dichotomy of 'theoretical versus practical' set forth in much scholarship in the field. I will argue that an enhanced 'practical' bent in medical education could, and in Montpellier did, entail as essential components not only the bedside and hands-on training ordinarily indicated by the term but also analytical, discursive and rhetorical shifts that promoted a more powerful engagement of medicine in society. As was true elsewhere in Enlightenment Europe, this goal was vigorously sought by pedagogues and practitioners alike in eighteenth-century Montpellier. Such a perspective on the practicality of medical training provides, I will argue, a useful alternative to measures of success or failure, mediocrity or 'excellence', that emphasises advances toward ideals of medical education that were realised only in later, markedly different historical contexts.

Medical Education in Montpellier

Montpellier's general historical background helps to illuminate some features of the medical education offered there in the early modern period. Unlike a number of the celebrated towns of the Midi – Nîmes, Orange, Marseille – Montpellier does not date back to Roman days. Rather, it emerged as a commercial centre in the tenth century, and it seems that some kind of medical teaching became part of

---

for Montpellier's advanced position in medicine, these authors reflected the self-assessment of Montpellier physicians; a founding text is Jean Astruc, *Mémoires pour servir à l'histoire de la Faculté de Médecine de Montpellier*, ed. A.-M. Lorry (Paris: P.G. Cavelier, 1767).

[3] For one discussion of the slow displacement of the 'theoretical' by the 'practical', see Laurence Brockliss and Colin Jones, *The medical world of early modern France* (Oxford: Clarendon, 1997), 166–9; a recent synthetic history of medical education indicates the wide range of meanings attached to the term 'practical,' including bedside instruction, apprenticeship training and other forms of extra-university instruction, the union of medicine and surgery, and applications of laboratory science; see Thomas Bonner, *Becoming a physician: Medical education in Britain, France, Germany, and the United States, 1750–1945* (New York: Oxford University Press, 1995), 1–11.

the life of the town early on. The medical faculty of Montpellier was first officially recognised in 1220, and it subsequently developed in loose association with the arts, law and theology faculties established in later years. By the late Middle Ages Montpellier enjoyed a leading position in medical education, in company with Paris and Bologna, as one of three 'major centers of medical education'.[4] Up to the first half of the sixteenth century Montpellier attracted large numbers of students from abroad: in the early sixteenth century the student population consisted of approximately 37 per cent 'foreigners', but by the 1590s this percentage had dropped to under 14.[5] This change, along with many others in the life of sixteenth-century Montpellier, reflects the ravages of the Wars of Religion. Before the era of religious conflict Montpellier had been a major centre of medical education for France's Catholic neighbours. By contrast, after the 1590s Montpellier was suspect to Catholics. Philip II reportedly forbade Spanish students to matriculate at Montpellier, given its post-Reformation reputation as a Protestant stronghold.[6]

In the long run, however, far from undoing Montpellier as a medical centre, the Wars of Religion and their outcome proved to be the making of the town in respect of medicine. The Montpellier faculty was closely identified with Henri IV and the Huguenot coterie surrounding him, and in consequence the king favoured Montpellier in ways that left a lasting imprint. It was during the king's ascendancy that chairs devoted to anatomy and botany (1593) and to surgery and pharmacy (1597) were established in addition to the four regents professorships (*régences*) that had been created at the end of the fifteenth century. After this era only two more permanent professorships were to be established during the *ancien régime* – the chemistry chair founded in 1676 and the professorship connected to the 'service for the poor' (*service des pauvres*) set up in 1715.[7]

In another, perhaps even more important way Montpellier's link to Henri IV determined its post-Reformation fate. It was during this period that Montpellier physicians first came to dominate the royal medical entourage. The medical household of Henri IV consisted solely of Huguenots trained in Montpellier, and from this point onward it was the Montpellier rather than the Paris faculty that

---

[4] On Montpellier through the late Middle Ages, see the pertinent essays in *Histoire de Montpellier*, ed. Gerard Cholvy (Toulouse: Privat, 1984); the quotation is from Nancy G. Siraisi, *Medieval and early Renaissance medicine: An introduction to knowledge and practice* (Chicago: University of Chicago Press, 1990), 55.

[5] Roger Chartier, et al., eds, *L'éducation en France du XVe au XVIIIe siècles* (Paris: Société d'édition d'enseignement supérieur, 1976), 269–73; Henri Dermigny, 'De Montpellier à La Rochelle: Route du commerce, route de la médecine au XVIIIe siècle', *Annales du Midi* 67 (1955): 31–58.

[6] Chartier, et al., *L'éducation en France*, 271.

[7] Louis Dulieu, *La médecine à Montpellier*, 7 vols (Avignon: Les presses universelles, 1975–90; Montpellier, 1994–99) 2: 13, 3: 26–27.

functioned as 'the nursery of court physicians' (*une pépinière des archiâtres*).[8] The patronage and influence of the court were exercised especially through the successive graduates of Montpellier who served as the king's First Physician. Of the eight First Physicians who held office between 1693 and 1792, four studied at Montpellier and one had important ties to Montpellier and sent his son to school there. As late as 1789 as many as half of the 200 or so physicians serving at Versailles were Montpellier graduates.[9]

At the opening of the eighteenth century, then, Montpellier was well established as a premier medical centre in France, the only medical school in the kingdom that contested the supremacy of the Paris faculty (Figure 10.1). The character of education at the University of Medicine of Montpellier, as it was called in the eighteenth century, was established first and foremost by the professoriate, which consisted of the four regents professorships and the four designated chairs mentioned earlier. As these professorial appointments were made for life, Montpellier had a stable core of teachers. The average tenure of professors in the eighteenth century was nearly two decades, and some chair holders remained in place for as much as a half century.[10] (In this respect Montpellier differed notably from Paris, where most teaching continued to be done by recent graduates holding two-year appointments).[11] The eight Montpellier chair holders who met regularly in faculty assemblies were responsible for routine decisions about curricular matters and the day-to-day governance of the school. Their decisions were carried out by a handful of officials and functionaries, including the dean, who was elected from among the faculty and who continued to teach while performing administrative

---

8 Hugh Trevor-Roper, 'The court physician and Paracelsianism', in *Medicine at the courts of Europe, 1500–1837*, ed. Vivian Nutton (London: Routledge, 1990), 79–94; the phrase 'pépiniêre des archiâtres', attributed to Louis XIV, appears in 'Mémoire concernant les abus', in Archives départementales de l'Hérault [hereafter ADH], Série C, Archives civils (Intendance), C524.

9 The four First Physicians who were Montpellier graduates included Pierre Chirac, François Chicoyneau, Jean-Baptiste Sénac and Joseph Lieutaud; J.-M.-F. Lassone studied in Montpellier for a time and sent his son there; see Williams, *Medical vitalism*, 132–3; Colin Jones, 'The *Médecins du Roi* at the end of the Ancien Régime and in the French Revolution', in *Medicine at the courts of Europe*, 209–61.

10 Calculating only professorial tenures that began in the eighteenth century (not those carrying over from the seventeenth to the eighteenth), the average is 18.6 years. If three professorships that were truncated by the coming of the Revolution (Henri Fouquet, Régence I, 1789–92; J.-B.-T. Baumes, Régence II, 1790–92; and Henri-Louis Brun, Régence III, 1788–92) are left out of the calculation, the average rises to 20.1 years. The two professors who were in place for over or nearly a half century were François Chicoyneau, anatomy and botany, 1701–52 and Antoine Magnol, Régence II, 1715–59. It should be noted, however, that both of these figures were sometimes away from their teaching posts for extended stints and replaced by temporary instructors.

11 Brockliss and Jones, *Medical world*, 511; Coury, 'Teaching of medicine in France', 128.

duties. Yet despite this structure of faculty governance, the professoriate was at all times subject to the will of overlapping local, regional and national authorities. At the top of the internal hierarchy stood the chancellor, who, from 1664 onwards, gained his office by purchase from the crown. The chancellor was a faculty member – attached to his office was the chair of anatomy and botany – but his chief role was to represent the interests of the university with the great personages outside the institution who had authority over it. These included the bishop of Montpellier, who was legally designated the 'guardian' of the university, and the intendant of Languedoc, who intervened on matters great and small on an almost daily basis. Ultimate authority rested with the crown and was exercised chiefly through the First Physician, resident at Versailles; until the last decade of the *ancien régime* he was consulted on every major decision affecting the institution. As will be seen, the actions of these sometimes competing, sometimes cooperating external authorities were often decisive in establishing the character of medical education.[12]

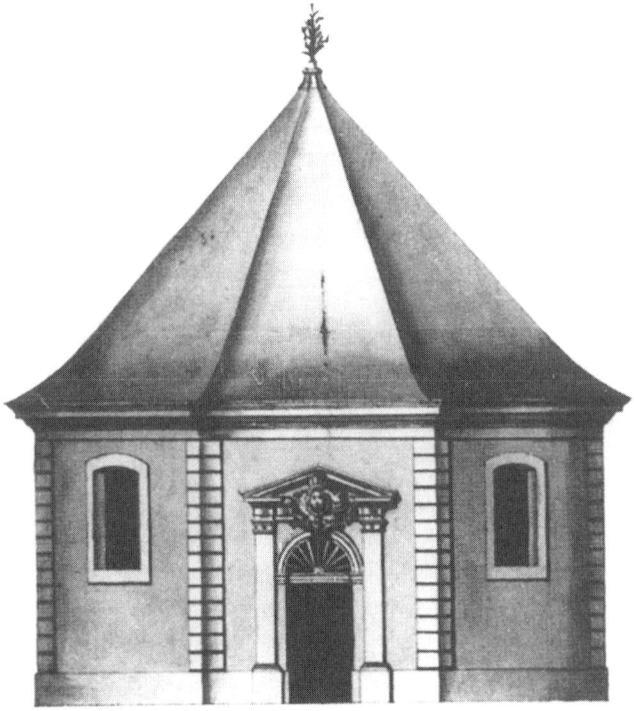

Fig.10.1 The amphitheatre of the Montpellier faculty of medicine in the eighteenth century

12 Williams, *Medical vitalism*, 52–6.

The medical curriculum in place in eighteenth-century Montpellier reflected the structure of the teaching faculty, with its mix of defined and general professorships. While the subject matter attached to the specially designated chairs – anatomy, botany, surgery, pharmacy and chemistry – was set, the regents professorships entailed no specified curricular responsibilities. Instead, professors were free to choose the subject matter of their courses in accord with their current interests.[13] In the later eighteenth century some students complained that the topics their professors took up were esoteric and their instruction was incomprehensible. In response, some professors began offering their own peculiar syntheses of the subjects – pathology, physiology and therapeutics – that had long dominated the curriculum.[14] A case in point is the physiology course offered in successive years in the early 1780s by J.C.M.G. Grimaud, which is extant in two posthumous editions published by Grimaud's students.[15]

Although it is of interest to know what the formal curriculum was in a given institution, it is of greater interest to know what was actually taught and how. In Montpellier, university statutes established in 1732 and reconfirmed in 1766 held that professors were to offer courses on a selected subject for six years in succession, but there is little evidence that this rule was enforced. The statutes also established that professors were to present at least 40 lectures per term, that they were to sign an attendance register signifying their presence, and that a fine of

---

13 Such was the case in the 1750s, for example, when Gérard Fitzgerald taught a course on 'venereal maladies and the ills of women and children', a subject on which he published a treatise in 1754; see Gérard Fitzgerald, *Tractatus pathologicus de affectibus foeminarum praeternaturalibus* (Paris, 1754).

14 On the establishment in 1665 of general courses of physiology and pathology, see A. Germain, *L'Ecole de médecine de Montpellier, ses origines, sa constitution, son enseignement: Etude historique d'après les documents originaux* (Montpellier: J. Martel, 1880), 99–100. Dulieu has counted the course offerings at Montpellier from 1601 to the Revolution and lists the following as those provided most frequently: 77 courses on maladies of the head, 1601–1762; 71 on fevers, 1603–1789; 68 on abdominal maladies, 1603–1758; 48 on therapeutics; 46 on *matière médicale*, 1635–1792; and 43 on gynaecology, 1601–1793. He observes further that personalised 'survey' courses increased in number as teaching based on Greco-Roman texts declined; the last course devoted specifically to a selection of Hippocratic texts was offered in 1771; see Dulieu, *La médecine à Montpellier*, 3: 229–34.

15 J.C.M.G. Grimaud, *Cours complet de physiologie, ouvrage posthume*, 2 vols (Paris: Méquignon Marvis, 1818); idem, *Cours complet de physiologie, distribué en leçons, ouvrage posthume*, 2 vols, 2nd rev. edn (Paris: Egron, 1824). The same was true for Grimaud's course on fevers, published in the following editions: idem, *Cours complet de fièvres*, 4 vols, ed. Charles-Louis Dumas (Montpellier: Jean-François Picot, 1791); idem, *Cours de fièvres*, 4 vols, 2nd edn, ed. J-.B.-E. Demorcy-Delletre (Montpellier: Veuve Picot, 1815). On Grimaud's theoretical stance, see Elizabeth A. Williams, 'Of two lives one? J.C.M.G. Grimaud and the question of holism in vitalist medicine', *Science in context*, forthcoming.

three *livres* was to be levied for each lecture missed. How commonly this occurred is impossible to know, given the patchy character of the attendance registers and the seemingly not uncommon practice of professors having the university beadle sign them in. In any event, the problem of professorial absenteeism does appear in student complaints and petitions, in remonstrations from Paris officialdom and in charges made on several occasions by professors about the slovenly behaviour of their colleagues.[16] Gaps in instruction were regularly filled by private courses offered by chair holders themselves, *docteurs ordinaires* resident in the town and recent graduates like Bordeu, who taught anatomy in 1745–46. As was true elsewhere, many disputes broke out over private courses given, that students paid for them separately and that the fees constituted an important part of the income of the instructors, including the regular chair holders. Professors objected when university facilities were made available to competitors – town doctors or students – or when such courses were offered at times conflicting with their own. Students objected that professors neglected their regular courses, or that the university failed to offer needed courses, so that money could be made from private courses covering the same material.[17]

Curricular offerings were of course dependent, in many cases, on facilities. Indeed Montpellier's reputation rested in good part on its provision of facilities that made possible practical training in anatomy, botany and, to a lesser extent, chemistry and in providing settings for clinical teaching; some historians have emphasised this theme in arguing that the medical education offered in Montpellier was superior to that provided by the Paris faculty.[18] The two most notable features of Montpellier's educational infrastructure were the Jardin des Plantes, established in 1593, and the diverse arrangements established in the town for clinical teaching. In both instances Montpellier's facilities provided grounds for local claims to pre-eminence in medical education while, nonetheless, manifesting weaknesses that characterised the school in the decades before the full-scale reorganisation effected during the French Revolution.

Montpellier's Jardin des Plantes was initially constructed under the direction of Pierre Richer de Belleval, the chair holder in anatomy and botany from 1593–1632 (Figure 10.2). In establishing a garden of this kind, Montpellier was preceded only by three Italian medical centres which had opened botanical gardens earlier in the sixteenth century: Padua in 1545, Pisa in1546 and Bologna in 1568. By the eighteenth century botanical teaching in Montpellier was concentrated in a section

[16] The 1732 statutes appear in Archives de la Faculté de Médecine de Montpellier [hereafter AFMM], Série S, Registres: S15, 52–9, those of 1766 in AFMM: S16, 103–8; see also Williams, *Medical vitalism*, 55, 57–9, 70, 189.

[17] Williams, *Medical vitalism*, 58–9; on the role of private courses in medical instruction offered in Paris and Montpellier, see L.W.B. Brockliss, 'Before the clinic: French medical teaching in the eighteenth century', in *Constructing Paris medicine*, ed. Caroline Hannaway and Ann La Berge (Amsterdam: Rodopi, 1998), 71–115, esp. 82–7.

[18] See the sources cited in n. 2 above.

of the gardens known as the Jardin du Roi, which housed the *école médicale*, structures and facilities reserved for teachers and students. Although a source of pride in Montpellier, the gardens were alternately the subject of careful attention and serious neglect. Control of the gardens was one of the perquisites of the university chancellor, the venal officeholder mentioned earlier, and this meant that the gardens were sometimes supervised by individuals who had knowledge of botany and sometimes not, depending on the interests of the men who purchased or inherited the office.[19] The gardens enjoyed a heyday in the middle of the eighteenth century, when they were managed not by the legal claimant to the intendancy, a child of the Chicoyneau dynasty, but by a replacement, the later much- celebrated François Boissier de Sauvages. The famous nosologist first filled a position as *démonstrateur* and then, from 1752 to 1758, occupied a temporary chair of botany created especially for him.[20] Sauvages, a lifelong correspondent and partisan of Linnaeus, introduced the latter's method and nomenclature in Montpellier, and also made a number of practical improvements to the gardens, including the construction of the first hothouse for exotic plants. He also routinely took students into the countryside surrounding Montpellier, conducting *herborisations* intended to acquaint them with the wealth of regional plants used in local therapeutics and to collect specimens (Figure 10.3). A recent study of the gardens has shown that much of the work of maintaining the them, building collections and teaching students was performed not by its intendant or any member of the medical faculty but instead by the gardeners, who struggled to establish in the institution a new kind of meritocratic authority.[21]

---

[19] The professorship in botany and intendancy of the gardens were for almost a century controlled by the Chicoyneau family, successive members of which served as chancellor from 1664 to 1759. The intendant and chairholder from 1732 to 1740, A.-F. Chicoyneau, a one-time student of Sébastien Vaillant in Paris, achieved some distinction in the field; see J.-F. Planchon, *La botanique à Montpellier, Etudes historiques, notes et documents* (Montpellier: Boehm et fils, 1884), 12–13, 20.

[20] The *démonstrateurs* in botany were as important for this activity as they were for the teaching of anatomy, though the position in botany was never formalised; see Dulieu, *La médecine à Montpellier*, 3: 408–11.

[21] Planchon, *La botanique à Montpellier*, 18–19 n. 1; Louis-Augustin d'Hombres-Firmas, *Notice biographique sur François Boissier de la Croix de Sauvages* (Nîmes: Ballivet et Fabre, 1838), 14; James Livesey, 'Botany and provincial enlightenment in Montpellier: Antoine Banal père and fils, 1750–1800', *History of Science* 43 (2005): 57–76.

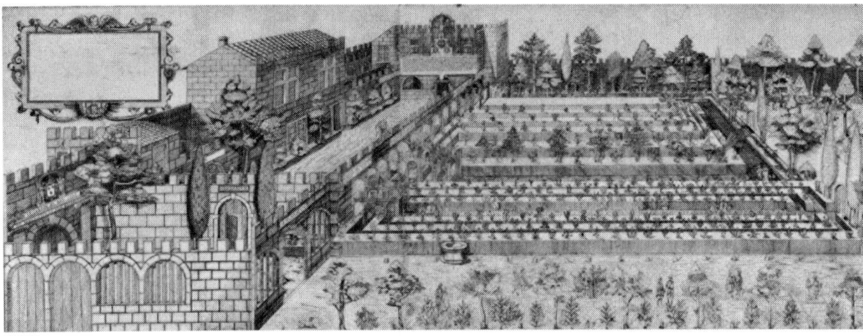

Fig. 10.2 The Jardin Royal, Montpellier, in the eighteenth century

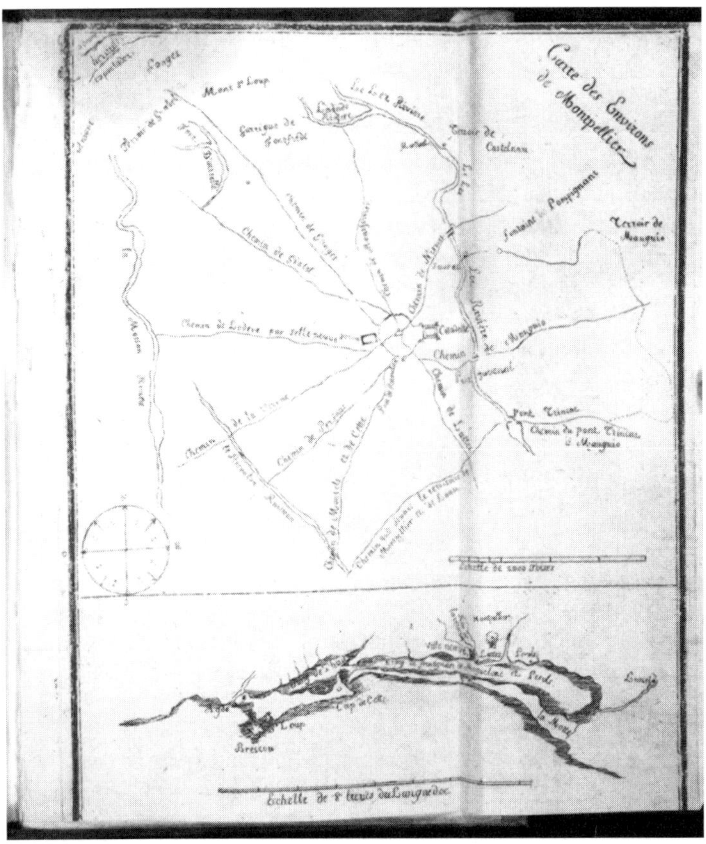

Fig. 10.3 'Herborisation' map, from Antoine Gouan, *Herborisations des environs de Montpellier* (1796)

The institutional ups and downs of the Jardin du Roi were, as with instruction in anatomy, the result of two chief factors. One was the venal system that attached control of the gardens to the chancellor's office and that, by definition, excluded knowledge and competence as criteria of appointment. The other was Montpellier's in other ways beneficial connection to the court, which ensured that key members of the institution were often away from Montpellier for long periods, pursuing, as the most important dimensions of their careers, service to king and courtiers at Versailles. Although it is clear that the teaching of botany within the Montpellier medical school rested on uncertain foundations, this matter became less pressing as the century wore on, given that botanists, even those who taught in medical schools, increasingly strove to establish the independence of their field in the face of medicine.[22] Of greater moment in assessing medical education, therefore, is the question of how Montpellier provided for clinical teaching, an increasingly critical element of professional training on which the pressures of the venal system and absenteeism were also brought to bear.[23]

The term 'clinical instruction' covers many dimensions of medical training; here I will focus on opportunities available to students in Montpellier for hands-on training in dissection and for bedside observation and treatment of patients. In Montpellier students did enjoy the benefits of a long-established tradition in anatomical investigation. Montpellier was the first of the French medical schools to build an anatomical amphitheatre, in 1556, and it was also the first to establish a designated chair in the field.[24] On the other hand, the chair in anatomy (the same chair, recall, to which supervision of the gardens was attached) was the preserve of the medical dynasties that held sway in Montpellier, and thus its occupants, just as with botany, were often ignorant of or uninterested in the field. This meant that in anatomy, as in botany, instruction by non-chair holders had to supplement or replace the teaching that was officially the responsibility of the designated professor. Already in the era of Richer de Belleval, anatomical teaching was in the

---

22 On this shift at the Jardin du Roi in Paris, see E.C. Spary, *Utopia's garden: French natural history from Old Regime to Revolution* (Chicago: University of Chicago Press, 2000), 15–17.

23 The most notable recent entry on this question is Othmar Keel's extensive survey of clinical training throughout Europe, a study intended to undercut the view that this innovation should be credited to the Paris Clinical School. In his zeal to overthrow the old view of Paris's leadership, Keel overstates his case, as when he claims that in Montpellier clinical instruction was 'well under way ... long before the Revolution'; see Keel, 'The politics of health and the institutionalisation of clinical practices in Europe in the second half of the eighteenth century', in *William Hunter and the eighteenth-century medical world*, ed. W.F. Bynum and Roy Porter (Cambridge: Cambridge University Press, 1985), 207–56, at 272; idem, *L'avènement de la médecine clinique moderne en Europe, 1750–1815: Politiques, institutions et savoirs* (Montréal: Les presses de l'Université de Montréal, 2001), 47.

24 The Basel native Felix Platter sent news to his father of the opening of the amphitheatre in January 1556; see *Félix et Thomas Platter à Montpellier, 1552–1559 – 1595–1599* (Montpellier: Camille Coulet, 1892), 126–8.

hands of a 'royal demonstrator', a position made official in 1595. For well over a century (1604–1726), the post was occupied by various members of the leading surgical clan of Montpellier – the Gariel-Haguenot-Nissolle family.[25] The three men who held this post between 1726 and the Revolution were all, at some phase of their careers, professors at the Collège royal de chirurgie founded in Montpellier in 1741 (one of them was the renowned lithotomist Thomas Goulard). If, then, as historians generally believe, appointment to the new colleges of surgery is a reliable index of knowledge and skill, these men who served as *démonstrateurs* at the University of Medicine and as professors at the College of Surgery were possessed of genuine expertise. No less a figure than Bordeu, whose own surgical skill belies the usual image of vitalist physicians as pure 'idea men', lauded Goulard's capacities as a pedagogue.[26]

Nonetheless, Montpellier students who sought to build expertise in dissection faced all the problems, especially difficulties in obtaining cadavers and inadequacies in dissecting facilities, that historians have long chronicled on this subject.[27] In eighteenth-century Montpellier the most important local hospitals – the Hôpital-Général, which as elsewhere housed all manner of social unfortunates as well as people suffering from physical ills, and the Hôpital Saint-Eloi, which was the town's 'elite' hospital in terms of funding and staffing – operated under a standing order to supply bodies to the medical school for use in dissection. But the faculty registers are filled with complaints about these institutions failing to meet their obligations in this regard.[28] Moreover, private instructors in dissection, like Bordeu, were obliged to purchase cadavers for use in their courses. This does not seem to have been difficult, but the practice was, so Bordeu complained, expensive.[29]

It is also worth pointing out, although to some extent even raising the question is anachronistic, that the training in dissection that was available in Montpellier entailed only in the rarest instances any kind of systematic practice of pathological

[25] Marie-André Haguenot, *Une famille de médecins à Montpellier (de 1605 à 1818)* (Montpellier: Firmin et Montane, 1900).

[26] The three anatomy demonstrators were Jean Soullier, who held the post from 1726 to 1749; Goulard, 1749–84; and Jean-Baptiste Laborie, 1784–92; Dulieu, *La médecine à Montpellier*, 3: 335–40; on the founding of the Collège de chirurgie, see idem, *La chirurgie à Montpellier de ses origines au début du XIXe siècle* (Avignon: Les presses universelles, 1975), 111–33, and François Granel, *Pages médico-historiques montpelliéraines* (Montpellier: Causse and Castelnau, 1964), 69–85; Bordeu's references to Goulard are in *Correspondance*, 1: 110, 135.

[27] Referring to his studies in Montpellier in the 1770s, J.-A.-C. Chaptal wrote that 'Les cadavres ne suffisent pas à Montpellier pour les besoins des amphithéâtres, et très souvent l'on est forcé de suspendre les cours jusqu'à ce que l'hospice puisse en délivrer'; J.-A.-C. Chaptal, *Mes souvenirs sur Napoléon* (Paris: Plon, 1893), 16.

[28] AFMM: S17, 2, 9; ADH, C526, extract, 'Registre des déliberations, Hôpital-Général'.

[29] For his 1745–46 course Bordeu used 13 cadavers, which cost him 26 *livres* each; Bordeu, *Correspondance*, 1: 105.

anatomy in which symptoms of the living were compared to the state of the body post-mortem. Indeed the only case in pre-Revolutionary Montpellier in which a skilled anatomist regularly had access to and knowledge of both the living patient and the corpse dates from the late seventeenth rather than the late eighteenth century, and involves the work of the celebrated anatomist of the nervous structures, Raymond Vieussens. As head physician (*médecin-en-chef*) at the Hôpital Saint-Eloi, Vieussens dissected hundreds of corpses, many of patients he had observed in the wards. Yet the example of Vieussens is isolated, and it is not clear even in his case how he managed to perform so many autopsies, given that hospital authorities regarded autopsy as the province of surgeons rather than physicians, a state of affairs mandated in regulations from 1704 onward. Post-mortems, they decreed, did not fall within the *métier* of the physician.[30]

It may be concluded overall, then, that while it was not impossible for students to obtain training in dissection that went beyond the formal experience of the standard anatomy course, neither was it easy. Hence the enthusiasm and crowding that Bordeu reported in respect of his private courses and the students' continuing complaints (surveyed below) that the anatomical instruction provided by the University of Medicine was inadequate.[31] Efforts made to provide students in Montpellier with bedside instruction were similarly vexed. From 1715, the University of Medicine had had a chair devoted to a 'service des pauvres', but it was not centred in one of the town's hospitals and it operated, at best, sporadically.[32] As in other medical centres, there was a prolonged conflict between hospital authorities and medical pedagogues over the presence of professors, students and clinical courses in the hospitals. By the eighteenth century medical professors in Montpellier did play a role in administration of the town's elite hospital, the Hôpital Saint-Eloi, and might then have been expected to promote clinical teaching within its walls. The professors' role in the hospital's governance, however, derived not from their capacity as members of the medical faculty but from other official positions that they concurrently held. Thus the long-time professor Henri Haguenot served on the Saint-Eloi governing board by virtue of a position he held as magistrate of the Cour des comptes, aides et finances.[33] Some professors did promote clinical

---

30 M.D. Grmek, 'Raymond Vieussens,' *Dictionary of scientific biography*, 16 vols, ed. C.C. Gillispie (New York: Scribner, 1970–80), 14: 25–26; Louis Dulieu, *Essai historique sur l'Hôpital Saint-Eloi de Montpellier (1183–1950)* (Montpellier: Charles Déhan, 1953), 49–50, 102, 104, 107; Bibliothèque de la Ville de Montpellier [hereafter BVM], Ms. 196, 'Extraits des archives hospitalières de Montpellier', 55–55r.

31 Bordeu, *Correspondance*, 1: 71–7, 104–5, 113. The importunate presence of students at autopsies may account for a new regulation promulgated in 1763 at the Hôpital Saint-Eloi that only physicians, surgeons and *garçons* employed by the house be admitted to dissections and that 'no strangers' be allowed; 'Extraits des archives hospitalières', 241r.

32 I survey the evidence in regard to its functioning in Williams, *Medical vitalism*, 62.

33 AFMM: S30.

instruction at St-Eloi, but not all, and indeed in the most concerted period of conflict over this issue Haguenot sided with the hospital board in resisting a strong medical presence in the institution. In any event, anecdotal evidence attests that medical students went into the town's hospitals before any formal provision was made for their doing so.[34] The first official arrangements for bedside instruction at Saint-Eloi were made in 1746, but the presence of students was hedged round with restrictions. Complaints from both professors and students about the inadequacy of bedside training mounted from the 1730s to the 1760s, when a determined effort was made by the medical faculty to regularise and extend such instruction by establishing a *salle* devoted specifically to medical instruction by a faculty member. At this point the hospital administrators turned to the crown for support against such an infringement of their traditional prerogatives, and the crown came down solidly on the side of the hospital.[35] After this contest came to a head in 1768, the medical faculty did not again make a strong effort to formalise instruction in the hospital. Reform plans continued to be developed, including one focused on the small, exclusively military hospital housed in the Citadel, but these plans came to nought.[36] Thus, far from constituting what Keel sees as a model case of long-functioning clinical instruction, Montpellier shows some success in meeting this goal but overall indicates the power of tradition, both in ways of thinking about the appropriateness and utility of clinical instruction and in institutional arrangements effected to pursue this goal.

A different gauge of quality, one that was much remarked upon in the eighteenth century, was the character of the examinations that students had to undergo, and in this respect Montpellier's reputation was formidable. While the examinations at some of the other faculties were perfunctory, or even nonexistent, Montpellier subjected students to what was, in principle at least, a rigorous round of examinations. As established in the university statutes, these exams included, in progression from the *baccalauréat* to the *licence* to the *doctorat*: a four-hour written exam; a thesis, ordinarily published; twelve public lessons, including three anatomical demonstrations spread across three months and attended by two professors; and the examinations called *per intentionem*, which consisted of responses to four questions put by four different professors on four different maladies. After an eight-day interval came the so-called *triduanes*, examinations administered for three hours in the morning and three in the afternoon, at each stage of which the student had to receive a vote of two-thirds of the examining professors; and, after another interval of eight days, a general examination (the *points rigoureux*) that began with an aphorism drawn from Hippocrates.[37] It is difficult to say whether

34 Bordeu stated in a letter of 27 December 1745 that he visited the sick regularly in the town's hospitals; Bordeu, *Correspondance*, 1: 92–3.

35 AFMM: S16, 160–65; 'Extraits des archives hospitalières', 304r–316r; see also Dulieu, *La médecine à Montpellier*, 3: 325–32.

36 ADH: C525.

37 AFMM, S15, Statutes of 1732; S16, 103–8, Statutes of 1766.

these examinations were ordinarily conducted at a high level, with seriousness and due attention to the regulations laid down in the statutes. As with the regularity of lectures given by professors, complaints were made about abuses in respect to examinations, but overall these do not seem to have been common. What is certain, unsurprisingly, is that there was considerable variation within this formal structure – in the length and timing of the examinations, in the number of professors who were in attendance, in the granting of exemptions to individual students, in the authorship and publication of student theses, and so on.[38]

Although overall this formal examination structure changed little between the Renaissance and the Revolution, two shifts involving issues of practical training and contact with patients merit attention. Both have to do with changes occurring during the seventeenth and eighteenth centuries that seem to belie, or at least complicate, the general impression conveyed in the literature of a linear movement away from theoretical and towards more practical training in this period. One is that in the seventeenth century Montpellier students were required, before becoming eligible for the *licence*, to arrange for a '*stage pratique*', a six-months period of work undertaken in company with a local physician.[39] This requirement does not appear in the eighteenth-century statutes and, although the evidence is uncertain, it seems that this way of assuring practical training by a kind of apprenticeship gave way fairly early in the eighteenth century to the idea that clinical training should be regularised within the institution itself (this was at least part of the thinking, along with a charitable impulse, for creation of the chair devoted to the *service des pauvres* in 1715). Another change was the elimination of the requirement, again found in the seventeenth-century statutes, that the *per intentionem* examinations conclude with the presentation of a sick person to the candidate, who would then render a diagnosis and propose a therapeutic response.[40] This requirement also disappeared from the eighteenth-century statutes, and there is no evidence that actual sick people figured in these examinations. Given the paucity of evidence on these points, it is hard to draw firm conclusions about their significance, but it seems at the least that we should be sceptical about reconstructions that suggest an uninterrupted progression from a strictly didactic and theoretical view of training to the ever more practical.

Another shift worthy of note is the change in the examination system that came in 1734 in Montpellier when students were given the option of undergoing examination in surgery as well as in medicine. This was the beginning of the mixed medical-surgical degree that was one of Montpellier's most important innovations.

---

38 On abuses, see J.-E. Gilibert, *L'anarchie médicinale ou la médecine considérée comme nuisible à la société*, 3 vols (Neuchatel, 1772), 1: 39–42; descriptions of the exam structure given in the following sources differ in some particulars: Dulieu, *La médecine à Montpellier*, 3: 96–97; Bordeu, *Correspondance*, 1: 31; Gaston Castaigna, *Etude sur Bordeu* (Thèse de la Faculté de Médecine de Montpellier, 1878), 78–9.

39 Germain, *L'Ecole de médecine*, 45.

40 Statutes of 1634, in ibid., 49.

The availability of this degree was probably one factor that made Montpellier increasingly attractive to students as the eighteenth century wore on. Certainly the numbers of graduates taking the degree, some 600 in the last three decades of the *ancien régime*, attest to its appeal.[41] Nonetheless the fact is that we know very little about these graduates, and indeed about the teaching of surgery generally in Montpellier, despite the existence of histories that provide a good deal of formal institutional detail.[42]

One final point to be made in respect of facilities in Montpellier concerns those of an institution that was of great importance to physicians but not part of the medical faculty. This was the Société royale des sciences de Montpellier, founded in 1706; in the eighteenth century over half of its members were medical people. Although it did not live up to its early promise to function as an important publisher of scientific papers, the society did serve as a major venue for discussion and it did confer prestige on Montpellier, since it was the only provincial society to enjoy formal parity with the Académie des Sciences in Paris and to confer automatic entree to the Academy's sessions for its members. The Society filled a number of functions in the learned world of Montpellier and was of benefit to both aspiring and established physicians in diverse ways. The chair holder, G.-F. Venel, took advantage of the forum provided by the Society to publicise his research into medical, industrial and agricultural applications of the science chemistry, in which he specialised but which he was not allowed to teach at the University of Medicine. In the 1770s the Society sponsored the creation of a private chemistry laboratory and the teaching of a private chemistry course by J.-A.-C. Chaptal. In the same decade Philippe Pinel delivered his first scientific papers before the society; one of these led to a major publication of 1803.[43]

---

[41] Toby Gelfand, *Professionalizing modern medicine: Paris surgeons and medical science and institutions in the 18th century* (Westport, CN: Greenwood Press, 1980), 153; Louis Dulieu, 'Pierre Chirac, sa vie, ses écrits, ses idées,' *Montpellier médical* 3rd ser., 51 (1957): 775–6.

[42] Dulieu, *La chirurgie à Montpellier*.

[43] Elizabeth Randall Kindleberger, 'The Société royale des sciences de Montpellier, 1706 to 1793', PhD dissertation, Johns Hopkins University, 1979; the society's publishing ventures are discussed in Williams, *Medical vitalism*, 29–31; Venel's activities within the society are traced in 'Eloge de M. Venel', *Assemblée publique de la Société royale des sciences de Montpellier, 2 Mars 1776* (Montpellier: J. Martel, 1776), 69–86; Chaptal's laboratory and course are discussed in Chaptal, *Mes souvenirs sur Napoléon*, 25–32; on Pinel, see Dora B. Weiner, *Comprendre et soigner, Philippe Pinel (1745–1826): La médecine de l'esprit* (Paris: Fayard, 1999), 47–8, 386.

The Quality of Montpellier Medical Teaching and Its Appeal to Students

Having described at least some of the basics of medical education in Montpellier, I turn now to the questions of its quality and appeal. As noted earlier, by around 1600 the percentage of students coming to Montpellier from abroad had dropped to under 14, thanks, it would seem, to the prolonged religious strife that ended only with the siege of the town by the forces of Louis XIII in 1622.[44] Even after the siege and the defeat of the Protestant municipal authorities, however, Montpellier continued for some time to be known as a Protestant centre and to draw students from Britain, Holland, Switzerland and Germany.[45] The Revocation of the Edict of Nantes in 1685 brought an end to this phase of Montpellier's history; once Protestants were legally barred from teaching, Protestant students largely ceased coming to Montpellier, though there were important exceptions such as Tissot, and the occasional medical student from England who came to Montpellier in the company of English tourists who favoured Montpellier in the late seventeenth and early eighteenth centuries.[46] To conclude on the confessional theme: by the eighteenth century the foreign students who did come were once again natives of Catholic lands, including a steady if small contingent from Ireland who were barred, as Catholics, from studying in British medical centres. It is a notable fact that the only foreign-born professor on the eighteenth-century Montpellier faculty, Gérard Fitzgerald, was a native of Ireland.[47]

Along with these confessional shifts, then, the other dramatic trend that set in from the mid- to late sixteenth century was the overall decrease in the numbers

---

44 On foreign students in Montpellier, see, in addition to the sources cited in n. 5, Dominique Julia and Jacques Revel, eds, *Les universités européennes du XVIe au XVIIIe siècle: Histoire sociale des populations étudiantes*, Vol. 2, France (Paris: Editions de l'Ecole des Hautes Etudes en Sciences Sociales, 1989), 328. The percentage of foreign students for the last decade of the sixteenth century given in this source, 10.5 per cent, differs from the 13.7 per cent cited in Chartier, *L'éducation en France*, because Julia and Revel used French boundaries of the 1790s rather than the 1590s in calculating the number of 'foreign' students in the latter decade; see, on this point, Dominique Julia, 'L'Université de Médecine de Montpellier à l'époque moderne', *L'Université de Montpellier, ses maîtres et ses étudiants depuis sept siècles, 1289–1989: Actes du 61e Congrès de la Fédération historique du Languedoc Méditerranéen et du Roussillon, Colloque historique tenu à la Faculté de Médecine de Montpellier les 23 et 24 octobre 1989* (Montpellier, 1995).

45 One event exemplary of the spirit of the Montpellier medical community in this period was the extended visit that John Locke made to the region in the 1670s; see *Locke's travels in France, 1675–1679, as related in his journals, correspondence and other papers* (Cambridge: Cambridge University Press, 1953).

46 Emch-Dériaz, *Tissot* (cited in n. 2); Constantia Maxwell, *The English traveller in France, 1698–1815* (London: G. Routledge, 1932).

47 'Gérard Fitzgerald', *Dictionnaire de biographie française*, 13 vols, ed. J. Balteau et al. (Paris: Letouzey et Ané, 1933–), 13: 1415; Liam Swords, ed. *The Irish–French connection, 1758–1978* (Paris: The Irish College, 1978).

of students coming to Montpellier from abroad. By the end of the eighteenth century the percentage of foreign students enrolled in Montpellier was very low – around 6 per cent.[48] Aside from religious strife, why exactly why this happened is not known: certainly other factors were at work than the local circumstances in Montpellier itself, especially the proliferation of new medical centres elsewhere in Europe and the decline of the whole tradition of student peregrination that came with greater use of the vernacular, the increased incidence and greater danger of warfare, emergent national loyalties and other factors.[49]

Finally, it is essential to point out that this drop in the number of students coming from abroad to Montpellier is the precise reverse of what was happening *inside* France. In the eighteenth century French medical students came to Montpellier in ever greater numbers, and by 1789 Montpellier had long had the greatest number of graduates of any of the French medical faculties.[50] This raises the question of why they came, and here four factors seem to be of special significance. One is Montpellier's continuing reputation as a centre of serious instruction. Another factor is cost: graduates of Montpellier paid a fraction of the cost of instruction and charges incurred by those who took degrees from the Paris Faculty. Also significant was the pull of family networks: in this respect growth was self-reinforcing, since the more students came, the more their kinsmen tended to follow.[51] Finally, a factor that might seem frivolous but that must have been important to some students was the round of pleasures available in the town. Colin Jones has documented the presence of Montpellier students in the taverns, gambling dens, brothels and other pleasure sites of Montpellier. Already in the 1660s Montpellier had this reputation; the son of the famed English physician Thomas Browne wrote to his father in October 1664 that 'this place is the most delightfull of all France, being seated upon an hill in sight of the sea; inhabited by a people ... the most handsome in the world'.[52]

---

48 Julia and Revel, *Les universités européennes*, 2: 328.

49 On the impact of the Thirty Years' War, see J.T. Hughes, 'The medical education of Sir Thomas Browne, a seventeenth-century student at Montpellier, Padua, and Leiden', *Journal of Medical Biography* 9 (2001): 70–76. In 1790 a response by the medical faculty at Perpignan to plans for centralisation of medical instruction in the capital stated directly that students were not willing to travel far to study medicine and would, instead, accept whatever was locally available; Académie nationale de médecine, Archives de la Société royale de médecine, 115–13, 'Mémoire de la Faculté de Médecine de Perpignan en réponse à la demande du Comité de Salubrité créé par decret de l'Assemblée Nationale le 12 7bre 1790'.

50 Julia, 'L'Université de Médecine de Montpellier', 87–9.

51 Evidence on costs is surveyed in Matthew Ramsey, *Professional and popular medicine in France, 1770–1830: The social world of medical practice* (Cambridge: Cambridge University Press, 1988), 51; on family networks, see Julia, 'L'Université de Médecine de Montpellier', 102–3.

52 Colin Jones, 'Montpellier medical students and the medicalisation of eighteenth-century France', in *Problems and methods in the history of medicine*, ed. Roy Porter and

So what, then, did the students who came to Montpellier think of the institution? Asking students about quality has become an entrenched method of evaluating instruction in our own universities, and historians have long tried to use student responses – found in memoirs, correspondence, or as stray comments in other kinds of publication – as a gauge of 'what really went on'. There are problems, of course, in using such documents to form a picture of the quality of medical education. First among these is the fact that the number of records is so small. Thousands of students moved through the medical school of Montpellier in the eighteenth century, and of those only a handful left first-hand accounts of their experience. Then there is the fact that the testimonials we have generally come from great and brilliant figures whose perceptions probably do not tell us much about preparation for success – however this may be gauged – in the ordinary medical practice or career of the time. These provisos made, however, it remains true that direct observations made by students provide some of the most interesting evidence available about medical instruction in the past, and the historical record of Montpellier is no exception.

Notable physicians who left comments on their training in Montpellier include Bordeu and Tissot, whose comments I cited at the outset, as well as J.-E. Gilibert in the 1730s; Pierre-Joseph Amoreux in the 1760s; Guillaume-François Laennec, Philippe Pinel and J.-A.-C. Chaptal, all in the 1770s; and Joseph Dulaurens and Pierre Roussel in the 1780s. The assessments of these figures are mixed. Of all of them, Tissot was perhaps the harshest, denouncing in a letter he wrote to J.G. Zimmermann in 1757 the 'ignorant and mercenary professors' of Montpellier and exempting from this judgement only Boissier de Sauvages, with whom he formed a lasting association.[53] Another more or less blanket condemnation of the instruction offered at Montpellier came from Dulaurens, who said of his time there: 'I did as the others; I copied much, I read much, I listened much, and, as the others, I profited little.'[54] Other student recollections included good points as well as bad. Pinel, for example, expressed great appreciation for the totality of his experience in Montpellier, while nonetheless indicating early on his desire to move to the capital, with its greater opportunities. Similarly, Chaptal had much good to say of Montpellier, though he lamented the fact that the professors there did not, in many cases, teach their best subjects.[55] Some testimonials are unequivocally positive: the famed theoretician of women's nature and ills Pierre

---

Andrew Wear (London: Croom Helm, 1987), 57–80; the quotation from Browne is cited in Hughes, 'Medical education', 72.

[53] Emch-Dériaz, *Tissot*, cited in n. 1.

[54] Joseph Dulaurens, *Essai sur les établissemens nécessaires et les moins dispendieux, pour rendre le service des malades dans les hôpitaux vraiment utile à l'humanité* (Paris: Royez, 1787), translated and cited in Gelfand, *Professionalizing modern medicine*, 140.

[55] On Pinel, see Pierre Chabbert, 'Les années d'étude de Philippe Pinel: Lavaur, Toulouse, Montpellier', *Monspeliensis Hippocrates* (Spring 1960), 15–21; Jan Goldstein, *Console and classify: The French psychiatric profession in the nineteenth century*

Roussel, for example, lauded the 'brilliance' of Montpellier's teachers, naming specifically the celebrated vitalist theoretician Paul-Joseph Barthez.[56] Roussel's testimony raises yet another problem in respect of anecdotal evidence of this kind: as a graduate of Montpellier and a member of what was increasingly known by the late eighteenth century as the 'Ecole de Montpellier' – a coterie of like-minded physicians promoting medical vitalism – he had a vested interest in describing the school in glowing terms. More generally, from at least the 1780s, we confront in student testimonials the effort Montpelliérains made to establish the distinctiveness and high reputation of their school in the face of intensifying centralisation, a process that eventually led to Montpellier's permanent relegation to a secondary position vis-a-vis Paris.[57]

The record of student responses to what they were offered in Montpellier is not limited to direct testimonials about quality. The archival record of the University of Medicine includes numerous student petitions and complaints, and student productions – theses, broadsides and placards – also give indications of their thinking. Most student petitions and complaints dealt with practical problems such as costs and scheduling, or with student prerogatives such as their claimed right to have a representative at faculty meetings, but some did speak seriously to fundamentals of pedagogy and training, including professorial absenteeism, the prevalence of private courses, the inadequacy of anatomical instruction and bedside training, and so on. Despite the difficulties involved in interpreting such complaints – did they express generally held student sentiments or just the views of a cantankerous few? – some patterns seem clear. Among these is the overall sense that the 'practical' training offered in Montpellier was inadequate.[58]

This survey of student assessments of Montpellier returns my discussion to the tendency in much of the literature on medical education to take the availability of 'practical training' as the best measure of a school's standing and accomplishment. Overall it is hard to quarrel with this approach – certainly the schools, in France and elsewhere, that continued to offer nothing but didactic lectures to students, as a number did, could not participate in the general forward

(Cambridge: Cambridge University Press, 1987), 67; Chaptal, *Mes souvenirs sur Napoléon*, 15–16; on Amoreux's assessment, see Brockliss and Jones, *Medical world*, 513.

[56] Pierre Roussel, review of Paul-Joseph Barthez, *Nouvelle méchanique des mouvements de l'homme et des animaux* (Carcassonne, 1798), in *La clef du cabinet des souverains*, 706 (6 nivôse, an VII): 6049–52, at 6049.

[57] Williams, *Medical vitalism*, 287–320.

[58] A petition signed by 58 students in 1762 called for a decrease in the material covered in courses other than physiology and pathology; fixed hours for registration; measures to prevent disruptions caused by surgical students at anatomical and botanical lessons; hospital-based instruction by the professor charged with the 'service des pauvres'; suppression of a circular to parents complaining of student behaviour; and re-establishment of the position of student *conseiller*; see AFMM, C63; other petitions from the 1760s and 1770s appear in AFMM: C61, 65, 72, 73, 76 and 100.

movement of medical science.[59] On the other hand, it seems advisable that in making such judgements we avoid embracing a whiggishness or 'presentism' that has been strongly challenged in other byways of cultural history. In particular it is important not to focus overmuch on methods that only much later, in the late nineteenth and early twentieth centuries, came to constitute the shared ideal of medical education. The vitalist medicine with which Montpellier came to be identified in the late eighteenth and early nineteenth centuries and whose influence was great, both in and outside France, depended in good part on the high development of a particular kind of discursive practice, one that linked medicine in a myriad of ways to the great intellectual and ideological struggles of the Enlightenment and the 'medical revolution'. The cultural authority that Montpellier vitalists wielded is perhaps best indicated by the dominant role they assumed in constructing the medical teachings purveyed by Diderot's *Encyclopédie*. Making use of that redoubtable forum, Montpelliérains asserted unique insight on such matters as the contest between Ancients and Moderns (Bordeu's famous article on 'crisis'), the applicability of the new chemistry to industry and agriculture (the 700-some entries of the University of Medicine chair holder Venel), and the indispensability of medical guidance in sexual and familial life (Joseph-Jacques Ménuret's many offerings on impotence, masturbation, marriage and related themes).[60] In so doing Montpellier physicians adopted strategies of 'practical' engagement – redefining the persona of the medical author, extending the venues of medical publication – that depended on strengths developed not only in the clinics and dissecting rooms for which students clamoured but also in the analytical, verbal, 'theoretical' instruction so assiduously cultivated in the traditional classroom setting. Adopting such a viewpoint on medical education does not discount the role of the 'practical' but, rather, insists on the interconnection of skills required for success in the eighteenth-century medical world. The earliest and arguably most brilliant of Montpellier's vitalist theoreticians, Bordeu, achieved his first celebrity with a work, his famed book on the glands, that rested both on anatomical expertise and on great analytical and rhetorical skill – his capacity to relate anatomical findings to a vexed problem of physiological 'theory' and to write persuasively about his proffered solution. Bordeu's case, of many that could be cited, should perhaps serve to remind us that just as the most insightful reformers of early modern medical education sought to blend the best of the old didactic pedagogy

---

[59] On instruction offered in the smaller French faculties of medicine, see Ramsey, *Professional and popular medicine*, 39–42, 49–50, 51; Julia, 'L'Université de Médecine,' 81, 88–90; Brockliss and Jones, *Medical world*, 499–516.

[60] On the Montpellier vitalists as Encyclopaedists, see Williams, *Medical vitalism*, 120–24, 147–84; an especially rich treatment of Ménuret's contributions to the *Encyclopédie* is offered in Roselyne Rey, *Naissance et développement du vitalisme en France de la deuxième moitié du 18e siècle à la fin du Premier Empire* (Oxford: Voltaire Foundation, 2000), 73, 154, 194, 258–69.

and the new clinical instruction, we too, in assessing their efforts, should not exaggerate the distinction to be drawn between skills of mind and hand, of the 'theoretical' and the 'practical'.

Chapter 11
Herman Boerhaave at Leiden: *Communis Europae praeceptor*

Rina Knoeff

It is a well-known fact that the Leiden medical faculty was *the* early eighteenth-century centre of medical excellence, attracting students from all over Europe. At the same time, however, it is hard to put a finger on what exactly made the Leiden medical faculty so very popular. The story usually told has it that Leiden was attractive due to its hands-on bedside teaching. And the famous medical teacher Herman Boerhaave (1668–1738) is generally considered the *spiritus rector* of a great increase in quality.

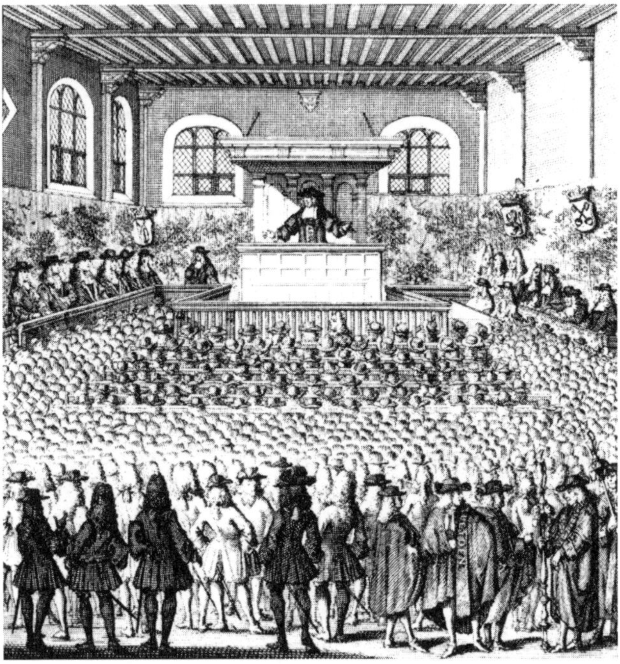

Fig.11.1 Frontispiece to Boerhaave's *Sermo academicus de comparando certo in physicis* (Leiden, 1715). Note the uncountable number of people hanging on Boerhaave's every word, thereby indicating his enormous popularity.

This narrative, however, smacks of a whiggish tendency to turn Boerhaave into a kind of scientific hero (even though he did not have any famous inventions or discoveries to his name).[1] Without denying that Boerhaave's teaching was very popular, I shall argue that this was primarily so because Boerhaave simply was *the right man in the right place*. The town of Leiden was attractive – it had excellent facilities for extracurricular activities such as theatre visits, pub crawls, horse riding and boating. Unlike most other universities, the University of Leiden welcomed students of all religious affiliations and it was praised for its 'great liberty, the freedom of thinking, speaking and believing'.[2] The medical curriculum, moreover, was significantly shorter than in other places. This more than compensated for Leiden's high living costs and made it an attractive place for poorer students. Boerhaave's teaching programme was anti-authoritarian, directed at teaching independence in practising medicine. His amiable character and manner of teaching, finally, made it a real privilege for students to attend his lectures.

This paper consists of two parts. It first takes a closer look at Boerhaave's partly unfounded reputation as an excellent clinical teacher. This reputation is traced to a nineteenth-century historiographic error that overestimated the value of bedside teaching for Boerhaave's eighteenth-century curriculum. It has no grounding in Boerhaave's own reflections, nor in the extensive notes of the students nor in the Leiden hospital records. The second part of the paper starts with Albrecht von Haller's description of Boerhaave as the *Communis Europae praeceptor*, the *teacher* of all of Europe.[3] It argues that Boerhaave's medical teaching was unique in its approach. Unlike other medical teachers, he stimulated his students to think, observe and experiment themselves, rather than to apply ready-made and generally accepted courses of action. I argue that precisely this aspect made Boerhaave's teaching attractive to students from all over Europe.

---

[1] Historians of medicine have already cast doubt on the hero-story. See, for instance: Charles Daremberg, *Histoire des sciences médicinales* (Paris, 1870), vol. 2, p. 890; Maarten Ultee, 'The politics of professional appointment at Leiden, 1709', *Journal for the History of Medicine and Allied Sciences* 9 (1990) 167–94; Harold Cook, 'Boerhaave and the flight from reason in medicine', *Bulletin for the History of Medicine* 74 (2000) 221–40.

[2] G.D.J. Schotel, *De Academie te Leiden in de 16e, 17e en 18e Eeuw* (Haarlem, 1875), p. 272.

[3] Albrecht von Haller, *Bibliotheca anatomica*, (Zurich, 1774–76), vol. 1, p. 756. Von Haller's description has become widely known and has been a model for many later publications recounting the attraction of Leiden for foreign students. See for instance R.W. Innes Smith, *English speaking students of medicine at the University of Leyden* (Edinburgh, 1932); E. Ashworth Underwood, *Boerhaave's men at Leyden and after* (Edinburgh, 1977); Gerrit A. Lindeboom, *Herman Boerhaave. The man and his work* (London, 1968), pp. 355–75; Gerrit A. Lindeboom, *Boerhaave and Great Britain* (Leiden, 1974).

Boerhaave's Bedside Teaching

Although historians of medicine have often claimed that bedside teaching in Leiden flourished under Boerhaave's inspiring leadership and that students were particularly attracted to his clinical instruction, which served as a model for the establishment of teaching hospitals all over Europe, the beds in the *Caecilia* hospital assigned to the *collegium medico-practicum* were empty most of the time (Figure 11.2).[4] Indeed, Boerhaave certainly advised patients medically in his extended private correspondence, but it is obvious that these paper patients had little to do with clinical instruction. It is doubtful whether students often *observed* Boerhaave treating patients.

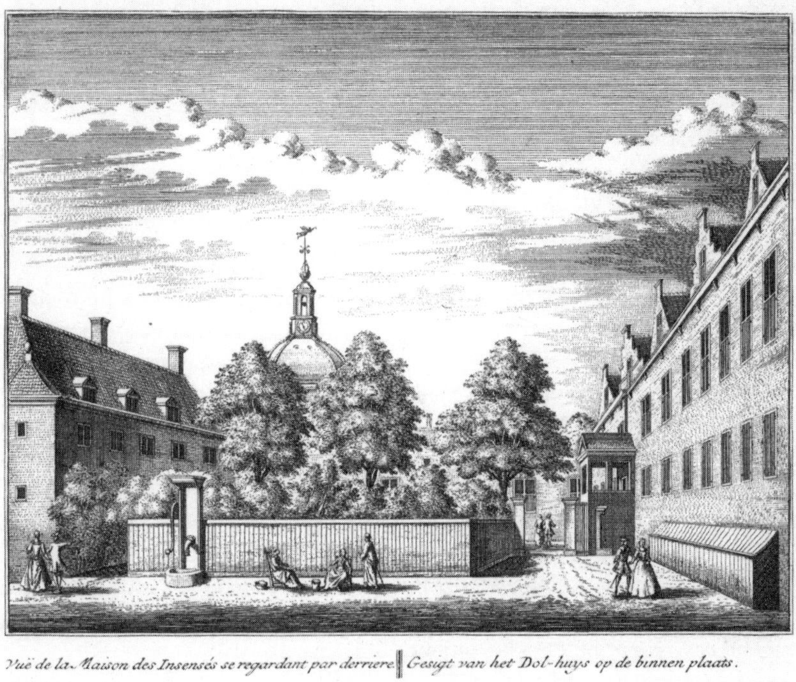
Vuë de la Maison des Insensés se regardant par derriere
Gesigt van het Dol-huys op de binnen plaats.
72

Fig. 11.2 The inner court of the Leiden Caecilia hospital. Engraved by A. Rademaker in 1732.

4 For accounts praising Boerhaave's clinical efforts see, for instance: Lindeboom, *Herman Boerhaave*, pp. 283–97; Günther B. Risse, 'Clinical instruction in hospitals: The Boerhaavian tradition in Leyden, Edinburgh, Vienna and Pavia', *Clinical Teaching Past and Present. Clio Medica* 21 (1987–88): 1–19.

In the period between 1711 and 1737, during Boerhaave's most successful years, there was a serious *decline* in the number of patients admitted to the hospital. Between 1721 and 1736 only three patients were admitted on average each year, and from 1732 to 1736 no patients were admitted at all! Presumably this has to do with Boerhaave's illnesses in 1731 and 1735, but the numbers nevertheless show that he cannot have been very active in the hospital. In 1737, one year before Boerhaave's death, the number of patients picked up again. Boerhaave started a lecture course on clinical practice, accompanied by visits to the hospital. He lectured on nervous diseases. Over the year 25 patients were admitted to the hospital. In February 1738, half a year before his death, Boerhaave wrote to his friend Bassand:

> … they [two physicians sent by the Duke of Tuscany to be educated by Boerhaave] were both able to accompany me on my rounds throughout the entire five months that I have been treating the patients in the hospital. They have, accordingly, not only followed my theoretical lessons, but they have also seen how I put teachings into practice.[5]

It is likely that the reputation of Boerhaave as a clinical teacher stems from this last year, not least because Gerard van Swieten meticulously noted down Boerhaave's lessons and published them later on.[6]

In spite of Boerhaave's absence from the hospital, he still has the reputation of a conscientious physician who would ride to the hospital every day to care for his patients. This narrative, however, is a nineteenth-century invention. It is partly based on Albert Schultens' exalted praises in his funeral oration of 1738 (the *Oratio academica: In memoriam Hermanni Boerhaavii*), and is furthermore derived from a series of articles on the early modern Leiden medical faculty written by the anatomist Bernard Suringar (1802–74). Suringar turned the medical faculty of Leiden University – as well as Herman Boerhaave – into a centre of excellence. More than Schultens ever did, Suringar emphasised Boerhaave's *practical* medical teaching, an interpretation that was followed by most medical historians up to the 1960s. Suringar's interpretation, however, reflects a nineteenth-century concern about the teaching of practical medicine.

---

[5] Boerhaave to Bassand, 21 February 1738, in Gerrit A. Lindeboom, *Boerhaave's correspondence* (Leiden, 1964), vol. 2, p. 365.

[6] The information on the hospital admissions is derived from Harm Beukers, 'Clinical teaching in Leiden from its beginning until the end of the eighteenth century', *Clinical Teaching Past and Present. Clio Medica* 21 (1987–88): 139–52. See also Rozemarijn Ramakers, 'Het Caecilia Gasthuis te Leiden. Onderwijsinsituut en Verpleeginrichting 1636–1799', MA thesis (Leiden 1989). For van Swieten's notes on Boerhaave's lectures see: B.P.M. Schulte, *Hermanni Boerhaave praelectiones de morbis nervorum 1730–1735. Een Medisch Historische Studie van Boerhaave's Manuscript over Zenuwziekten* (Leiden, 1959).

All his life Suringar was passionate about clinical teaching: he trained at the Hôtel Dieu in Paris and at the Charité in Berlin, after which he taught at the Amsterdam Clinical School and Leiden University. Most notably, he changed the emphasis of medical teaching at the Amsterdam Athenaeum, as well as at the Leiden medical faculty, towards practical medicine and bedside teaching.[7] Suringar's medical historical papers, published in the *Nederlands Tijdschrift voor Geneeskunde* [*Dutch Journal for Medicine*] between 1862 and 1870, not only reflect his personal interest in bedside teaching, but also respond to general concern about the union of medical theory and clinical practice. In 1865 an Act was passed in Parliament by which the classification of medical jobs was abolished and only doctors licensed by a state committee for medicine were to be allowed to practise. All medical students had to pass two exams: one in physic (medical theory) and one in practical medicine. It was, furthermore, considered irrelevant whether the candidate was originally trained at university or at a clinical school.[8] Unsurprisingly, the Act caused great unrest in the oldest Dutch medical faculty, with its long tradition in medical teaching. The supposed 'devaluation' of its medical curriculum to the level of what was formerly done by surgeons, apothecaries and midwives seriously threatened Leiden's status as a 'centre of excellence'.

Suringar's history of Leiden medicine was geared to the problems of his time. The modern emphasis on practical medicine, he argued, was by no means an innovation – in Leiden it had always been there. Suringar assured his readers that there was, in fact, no problem. The Leiden professors of medicine had practised bedside teaching all along. In line with the nineteenth-century ideal of medical teaching, Suringar invented an image of the Leiden medical faculty, from the seventeenth century onwards, in which theoretical medicine and bedside teaching always went hand in hand. He devoted much attention to the close connections between the supervisors of the Caecilia hospital and the Curators of the University, and in his descriptions of the Leiden professors of medicine he always judged them on their practical skills. In Suringar's descriptions the most successful professors were also the most skilled and popular practical medical teachers. And in his view it was the immensely successful Boerhaave who embodied the true unity of theoretical and practical medicine as he walked along the beds in the Caecilia hospital.[9] Suringar's story was adopted by Gerrit Arie Lindeboom, who, for a long time, was considered the Boerhaave scholar *par excellence*. His opinion that

---

7 For a biography of Bernard Suringar see: P.H. Suringar, 'Bijzonderheden betreffende het Leven van Dr. G.C.B. Suringar', *Nederlands Tijdschrift voor Geneeskunde* 10.2 (1874): 66–93.

8 Willem Otterspeer, Groepsportret met Dame III. De Werken van de Wetenschap. De Leidse Universiteit, 1776–1876 (Amsterdam, 2005), pp. 33–5.

9 Gerard Conrad Bernard Suringar, 'De Leidsche Geneeskundige Faculteit in het Begin der Achttiende Eeuw. Boerhaave en zijne Ambtgeuoten', *Nederlands Tijdschrift voor Geneeskunde* 2 (1866) 1–39.

'there is no doubt that Boerhaave was at his best at the bedside' became generally accepted among historians of medicine.[10]

Yet, Boerhaave's practical medicine had little to do with hospital and bedside teaching. Rather, it was directed at diagnosing some internal conditions and was followed by advice on diet, lifestyle and remedies. This could be done by letter just as well as at the bedside. Boerhaave hardly ever got his hands dirty – he always called in a surgeon if he needed to touch or cut into his patients. Even more, in letters to his friend Bassand, Boerhaave regularly complained about his tiresome medical practice. In May 1723 he wrote:

> … the expectations of both my patients and my pupils stand in the way of my wishes and pursue me everywhere, even when I flee. In the summer holidays I twice left my native town for a month in order to let it be known that *I wished to have nothing more to do with practising medicine.*[11]

Although patients kept knocking at his door and Boerhaave claimed never to have been more busy, he 'retired from the turbulence of medical practice' (i.e. he gave up doing rounds) in the same year.[12] Moreover, he wrote to his friend that he would not be able to provide one of Bassand's protégés with clinical experience.[13] In his letters Boerhaave mentions the hospital only once.

Indeed, Boerhaave's practical medicine had so little to do with medical practice that he was severely criticised by contemporaries and even by his pupils. His good friend Frederik Ruysch, for instance, could get very annoyed about Boerhaave's armchair medicine, which, in Ruysch's view, often had no grounding whatever in what could really be seen in bodies and body parts.[14] Boerhaave's lack of anatomical and physical knowledge was apparently so obvious that soon after he died a new medical system was called for. William Cullen, for instance wrote:

> When I First applied to the study of physic, I learned only the system of Boerhaave; and even when I came to take a Professor's chair in this university, I

[10] See Lindeboom, *Herman Boerhaave*, p. 291. Paradigmatic for this story is also J. Dankmeijer's oration entitled 'Is Boerhaave's fame justified', to which the answer, of course, was 'yes'. See: J. Dankmeijer, *Is Boerhaave's Faam Gerechtvaardigd?* (Leiden, 1968).

[11] Boerhaave to Bassand, 6 May 1723, in Lindeboom (ed.), *Boerhaave's correspondence* (Leiden, 1964), vol. 2, p. 199. My italics.

[12] Boerhaave to Bassand, 9 September 1726 and 7 November 1727, in Lindeboom, *Boerhaave's correspondence*, vol. 2, p. 239, 251.

[13] Boerhaave to Bassand, 23 January 1728, in Lindeboom, *Boerhaave's correspondence*, vol. 2, p. 253.

[14] I have looked at the relationship between Ruysch and Boerhaave before, in Rina Knoeff, 'Chemistry, mechanics and the making of anatomical knowledge. Boerhaave vs. Ruysch on the nature of the glands', *Ambix* 53 (2006): 201–19.

The eighteenth century was of great significance in medical education in Europe, described by Bonner, probably correctly, as 'a more critical watershed' than previously acknowledged.[2] There were differences among European countries, for example in Germany with its academic hospitals,[3] and France, which had the first nationwide scheme for clinical teaching.[4] Students were also becoming – or wished to become – more than mere spectators at the feet of the university teachers, desiring more practical, 'hands-on' training by the end of the century, at least. Edinburgh benefited from Scotland's historically strong European links and, like Leiden, Edinburgh's university, the Toun's College, was under the control of the Town Council, which freed it from any possibly damaging religious constraints.

The Edinburgh Medical School finally emerged as an entity, rather than an amorphous collection of individuals, in 1726, following the alleged 'flight' of Alexander Monro *primus* and his anatomy class into the protection of the university after accusations of grave-robbing the previous year, though it may also be argued that this was just part of longer-term strategies by the Town Council and other interested parties.[5] The Town Council had appointed three of the most prominent Edinburgh physicians (James Halket, Archibald Pitcairne and Robert Sibbald) as 'professors of medicine' in 1685, but they had no stipend or accommodation in the College, and there is no evidence that they did any systematic teaching at all. James Sutherland was appointed Professor of Botany in 1695 and took charge of the physic garden; the Town Council elected Robert Elliot as the first 'professor' of Anatomy in 1705; and James Crawford became Professor of Chemistry and Physic in 1713 (though his teaching was primarily of chemistry rather than medicine), so there was clearly a wish on the part of local political leaders to enhance the teaching of medical and scientific subjects in the town.[6] By 1720, and as a result of blatant political manoeuvring (typical of the time), the incumbent joint professors of Anatomy, Adam Drummond and John McGill (or M'Gill), demitted office and were succeeded by Alexander Monro *primus* (Figure 13.2). Monro moved to the

---

[2] Bonner, T.M., *Becoming a physician: medical education in Britain, France, Germany, and the United States, 1750–1945* (Baltimore, 2000), 6.

[3] See Lindemann, M., *Health and healing in eighteenth century Germany* (Baltimore, 1996).

[4] Gelfand, T., *Professionalizing modern medicine. Paris surgeons and medical science institutions in the eighteenth century* (London, 1980). See also Brockliss, L. and Jones, C., *The medical world of early modern France* (Oxford, 1997). For a masterly account of the evolution of medical hospitals, see Risse, G., *Mending bodies, saving souls. A history of hospitals* (New York, 1999).

[5] Accusations of grave-robbing for anatomical purposes were levelled against the surgeons in 1720 and again in 1724–25, which prompted the Incorporation of Surgeons to issue vehement denials and threaten its members with severe penalties if found guilty.

[6] Dingwall, H.M., *A famous and flourishing society: The history of the Royal College of Surgeons of Edinburgh 1505–2005* (Edinburgh, 2005), 55.

university in 1725 and delivered his inaugural lecture, entitled *De Origine et Utilitate Anatomiae* on 3 November.[7] In 1726 John Rutherford (grandfather of Sir Walter Scott) and Andrew Sinclair were established as professors of Theory and Practice of Medicine, while John Innes and Andrew Plummer became professors of Medicine and Chemistry. All four had studied at Leiden, thus establishing a clear 'Leiden link'. By 1726 the university was able to offer teaching in anatomy, surgery, chemistry, medicine, botany and midwifery, and the desire was expressed that this 'medical school' would have powers to 'examine candidates and do every other thing requisite and necessary to the graduation of doctors of medicine as amply and fully and with all the solemnities that the same is practised and done by the professors of medicine in any College or University whatsoever'.[8] The university had awarded a small number of MD degrees from 1705 (around 20 in total), but candidates had been examined externally by fellows of the Royal College of Physicians of Edinburgh, as the university had no examining powers of its own in this area. A key requirement for designation as a 'school' was the ability to award its own qualifications, and 1726 marked the completion of all the required elements. It is possible, therefore, to view 1726 as the culmination of a cumulative process as well as the start of a new phase in Scottish medical education. It has been claimed that Edinburgh was always careful of its 'particular',[9] and it would seem that this particular 'particular' was a crucial backdrop as well as stimulus.

Part of the important background context to all of this was the structure and functions of the university as a whole. Morrell's work, though a little dated, is still of value here.[10] He emphasises the non-collegiate nature of the university and its municipal origins and control, as well as its prominence in science, lack of religious barriers and the dominance of the moderate wing of the Church of Scotland.[11] These were all important facets in a complex social, political and intellectual situation, and perhaps the Town Council-dominated background was the key element, despite the importance of religion and the church in all aspects of life. The economic structure of the university meant that the livelihoods of the professors depended directly on student fees. Subjects which were necessary for graduation, or were taught by the more charismatic professors, quite naturally drew the largest numbers of students. The standard class fee remained at 3 guineas (£3 3s) for much of the eighteenth century and, with some classes attracting several

[7] *Dictionary of National Biography.*

[8] Harrison, J., *Oure tounis college. Sketches of the history of the Old College of Edinburgh* (Edinburgh, 1884), 95–6.

[9] Makey, W., 'Edinburgh in mid-seventeenth century', in *The early modern town in Scotland* (ed.) Lynch. M. (Edinburgh, 1987), 196.

[10] Morrell, J.B., 'The University of Edinburgh in the late eighteenth century: its scientific eminence and academic structure', *Isis* 62 (2) (1971), 158–71.

[11] Morrell cites the work of Hans, who analysed the careers of individuals who made a contribution to new science, showing that a significant proportion had studied at Edinburgh. Ibid., 158–9.

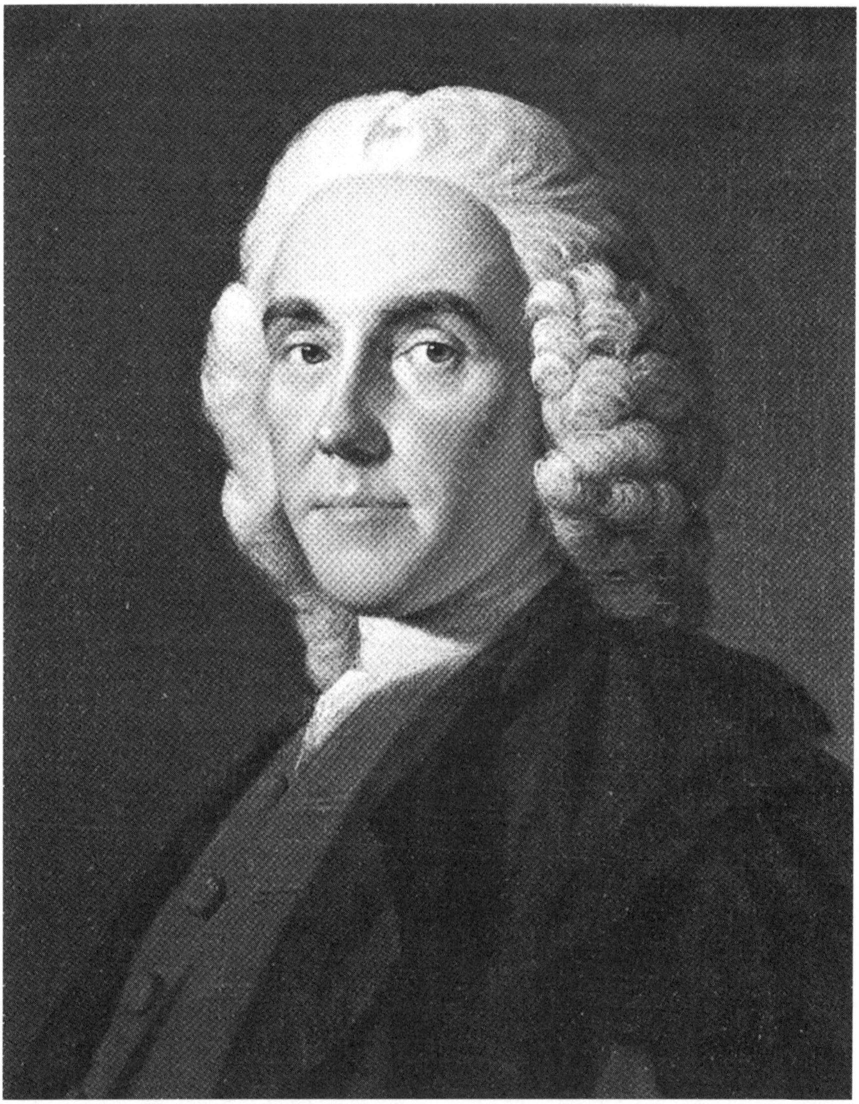

Fig. 13.2 Portrait of Alexander Monro ***primus*** – one of the key early figures in the Edinburgh Medical School

hundred students, an individual's income could be quite considerable. Of the 25 chairs in operation at the university by the end of the eighteenth century, 7 were in the faculty of medicine, some having been occupied by the so-called 'great doctors' of the Enlightenment era, such as William Cullen. Of considerable significance also was the concurrent burgeoning of Edinburgh's printing and publishing trades, which helped to service the growing requirements of the university and its students and enabled more local publication of medical books and articles, though many authors continued to publish in London or Europe during this time. The important factor was perhaps not where books were published, but that they were being produced by Edinburgh medical men both within and outside the walls of the university. One example, which illustrates both local publication and the aim of providing works for medical students which emphasised the practicalities as well as the philosophy of medicine is Cullen's *First lines of the practice of physic. For the use of the students in the University of Edinburgh*, published in Edinburgh in 1783.

The foundation and progress of the medical school were based, it seems, on a fortuitous and eclectic combination of circumstances. It has been claimed that the school owed its ethos to a desire for 'peace' after the upheavals of the union of the Scottish and English parliaments 1707, and that the eirenic philosophy of the school reflected this, though the timing of the various stages owed more, perhaps, to coincidence than to a conscious desire to channel Edinburgh's energies into more intellectual pursuits.[12] A longer-held but probably over-simplistic view has been that the school owed its existence almost entirely to the efforts of John Monro (surgeon and father of Alexander Monro *primus*) and the prominent Edinburgh politician George Drummond, who shared a vision for the intellectual progress of Edinburgh.[13] It may be more correct to assert that Monro's vision was perhaps less broad, his main desire being to boost the status of Edinburgh surgeons in general and of his son in particular.[14] These were influences, certainly, but what was perhaps equally important was the fact that after the union of 1707, and for most of the eighteenth century, Scottish politics was 'managed' on behalf of the Westminster government by a small band of elite Scots, notably the second and third dukes of Argyll (members of the prominent and ever-loyal clan Campbell, which had long exercised an opportunistic political support of the government), and Henry Dundas, who was not born an aristocrat but rose to political prominence through the legal profession (confirming the increasing acceptance of professions as part of elite society). The management of Scottish politics meant that the patronage which was necessary for the establishment of any institution at that time was channelled through a clear and fairly direct network.[15] As Emerson states, most of the university

---

12 Cunningham, A., 'Medicine to calm the mind: Boerhaave's medical system and why it was adopted in Edinburgh', in *The medical Enlightenment of the eighteenth century*, (eds) Cunningham, A. and French, R. (Cambridge, 1900), 40–66.

13 Chitnis, A.A., 'Provost Drummond and the origins of Edinburgh medicine', in *The origins and nature of the Scottish Enlightenment*, (eds) Campbell, R.H. and Skinner, A.S. (Edinburgh, 1982), 86–97.

14 Anderson, R.D., Lynch, M. and Phillipson, N., *The University of Edinburgh. An illustrated history* (Edinburgh, 2003).

15 For full account of this topic, see Shaw, J.S., *The political history of eighteenth century Scotland* (Basingstoke, 1999); Whatley, C.A., *Scottish society 1707–1830* (Manchester, 2000). More dated, but still useful, is Murdoch, A., *The people above. Politics and administration in eighteenth century Scotland* (Edinburgh, 1980).

hairs were, on the surface, in the gift of the Town Council, but the council itself had long relied on political patronage for survival[16]. This was no less the case in the middle of the Enlightenment century, and may even have been more important, given the changed political environment following the events of 1707.

However, despite any political influence, overt or covert, it does seem that in the Edinburgh Medical School what was taught and the ways in which it was taught were not dictated by political managers. Chairs may have been given to political allies but, however erudite or influential the politicians, the day-to-day teaching was carried out according to the philosophy and intents of the individual professors. Once appointed to a chair, the first priority of any incumbent was to earn a living, and this he had to do by attracting sufficient numbers of students to his classes to meet his costs and provide a modest profit on which to live. Economics were just as important as politics here, and if a political appointee could not deliver teaching in line with student expectations, political connections were of little value.

The medical school was in some ways curiously contradictory as well as uniquely flexible. There was a clear desire to show that students who did eventually graduate with an Edinburgh MD had followed a rigorous programme of required subjects, including at least one year spent in Edinburgh. That was the top of the pyramid, though. All other levels were catered for and, since medical graduates were a significant minority of medical students, this was – at least for the time being – to the advantage of all, economically as well as educationally.

The Students

Historians in the past have acknowledged the huge popularity of the Edinburgh Medical School and the ability of its professors to attract large numbers of students, from both home and abroad.[17] What has not been emphasised enough, perhaps, is the role of the students themselves as consumers with considerable powers, given that the professors' only source of remuneration for their teaching was the fees paid by the students. In simple terms, they must have 'got what they wanted', at least in the high days of the school in mid-century. Students were not obliged to take their courses in any order, nor were they required to spend their whole period of study in Edinburgh. Although graduation requirements were stipulated and enforced, there was as yet no full residence requirement. This gave considerable flexibility and allowed students to study according to individual circumstances and aims. Quite naturally, the 'required' classes were those which attracted the highest numbers of students, and this open choice would eventually help to bring about the relative decline in the reputation of the school, as the students sought more

---

[16] Emerson, R., 'The founding of the Edinburgh Medical School', *Journal of the History of Medicine and Allied Sciences* 59 (2) (2004), 183–218.

[17] Full account in Rosner, L., *Medical education in the age of Enlightenment* (Edinburgh, 1991)

'modern' teaching and greater participation in classes, often outside the walls of the university.

Students came from many places, including America, where significant links were forged. For example, 321 students came from the nine seaboard states of North America in the 25 years around the end of the eighteenth century, and during the last quarter of the century around 12 American students enrolled each year.[18] These included three generations of some families, many of whom were descendants of Scots emigrants. On their return to America they were often involved in setting up private medical training, and the influence of Edinburgh on the early American hospitals and medical schools is well documented.[19] Edinburgh also attracted students from Oxford and Cambridge who wished to find some practical clinical teaching to complement the theoretical approach of their home universities. Evidence from research on a number of American students coming to Edinburgh – many of whom expressed deep admiration for the teaching of William Cullen in particular – shows that they took an eclectic variety of courses and studied in Edinburgh for widely varying time periods. Some attended only one session, in order to partake of Cullen's chemistry course, while others, as in the case of one student from Barbados who subsequently practised in Charleston, South Carolina, took a full-blown and apparently carefully planned programme of study in what would seem to be the 'correct' order of courses. He, though, was in the minority.[20]

One of the main economic backbones of the school was the large cohort of 'occasional auditors', or students who enrolled for classes but did not intend to take the whole medical degree. From 1760 to 1826, no less than 64 per cent of medical students came into this category, and of these, 70 per cent attended for only one year.[21] This phenomenon has long been recognised, but one recent paper has confirmed that some of these individuals were able subsequently to pursue significant medical careers. One such was Abraham Sutcliff (1721–98), who was an occasional auditor during at least two academic sessions. He did not graduate but went on to have a successful career as an apothecary in Yorkshire. One of his apprentices, John Lettsom (1744–1815) would become an eminent London physician, who showed his esteem for his former master by purchasing him an MD degree from Aberdeen – a little ironic to say the least.[22] This does show, though,

[18] Entin, M.A., 'Edinburgh Medical College at the end of the eighteenth century and the training of North American doctors', *Proceedings of the Royal College of Physicians of Edinburgh* 28 (2) (1998), 219.

[19] Rosner, 'Thistle on the Delaware.'

[20] Bell, W.J., 'Some American students of "That Shining Oracle of Physic", Dr William Cullen of Edinburgh, 1755–1766', *Proceedings of the American Philosophical Society* 94 (3) (1950), 275–81.

[21] Rosner, *Medical education*, 105.

[22] Swan, H.T., 'Edinburgh medical students peculiarly described as "occasional auditors"', *Journal of Medical Biography* 13 (2005), 207–17. Lettsom had been born in the Virgin Islands, was sent to England to be educated, and practised subsequently in London,

that it was possible for non-graduates to build medical careers on the basis of their occasional auditing, thus helping to alter the view that occasional auditors were merely attending out of personal interest or as part of the general education of a gentleman of the Enlightenment. In other words, the particular form and ethos of the school allowed these individuals to follow more deviant paths to a medical career, but to careers nonetheless. This would of course come to an end in the aftermath of the entrance of big government and the effects of the Medical Act in 1858.

Lawrence has argued that the Edinburgh Medical School underwent significant changes during the course of the eighteenth century and that its life can be viewed in three main phases: in the early years what was on offer was a replicated European (Leiden) model; by the middle two decades of the century there were 'distinctive local elements' (such as midwifery) and by the mid-1760s there was an 'authentic' Scottish medical school.[23] In other words, Leiden's daughter had Dutch parents but produced Scottish offspring. The 'Scottishness' of Scottish medicine and medical education is difficult to define, and Lawrence's model may be a little too convenient, but certainly there is a case to be made for claiming a Scottish Enlightenment, as opposed to an Enlightenment in Scotland, and this was the background to medical change. This may be best related to the practical application of Enlightenment thought (in areas such as agriculture and chemistry), which seems to have been a particularly Scottish trait. However, these changes were not enough to sustain the dominance of the school in the longer term, and the 'Scottishness' would diminish by the early decades of the nineteenth century, when more 'British' influences, not least in terms of the growth of 'big government', began to take effect.

Lawrence also claims that the main aim of the school was to produce elite physicians who would tend to the medical needs of elite Scottish society, of which the professors themselves were part.[24] This may indeed be partly true, but, in addition to the many occasional auditors, a significantly Scottish factor here was the attendance by many surgical apprentices at anatomy classes in the university (a number of Edinburgh surgeons had also studied at Leiden, and the Incorporation was always keen to be seen to pursue academic studies. The College of Surgeons' diploma – see below – also required courses in physic). The elite physicians produced by the Medical School may have been those few who fulfilled the entire curriculum, but it was perfectly possible at this time to follow a medical career without this full qualification. One point made by Lawrence, which may not have been considered fully enough in the past, is that many students who attended classes within the walls of the Toun's College did so because of the individual teachers and their reputations, not necessarily because they taught in a

having also taken possession of a plantation in the West Indies, where his first act was to free the slaves. *Dictionary of National Biography.*

23 Lawrence, C., '"Ornate physicians and learned artisans". Edinburgh medical men, 1726–1776', in *William Hunter and the eighteenth-century medical world* (eds) Bynum, W.F. and Porter, R. (Cambridge, 1985), 153–76.

24 Ibid., 156.

university.[25] This would appear to be a key point, and emphasises the openness and non-regulation of medical education in the days before the Medical Act of 1858. It also helps to explain the rise in extramural teaching in Edinburgh later on in the century, discussed below.

Clinical Teaching

One area where Edinburgh was also pioneering was in clinical teaching, and though the initial Leiden connection is important here, the particular ambience of Enlightenment Edinburgh enhanced this influence. Described, with justification, by Risse as 'one of the most critical developments in the history of medical education',[26] this was one area where the confluence of 'Edinburgh factors' helped. Boerhaavian clinical teaching did not focus necessarily on the particular circumstances of the individual (as it was beginning to do in other European centres) – rather, Boerhaave was concerned to show how the individual fitted neatly into the current general view on disease processes – colourfully described by Risse as 'performances in a nosological theatre'.[27] But any new teaching method, and one based on a new philosophy of consultation and diagnosis, has to start somewhere, and what Boerhaave had begun was the long journey towards detailed clinical assessment of the individual in the more modern sense, and the many Edinburgh medical men who experienced his teaching had gained a basis for more individual assessment as diagnostic techniques developed.[28] The first Edinburgh infirmary, which opened in 1726, was too small to make a great contribution, but the significance of clinical observation was soon recognised. The opening of the second infirmary in 1741 eased the congestion somewhat, though it too became overcrowded. Facilities for clinical observation were utilised more by surgical apprentices at the beginning, but perceptive medical students soon began to realise the opportunity – and the need – and in 1748 formal clinical teaching was instituted by John Rutherford, including bedside demonstrations as well as lectures. Rutherford, interestingly, had started his medical career as an apprentice to an Edinburgh surgeon, before moving on to study in London and Leiden, gaining his MD at Reims in 1719, so this may have influenced his views on the more practical

---

25 Ibid., 162. Lawrence also makes the point that, despite the apparent emphasis on clinical teaching, the shortage of facilities meant that many students went to London during the summer vacation to study anatomy.

26 Risse, G., 'Clinical instruction in hospitals: the Boerhaavian tradition in Leiden, Edinburgh, Vienna and Pavia', *Clio medica* 21 (1987–8), 1–19. See also Risse, G., *Hospital medicine in Enlightenment Edinburgh. Care and teaching at the Royal Infirmary of Edinburgh* (Cambridge, 1986).

27 Ibid., 4. See also Risse, 'Clinical instruction in hospitals'.

28 Underwood, E.A., *Boerhaave's men at Leiden and after* (Edinburgh, 1977).

elements of medicine.[29] Beds at the infirmary were allocated specifically for the clinical teachers, and students were also afforded the opportunity of copying out entries from case notes and ward journals – observation and recording in the true sense of the Enlightenment. By 1783 the university ordained that MD graduates must prove attendance at clinical lectures as part of their qualifying curriculum, and following Rutherford in clinical teaching were some of the 'great names' of the period, including William Cullen, John Gregory and Andrew Duncan senior.

This flourishing of clinical instruction was of necessity limited to the patients who happened to be in the infirmary. Those admitted were mostly poor and suffering from a limited range of conditions, such as fevers and consumption. Accident cases were not admitted, nor were patients who were not expected to recover – favourable statistics are not just a feature of politicised twenty-first-century medical services. Individuals of high social status would not dream of entering a hospital for treatment. Despite this relative narrowness of opportunity, there is evidence that clinical training was being translated – gradually – into clinical practice, as shown by Macdonald's analysis of the medical casebooks of a late eighteenth-century Glasgow physician, Robert Cleghorn.[30] Cleghorn was, apparently, somewhat ahead of his time, and ahead of many of his fellow practitioners, in that he was very much in favour of clinical examination and physical contact with patients, using palpation to assist diagnosis and taking careful notes of post-mortem findings as a test of his diagnostic powers. Cleghorn noted in his diary, about a patient with kidney disease confirmed at post-mortem, that the case was 'another proof of the necessity of attending to local symptoms & to the feelings of the patient, no matter how bizarre these may appear & however contrary to nosology!'[31] Lawrence takes the view that the 'clinical encounter' was at the heart of medical change from the early eighteenth century, and Cleghorn seems to be a good example to confirm this.[32] The clinical encounter had always been important, but hitherto perhaps had been more conversational and philosophical in nature, and also frequently at a distance, by correspondence. Cleghorn was a Glasgow graduate, but the example is valid in terms of demonstrating that the changing ethos of the clinical encounter did influence medical practice, however gradually.

The increasing availability of midwifery teaching was a further important 'Edinburgh factor'. The first two incumbents of the Chair of Midwifery were mainly involved in training female midwives, but Thomas Young, appointed in 1756, also taught medical students and gave clinical instruction in obstetrics in a

29 *Dictionary of National Biography.* It was quite common at that time for individuals to study in one location and take final examinations at another, and the combination of study in Leiden and examinations at Rheims was quite common.

30 Macdonald, F.A., 'Reading Cleghorn the clinician: The clinical case records of Dr Robert Cleghorn, 1785–1818', in *Science and medicine in the Scottish Enlightenment*, (eds) Withers, C.W.J. and Wood, P. (East Linton, 2002), 255–79.

31 Ibid., 260–1.

32 C. Lawrence, *Medicine in the making of modern Britain* (London, 1994), 3.

separate eight-bed ward on the top floor of the infirmary set aside for maternity patients. This was technically outside the remit of the hospital and the nurses were paid by the professor himself. After 25 years, Alexander Hamilton was appointed co-holder and succeeded on Young's death in 1783. Hamilton had been Deacon of the surgeons' Incorporation from 1776to 1778, thus further enhancing the academic profile of the surgeons and their links with formal teaching (Young did eventually obtain Fellowship of the Royal College of Physicians of Edinburgh also). Young's course was optional, but increasingly popular. Lecture courses were given to medical students and midwives separately, and eventually Hamilton was obliged to open a separate midwifery institution, which he did in 1791.[33] All of this was very much in line with the Scottish Enlightenment ethos of the practical application of the fruits of intellectual endeavour.

The Role of the Surgeons

What is also significant in the particular circumstances of Edinburgh is that the Incorporation of Surgeons had long experience in politics and patronage at local and at national and royal levels. The Edinburgh surgeons were incorporated in 1505, well before the foundation of the university in 1583, and even longer in advance of the College of Physicians, which did not appear till 1681. This gave them a good start and much practice in the art of local politics. The Incorporation had a permanent seat on the Town Council, following the Decreet Arbitrall of 1583, which altered the 'sett' of burgh government, and was recognised as the leading burgh craft, though one of the smaller in numerical terms.[34] This gave the surgeons close insight and influence in local politics. Before 1707, Edinburgh surgeons represented the burgh at sittings of the Scottish parliament and at the unique Convention of the Royal Burghs of Scotland (an organisation which afforded the burghs a corporate political voice).[35] Master surgeons served successive monarchs and regiments and, not least, the Incorporation had the foresight – or insight – to begin awarding honorary membership of the Incorporation, and later Honorary Fellowship of the Royal College, to high-status individuals who would be potential sources of political support and patronage – the first recipient, in 1671, was Sir

33 This provided a high level of care, funded by appeals and private practice. Separate diplomas were awarded to male and female pupils. Simpson, A.D.C., 'James Hamilton's Lying-in Hospital at Park House and the status of midwifery instruction in the Edinburgh Medical School', *Book of the Old Edinburgh Club*, New Series 3 (1994), 131–41.

34 Following the Decreet Arbitrall, the burgh crafts were guaranteed six seats on the Town Council – very much in the minority in a merchant-dominated system, but this was, nonetheless, significant. The Edinburgh model was subsequently adopted in other Scottish burghs.

35 Dingwall, *Famous and flourishing society*, 67.

Andrew Murray, Lord Provost, Privy Councillor and Lord of the Exchequer.[36] The Edinburgh surgeons knew very well how to use patronage to their benefit, and this was no less the case in the eighteenth century. Another significant factor was that surgical apprentices were required to be literate in Latin from the start, and this also assisted their determined drive towards acquiring the trappings and ethos of a 'learned society' (there is some evidence that attainment levels were occasionally patchy, but this does not detract from the main point). Literacy and knowledge of Latin also meant that the surgeons, individually and corporately, could develop and foster potentially profitable contacts at relatively high social levels, in turn perhaps enabling the academic acceptance of individuals with a surgical pedigree.

The Royal College of Surgeons had another significant asset by the latter part of the eighteenth century – a surgical diploma. A lesser qualification than full Fellowship of the College, into which the Incorporation had been translated in 1778, this examination was taken by increasing numbers of medical students who required a surgical qualification and licence to practise surgery in the armed services or East India Company.[37] As well as being economically useful to the College, it was another pulling factor in the complex attraction of Edinburgh for medical study in the broadest sense. The regulations were extended in 1809, after which the required curriculum bore close similarities to the university medical curriculum and included hospital practice. By 1815 the various diplomas which had been created for army surgeons, country surgeons and – for a brief period – slave ship surgeons, were rationalised into a single qualification, and this was designated Licentiateship from 1816.[38] This qualification was perhaps more significant in its effects on Edinburgh medical training as a whole than may have been recognised previously.

Another factor in this multifaceted situation, and one which contributed significantly to the decline in the popularity of the Medical School and concomitant blossoming of extramural teaching, was the 'battle for anatomy and surgery' which raged between the university and the Royal College of Surgeons. Since the foundation of the Medical School, surgery had been subsumed within the remit of the professor of Anatomy, in other words, the Monro dynasty. Things would come to a head by the turn of the nineteenth century, but for most of the eighteenth century the Monro monopoly dominated anatomical and surgical teaching. This may have been appropriate at the start – Monro *primus* was a master of the Incorporation of Surgeons, but his son and grandson were physicians by inclination and institutional affiliation (*Primus* was awarded the degree of MD *Honoris Causa* by the University of Edinburgh in 1756). As the Edinburgh surgeons began to enjoy increasing

---

36 Ibid., 65–6.

37 Ibid., 111–15.

38 Ibid., 115–20. The College advertised that it had been granted powers to 'give certificates to surgeons of ships employed in that [African slave] trade'. *Edinburgh Advertiser*, 20 October 1789. Around 20 such certificates were awarded and were occupation specific, entitling their holders to work aboard slave ships only.

status and power, they started to push for the establishment of a separate Chair of Surgery at the university. The move was blocked successfully by the Monros, mainly due to their political contacts and influence, and eventually the College established its own professor, the first incumbent being John Thomson, in 1804. The post would be discontinued in mid-nineteenth century in the light of changes in the university, but at that time the surgeons were able to 'go it alone', perhaps because of the 'background acceptance' of non-university teaching as legitimate. Indeed, it was not unknown for an extramural teacher to achieve an intramural chair later, as in the case of Andrew Duncan, who offered an extramural winter course on Practice of Medicine and a summer course on Materia Medica in the early 1770s, and was thereafter elected to a professorship in Institutes of Medicine in the University in 1789, as successor to James Gregory. J.W. Turner, who held the College of Surgeons' Chair of Surgery from 1821, was the first occupant of the university's new Chair of Surgery, established in 1831. This ability to 'leap over the wall' may be seen to have lent continuing legitimacy to extramural teaching, which could develop without academic or political constraints.

Practical surgery was still severely limited by the lack of anaesthesia (though attempts were made in some areas such as the performance of Caesarean sections on live mothers),[39] but considerable progress had been made in the elucidation of the structure and function of the body – not least by Monro *secundus*. However, within the confines of the anatomical lecture theatre, what was taught was seen to be increasingly old-fashioned in the light of these new advances, and not geared towards the practicalities of surgery. This was a major stimulus to the blossoming of extramural education and the relative decline of the Medical School itself.[40] So the factors that helped to found and sustain the school initially proved also to contribute to its relative decline in popularity. In the world of Edinburgh medicine, the 'best' education was still available, but not necessarily within the walls of the Medical School. Two physicians from St Andrews, Dr George Martine and Dr William Graeme, had tried to establish a medical school in Edinburgh in the 1720s. This was not successful, but the enterprise had been encouraged by Monro *primus*, who considered that extramural lecturers would add to the reputation of Edinburgh as a focus of medical excellence – the implication being that he considered the university to be only a part of a wider sphere of medical teaching

[39] Kaufman, M.H., 'Caesarean operations performed at Edinburgh in the eighteenth century', *British Journal of Obstetrics and Gynaecology* 102 (3) (1995), 186–91. Research showed that of eight operations performed on live subjects, all the mothers died, but three of the infants survived.

[40] Lawrence, C., 'The Edinburgh Medical School and the end of the "Old Thing", 1790–1830', *History of Universities* 7 (1988), 259–86. For a full account of extramural teaching see Kaufman, M.H., *Medical teaching in Edinburgh during the eighteenth and nineteenth centuries* (Edinburgh, 2003).

– in effect a teaching marketplace alongside the medical practice marketplace.[41] This seems to have continued throughout the period.

During this time, medical individuals and institutions made increasing use of the press to advertise their expertise and lecture courses, and this was one of the ways in which extramural teachers were able to run classes and draw in students. In May 1699 surgeon Alexander Monteith announced in the *Edinburgh Gazette* that he would 'begin a course of Chymie [chemistry] in which all the useful operations and preparations will be performed'.[42] On 24 September 1771 the *Edinburgh Advertiser* announced that: 'It is with pleasure we inform the public that the University here daily increases in its reputation for medical knowledge; and indeed, what university has been able to boast of having at the same time, four such great professors as Cullen, Monro, Gregory and Black?' The press was recognised as a potentially powerful tool in the eighteenth century, just as much as in modern times, and there were no constraints on the advertising of medicine in all its forms. Newspapers such as the *Caledonian Mercury* contained frequent medical announcements, such as the course of lectures to be run by surgeon James Rae, who offered a course on surgery, illustrated by plaster of Paris casts and wax models.[43] Rae also delivered clinical lectures on surgery in the Royal Infirmary, and was one of the first to focus on dentistry, stating in 1784 that he 'continues to transplant teeth and to perform every other operation relative to natural teeth' as well as offering high-quality false teeth.[44]

The pages of the newspapers were also used to advertise the formal curricula of the university and the surgeons' diploma, and the use of the press to publicise individuals and their teaching seems to have been an important feature in the rise of both the Medical School and the wider extramural teaching sphere.

Surgeons' Square – the Hotbed of Extramural Anatomy

The second Royal Infirmary and Old Surgeons' Hall (the 1697 building) formed two sides of what became known as Surgeon's Square (see Figure 13.1). This set of buildings housed the anatomical schools of several well-known Edinburgh names, including the infamous Robert Knox of Burke and Hare notoriety. One of the earliest establishments here was the anatomical school of John Bell (Figure 13.3), set up around 1790 – Bell had lectured within the College of Surgeons till it was completed. Described by Cathcart as 'the founder of surgical anatomy',

41 Guthrie, D., *Extramural medical education in Edinburgh and the School of Medicine of the Royal Colleges* (Edinburgh, 1965, 11).

42 *Edinburgh Gazette*, 8–11 May 1699. This came a short time after the opening of the surgeons' new Hall. Monteith had rented a room in the basement to use as a laboratory.

43 Dingwall, H.M., '"To be insert in the *Mercury*". Medical practitioners and the press in eighteenth century Edinburgh', *Social History of Medicine* 13 (1) (2002), 36.

44 *Edinburgh Advertiser*, 12–16 January 1784.

Bell taught in conjunction with his brother Charles, and concentrated on teaching anatomy in ways that were appropriate for practical surgery.[45] Bell's view that surgery must relate closely to practical anatomy was opposed by some members of the medical establishment, including James Gregory,[46] and he eventually stopped teaching at the turn of the nineteenth century, while maintaining his surgical practice in Edinburgh. His legacy included the influential *Principles of Surgery*, which combined detailed anatomy with illustrations and descriptions of surgical procedures, and his work on arterial surgery led to his being described as the father of vascular surgery.[47]

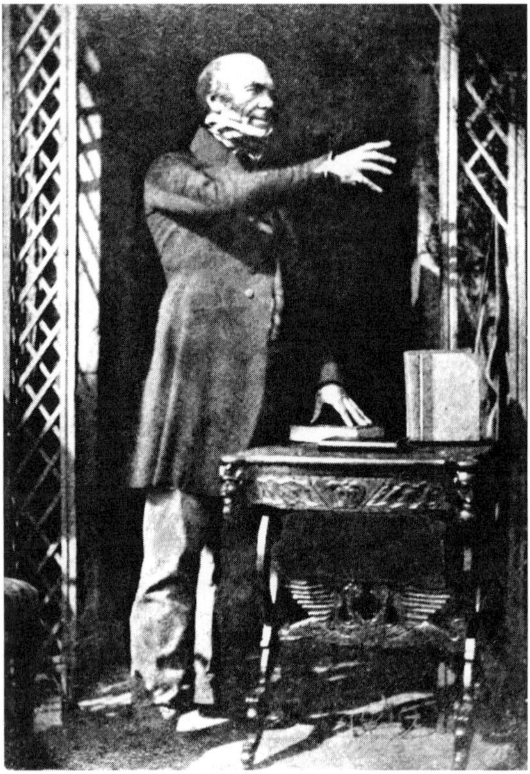

Fig.13.3 Portrait of John Bell, extramural teacher and pioneer of vascular surgery

45 Cathcart, C.W., 'Some of the older schools of Anatomy connected with the Royal College of Surgeons, Edinburgh', *Edinburgh Medical Journal* (March 1882), 774; Kaufman, *Medical teaching in Edinburgh*, 73–4.

46 Gregory waged a pamphlet war against Bell, warning students against attending his lectures.

47 *Dictionary of National Biography*. Bell, J., *Principles of surgery*, 2 vols (Edinburgh, 1801).

Another notable occupant of Surgeons' Square was John Barclay, eminent collector and pioneer of comparative anatomy. Barclay ran his anatomical school there from 1800 until his death in 1826 and was assiduous in his collection of museum specimens.[48] His teaching was popular and his collection of museum items formidable. Barclay's lecture room was well placed, adjacent to the home of the Royal Medical Society (the main medical student society) and very close to Surgeon's Hall. Lectures were popular and delivered twice a day in the winter session, while in the summer session Barclay offered a course on comparative anatomy.[49] Barclay also took advantage of the press by advertising his courses and claiming that his work on comparative anatomy was 'not only calculated to throw much light on the form and structure, but an accurate knowledge of the organs which produce them is of much more importance than is generally imagined both in the Practice of Surgery and Physic'.[50] The nuances of this comment would not be lost on either side of the anatomical debate, and indeed Barclay was the subject of opprobrium in the ongoing pamphlet wars. One such attack stated: 'from the time of Eristratus to that of Dr Barclay, there have not been wanting men to totally devoid of principle as to perform divers cruel, and no doubt *painful* incisions upon dead bodies'.[51] This pamphlet also bore clear witness that the Enlightenment could not wholly change long-held views, with the acid remark: 'I see no necessary connection between presenting a dose of salts, and dissecting a dead body'.

In common with many of his colleagues, Barclay also published widely, thus contributing to the academic advancement of his subject without the need to occupy a university chair in order to gain academic legitimacy, at least in the eyes of the medical students. Among his main publications were *Muscular Motions of the Human Body* (1808) and *A Description of the Arteries of the Human Body* (1812).

By 1825, in failing health, Barclay made an association with Robert Knox (Figure 13.4), who succeeded him on his death[52]. Knox seems to have been even more popular than Barclay, regularly attracting over 150 students to his lectures, with the result that he had to give each lecture twice because of lack of space in his teaching rooms.[53] Knox was implicated in the murderous acquisition of anatomical subjects – one anonymous writer claiming that if Knox were really unaware of the source and manner of death of these bodies, then he was 'equally

48 For a full account of Barclay's teaching see Kaufman, *Medical teaching*, 83–9.

49 For a biographical account see *Dictionary of National Biography.*

50 *Edinburgh Advertiser*, 3 October 1800.

51 Pasquin, P., *Tubs for whales, or a plan for regulating the study of anatomy in Edinburgh* (Edinburgh, 1819), 6–8.

52 For a full account of Barclay's work and relationship with Knox see Kaufman, M.H., *Dr John Barclay (1758–1826), extra-mural teacher of human and comparative anatomy in Edinburgh* (Edinburgh, 2007).

53 Dingwall, *Famous and flourishing society*, 112–13.

as ignorant as his students'.[54] Ironically, however, the very success of extramural anatomy can be put forward, at least in part, as explanation as well as consequence of the murderous activities of Burke and Hare. Bodies for dissection would be the subject of the Anatomy Act of 1832, which oversaw and regulated their acquisition and treatment by anatomists.

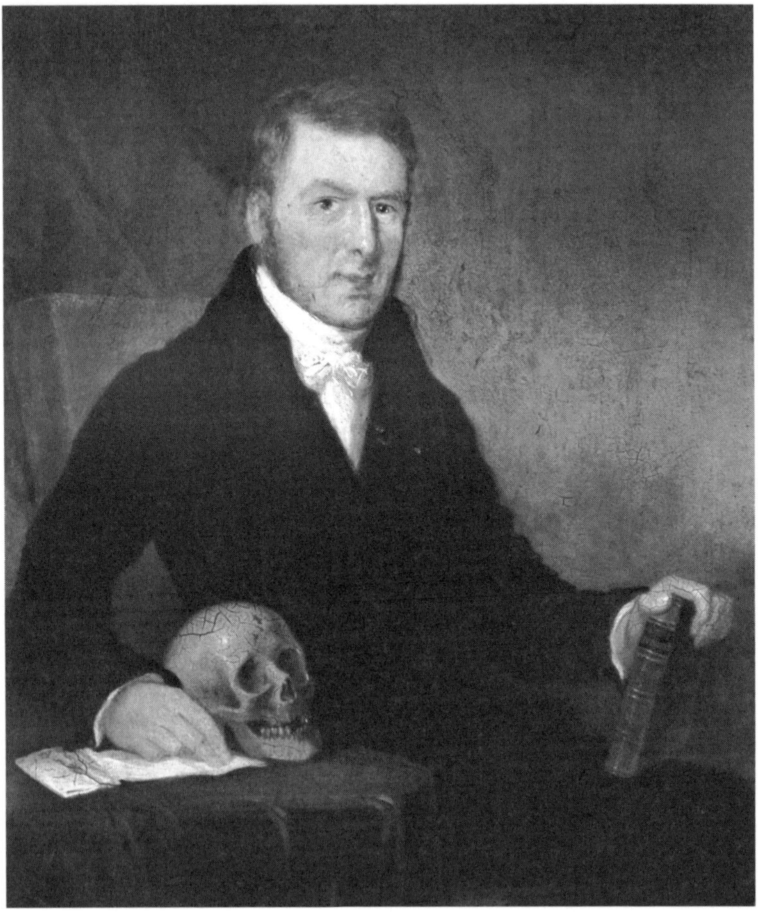

Fig.13.4 Portrait of Robert Knox, popular extramural teacher but notorious for his alleged links to the Burke and Hare murders

One of Barclay's students, John Gordon, offered classes in anatomy and also physiology from around 1808, but died young, thus being unable to establish a reputation on a par with his mentors. William Cullen, great-nephew of the

[54] National Library of Scotland, Ry.1.3.1(2), Aristides, *Letter to Sir William Rae of St Catharines, Baronet, Lord Advocate of Scotland* (Edinburgh, 1829).

more famous Cullen, gave lectures on anatomy in the 1820s and also lecture/demonstrations on the use of the stethoscope. René Laennec, a young French physician credited with inventing the device, had begun his experiments only around 1816, so Cullen was clearly interested in and in favour of incorporating new equipment and examining techniques into his medical teaching and, by implication, medical practice.

By the late 1830s there was a considerable clustering of expertise in two extramural schools – Argyle Square and Queen's College. Tuition was available in Physic, Anatomy, Medical Jurisprudence, Surgery, Midwifery, Materia Medica, Botany, Operative Surgery, Forensic Medicine, Practical Chemistry, Natural Philosophy, Mathematics – together with Greek, Arabic and Persian, French, Italian and German.[55] The School of Medicine of the Royal Colleges was founded in 1895, and housed adjacent to the Royal College of Surgeons. It lasted as an undergraduate teaching unit until the mid-1940s, when the Goodenough Report concluded that the universities should form the main entry portal at undergraduate level.[56]

Conclusions

There are many potential explanations for the rise and relative decline of the reputation of the Edinburgh Medical School, but an angle which may not have been emphasised sufficiently is the status and role of the Edinburgh surgeons at this time. Edinburgh surgeons were held in higher regard than their counterparts in London – the situation was rather different in Paris, with the division between academic and non-academic surgeons. Edinburgh surgeons were literate, some had studied in Leiden, and many apprentices took courses at the Edinburgh Medical School. A number of individual surgeons came from relatively high-status social backgrounds and several took a prominent role in the development of medical education in the eighteenth century. There were many squabbles and confrontations among the Incorporation of Surgeons (Royal College from 1778), the Town Council, the Royal College of Physicians and the university, not to mention the managers of the Infirmary, but these clashes and disagreements did not prevent the surgeons from contributing actively to the totality of the medical education sphere of Edinburgh.

Another perhaps indirectly relevant point to make is that the beginning of the end of the dominance of the Medical School towards the end of the eighteenth century coincided with the apparent reversal within the two wings of the Scottish church. The moderate literati who had dominated intellectual discussion and the General Assembly of the Church of Scotland began to be accused of reactionary

[55] Guthrie, *Extramural medical education*, 16–18.

[56] Goodenough, W., *Report of the Interdepartmental Committee on Medical Schools* (London, 1944).

tendencies, and the previously reactionary evangelical wing was perceived to be more liberal. This is perhaps a general phenomenon with movements which start out as free and liberal but, once they gain dominance, reaction sets in and the desire to propagate change fades in favour of the wish to maintain personal or dynastic status. What happened in the Medical School seems to mirror this somewhat. It started life in the glow of religious moderatism, and the church had significant effects on the general ambience of the time. By the turn of the nineteenth century the established church was perceived to be less moderate, and the university was seen by some to be reactionary and old fashioned. There may or may not be a direct connection here, but context is key to most aspects of the historical process.

At the start of the period, the Edinburgh Medical School had no real competition. There were considerable problems in Glasgow because of the tensions between the university and the Faculty of Physicians and Surgeons, and Aberdeen was rather too remote to provide serious competition. Although the school rose and then stalled because of a complex and shifting pattern of influences, the key to initial success, at least, seems to have been the role of the surgeons, who were very experienced in politics and had long had a voice on the Town Council. By the early decades of the nineteenth century other factors were coming into play, including the increasing desire of the university to dominate medical teaching, the influence of national as opposed to local politics, and the growing desire for some sort of standardisation and regulation of medical training. The best education may still have been available in Edinburgh, but it was, by the end of the century, a different best, affected by changing circumstances and changing times. Students who sought what they considered to be the best were able to go wherever they thought they could get it, and this was increasingly outside the university's medical school.

It is perhaps unsurprising that such a variety of educational opportunities existed in Enlightenment and post-Enlightenment Edinburgh. The university medical school was only one of a range of establishments offering the same subjects. This, it seems, was due in no small part to the strong tradition of medical institutions in the town, and to the close contacts which had existed between the surgeons in particular and the Town Council. By the turn of the nineteenth century and the end of the 'old thing',[57] the best medical education could still be found in Edinburgh, but not necessarily within the walls of the university. It would be another half century before national legislation intervened, but even after 1858 many doors led to medical qualification in Edinburgh and the United Kingdom as a whole.

---

[57] This is how Lawrence describes the situation with anatomy towards the end of the period – the 'old thing' being the classical approach to anatomical teaching.

Index